Cardiovascular Essays, 1983–2024

By

Charles Stewart Roberts, MD

"I certainly agree with you about freedom, only more so. It is why I could never tie myself up with church or educational institution and bend my back to their limitations."

—Stewart R. Roberts, MD
The First Cardiologist in the South
Letter to Dr. W. R. Houston, UT-Austin
June 17, 1936 (58 years of age)

Preface

The fourth quarter of life may be considered age 60 to 80. It is a period perhaps to add organization and reflection to present goals. With this consideration in mind, I decided to collect various articles pertaining to cardiovascular medicine, surgery, and history into one volume, excluding purely scientific or patient-specific research studies, which usually involve multiple authors. These articles were written across a 40-year span, from medical student to senior surgeon. No grand expectation attends this publication, but the author will be gratified if a reader profits from a single article, or a single paragraph, or even a single sentence in this volume.

Contents

Appendices

1

On The Darsee Affair

By Charles S. Roberts
EUSM '86

I arrived at the Cardiac Research Laboratory of Harvard Medical School in late January 1982, a month after Dr. John R. Darsee left. Many of his belongings were still there, including journals, degrees on the wall, and a few books. There was a photograph of him on a wall which one of the technicians had turned upside down. This was not the same lab I remembered from two summers before.

While in another laboratory at Harvard during the summer of 1980, I happened to work on a project which involved a myocardial staining technique being used daily by Darsee and by the chief of the Cardiac Research Laboratory of Harvard, Dr. Robert A. Kloner. Consequently, I was instructed to go see them and learn the method. There was never a time when either Kloner or Darsee would not stop to explain anything to me. If I called to ask if I might come over with a few questions, one or the other would often meet me at the front door of the building to let me in. Darsee smoked a pipe, was full of warm humor, and kept a dog named Snoopy for a pet in the laboratory. One was immediately struck by the harmony with which Kloner's lab operated at the time. For this reason, I wished to return there.

After reacquainting ourselves on my first day, I sat with Kloner in his office at the large conference table and listened in dismay while he said that, not only had Darsee been caught once falsifying data, evidence suggested that this incident was part of a pattern. I cannot adequately describe the tension that pervaded the Cardiac Research Laboratory in the early months of 1982. Some members of the lab took offense at any derogatory comment on Darsee in their presence; others cultivated a sardonic attitude, while others were still uncertain what to think. Whenever Kloner referred to Darsee, it was with perfect seriousness and always a touch of absolute bewilderment.

Dr. Kloner now stresses 'defensive research'. . . just be able to defend with 'raw data' everything that you say.

Laboratory meetings were held every week around Kloner's conference table. Attended by the research fellows and technicians, and occasionally by Dr. Frederick J. Schoen of the Department of Pathology, these meetings were conducted by Kloner. The first one of the year was memorable. I copy this from a journal I kept during those months: "Dr. Kloner now stresses 'defensive research.' One does not have to be paranoid --just be able to defend with 'raw data' everything that you say-- first lab meeting."

One always heard when Dr. Eugene Braunwald, Chairman of the Department of Medicine at the Brigham and Women's Hospital, was coming over to the lab. Braunwald, in his mid-fifties, would come walking through the snow with a tremendous briefcase, usually after 5 p.m., then through the door and directly to Kloner's office where, as I understand, the Darsee affair was discussed. I was told that Braunwald described these months as the worst in his life. I recall Kloner mentioning that he spent as much as 75 percent of his time on this issue and Braunwald as much as 50 percent of his time. Nevertheless, Kloner would stop by my desk a few times every day to inquire how things were, answer questions, or discuss the project on which I worked.

In late January 1982, I saw Darsee for the first time since my arrival. It was around six o'clock one evening. He was coming to the lab to meet with Kloner for what I believe was their last formal meeting. I recorded this from my journal: "When he walked into Kloner's lab as I was typing a protocol, I stood up and we smiled, joked, and shook hands. His eyes showed signs of heavy crying, and there was a sense of depression or

Continued on page 14

Roberts: *defensive research*

Continued from page 8

despair in his appearance." I had dinner with him and his girlfriend a week or so later and, that evening, recorded this: "His message today-- do not work so hard that you make mistakes and can't see the forest for the trees."

There can be no doubt that for Kloner, who is 32 years old and about a year younger than Darsee, these few months were far from pleasant and, indeed, an unfortunate challenge. While the pressure he must have felt was great, his graciousness never waned during this time. With committees hovering over him, it was not uncommon for Kloner to leave a fellow a note on his desk Monday morning like this one: *Dear ---, The N.I.H. is returning April 12th. I wish to have all notebooks, gamma counter sheets, hemodynamic strip charts, slides (please obtain from pathology), echo tapes, etc., all organized and ready to show them.* **Copies of gamma counter sheets** *must appear in your notebooks as well as the weights of each individual piece of heart tissue. THIS MUST TAKE PRIORITY OVER ALL other work this week. I would like to inspect all notebooks by Wednesday....*

Thank you, Bob

To prepare for one meeting, a former research fellow was asked to return to the lab to organize data with his undergraduate assistant. They spent the weekend at a table poring over notebooks and, at one point, the two came bursting out of the room and started jumping, cursing, yelling, and laughing. Evidently, before leaving the laboratory the previous May, the fellow had xeroxed the daily log book of all dog experiments done while he was there. As he was comparing his xerox copy with the old log book, he found pages on which Darsee had apparently gone back and added more notes or drawings.

In June 1983, I returned to the Cardiac Research Laboratory for the summer to find fellows who had never met Darsee. While "defensive research" was quietly emphasized by Kloner, the original harmony of the laboratory was restored. To sit with Kloner at his table while he, in a burst of creativity, drew out a scientific hypothesis on paper and outlined a simple experimental protocol, was an experience no different, I suspect, than it would have been for a student with him three years earlier. Braunwald attended the lab meetings occasionally around Kloner's table. Data were presented and discussed; questions were posed.

Roberts CS. On the Darsee affair. *Anlage*, Newspaper of the Emory Medical Community, Vol. 16, No. 2, December 1983.

Addendum to "The Darsee Affair" article

The essay appeared in *Anlage* ("Newspaper of the Emory Medical Community") in December 1983, together with five other articles (four by faculty and two by students in all) in a section called "Perspectives on the Darsee Affair." Andreas R. Gruenzig, MD, the first to perform coronary angioplasty, wrote in his article:

> Any one of you who is considering a career in research in medicine should examine the case of John Darsee very carefully, as you examine yourself. We all have some of his qualities of ambition and determination. Acknowledging that fact and using these abilities properly are essential in building the foundation of a productive career in research.

My article was simply an account of one medical student's interaction with Dr. John Darsee in the Harvard research laboratory in which he had worked. A brief chronology of the major events is presented.

Chronology of Research Events of Dr. John Darsee

1966-1970 Notre Dame University

1970-1974 Indiana University School of Medicine

1974-1979 Residency at Emory University
Chief Resident in Medicine, Clinical Fellow in Cardiology
45 Abstracts and 10 Papers

July 1979 Begins at Cardiac Research Laboratory, Brigham and Women's Hospital, Harvard Medical Center; directed by Dr. Robert Kloner

1980 Offered faculty appointment to begin July 1981 as Assistant Professor of Medicine by Dr. Eugene Braunwald, Chairman of Medicine

May 21, 1981 Data irregularities brought to attention of Dr. Koner by laboratory personnel

May 26, 1981 Faculty appointment offer withdrawn and fellowship terminated, though allowed to complete ongoing studies in the laboratory through 1981. The data irregularities were considered "a single act of scientific dishonesty." Detailed reviews initiated.

Oct 1981 Harvard notified of discrepancies in federally funded experimental heart drug study in which Darsee participated.

Nov 1981 Emory notified of Harvard investigation. Emory initiates investigation under direction of Dr. Neil C. Moran, appointed by Dean Glenn.

Dec 7, 1981 First formal meeting of Ad Hoc Advisory Committee to the Medical Dean at Harvard on "Dishonesty in Scientific Research." Dr. Darsee meets with committee members on December 7 and 24 and January 11.

Jan 25, 1982 Report of Harvard Committee completed, concluding that "there are serious questions of credibility in three recent studies in which Dr. Darsee was significantly involved."

Oct 1982 Emory Committee reports "serious problems."

March 1983	Emory Committee (Moran Report) concludes that 2 of 45 abstracts and 2 of 10 papers from Emory stood up to scrutiny. Retraction of publications was recommended. "Many abstracts appear to be completely ficticious."
Spring 1983	National Institutes of Health asks Harvard to return $122,371 it had received in federal study in which Darsee participated. Federal officials bar Dr. Darsee from applying for an NIH grant or participating in an NIH peer review committee for 10 years.
June 9, 1983	Two retractions, two corrections, one editorial, and one letter-to-the-editor by Darsee appear in the *New England Journal of Medicine* (see below).

NEJMAG 308(23) 1373–1432 (1983) JUNE 9

Abstracts in the advertising section

The New England Journal of Medicine

Established in 1812 as The NEW ENGLAND JOURNAL OF MEDICINE AND SURGERY

VOLUME 308 JUNE 9, 1983 NUMBER 23

2

The Case of Richard Cabot

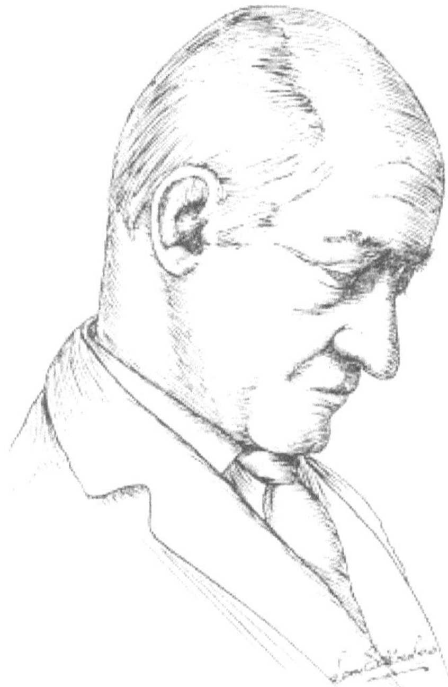

Paul Dudley White, the distinguished cardiologist, wrote of Richard Cabot after his death:

> In every generation there are restless souls who cannot be made to fit the common mold. A few of these are valuable in keeping their communities and professions in a ferment by their constant challenge to the existing order of man's thought and action. But when, in addition to possessing these attributes, a rare individual is endowed with the divine fire and makes important contributions to the pioneering progress of humanity, then indeed we recognize a great leader. In the thick of the fray such recognition comes slowly but as soon as the smoke of the battle clears the acclaim is universal. (1939)

Born into an old Bostonian family in 1868, Cabot was graduated from Harvard College in 1889 with a major in philosophy, his father's pursuit. After considering a career in the Unitarian ministry, he chose medicine and was graduated from Harvard Medical School in 1892 at age 24. His senior thesis was on "The Medical Bearing of Mind-Care," a study of healing by Christian Science.

During his internship at Massachusetts General Hospital, Cabot published a paper entitled "Leucocytosis as an Element in the Prognosis of Pneumonia" (see White, 1939), in which he described the elevated white blood cell count in pyogenic infections. Cabot spent the following year in hematologic research. His studies of blood culminated in his first book, A Guide to the Clinical Examination of the Blood, which was published in 1896 and went through five editions. In its preface he wrote, "the first book of its kind, so far as I am aware." Despite a busy private practice and service to outpatients at Massachusetts General Hospital, Cabot published a monograph, The Serum Diagnosis of Disease, in 1899, and another, Physical Diagnosis of Diseases of the Chest, in 1901. He expanded the latter book to include the rest of the body, writing twelve editions from 1901 to 1938. His book, Differential Diagnosis, published in 1938, went through seven editions. He emphasized errors of omission and commission in clinical diagnosis.

Cabot devoted much time to clinical research, gathering data from a large number of cases and then applying statistical analysis. He sought facts. After examining autopsy reports of 3000 cases, Cabot wrote in 1912 a controversial paper in which he pointed out "a goodly number of "classic" time-honored mistakes in diagnosis." In response to a Chicago physician who criticized his pessimism, Cabot wrote:

> When he has had three thousand clinical diagnoses criticized at autopsy by an independent and unprejudiced pathologist who makes full bacteriologic and histologic examinations of every case, he will find, I believe, that the facts are not less unpleasant than I have stated them to be. He will know that his most scrupulous and careful examination of the precordia often fails to reveal acute pericarditis when it is present; that his examination of the urine will not always distinguish either acute or chronic nephritis from other conditions resembling them, and that mitral stenosis and aortic stenosis are sometimes overlooked by the best diagnosticians. (1913)

Cabot's paper on "The Four Common Types of Heart Disease" appeared in 1914 and is a landmark in medical history. For the first time, heart disease was classified according to its cause, which was a revolutionary point of view. He reported that 93% of 600 cases of heart disease were of either rheumatic, atherosclerotic, syphilitic, or nephritic etiology. Paul Dudley White (1939) described Cabot as the greatest contributor to cardiology in his generation.

After Walter B. Cannon introduced the idea of case teaching in medicine in 1900, Cabot became its most ardent advocate. His Exercises in Differential Diagnosis, published in 1902, consisted of 43 case summaries, each ending with the questions "Diagnosis? Prognosis? Treatment?" Cabot stressed the importance of deciding on a diagnosis and writing it down. He believed that "after the student has learned to open his eyes and see, he must learn to shut them and think" (1908). He considered the case method superior to other methods of teaching medicine. Wrote Cabot,

> By using this method a single teacher can keep a large class of students actively busy. They are not merely listening or watching; they are doing the work of construction themselves. In lectures or large amphitheatre clinics the whole class is managed by one teacher, but the teacher does the work and hence the student's gain is relatively slight. (1908)

Cabot believed strongly in student participation, that the case method of teaching succeeds when the students are called on by name, that "only if no one in the class knows the answer should the teacher give it himself; for the process of answering serves to fix the fact in the student's mind and he should never be deprived of this benefit" (1908). The clinicopathologic conference, or CPC, was originated by Cabot in 1910, a result of his emphasis on the case study and the confirmation of a diagnosis by autopsy. His regular conference was held at

Massachusetts General Hospital, a record of which was edited by him and published in the Boston Medical and Surgical Journal (now the New England Journal of Medicine) from 1924 to 1935.

Apart from his medical activities, Cabot gave much attention to social services, which he founded at Massachusetts General Hospital in 1905. His book, Social Service and the Art of Healing, appeared in 1909. Cabot's lifelong interest in ethics resulted in several books on the subject, and in 1919 at age 51, he was appointed professor of social ethics in addition to professor of clinical medicine. He was working on a philosophical treatise called "Creation" when he died in Boston in 1939.

References

1. Cabot RC. Case teaching in medicine. Boston: D.C. Heath, 1908.
2. Cabot RC. Diagnostic pitfalls identified during a study of three thousand autopsies. JAMA. 1912;59:2295–98.
3. Cabot RC. Letter. JAMA. 1913;60:145.
4. White PD. Richard Clarke Cabot 1868–1939. New Engl J Med. 1939;220:1049–52.

Roberts CS. The case of Richard Cabot. In: Walker HK, Hall WD, Hurst JW, eds. *Clinical Methods: The History, Physical, and Laboratory Examinations.* 3rd ed. Boston: Butterworths; 1990. https://www.ncbi.nlm.nih.gov/books/NBK702/

3

Herrick and Heart Disease

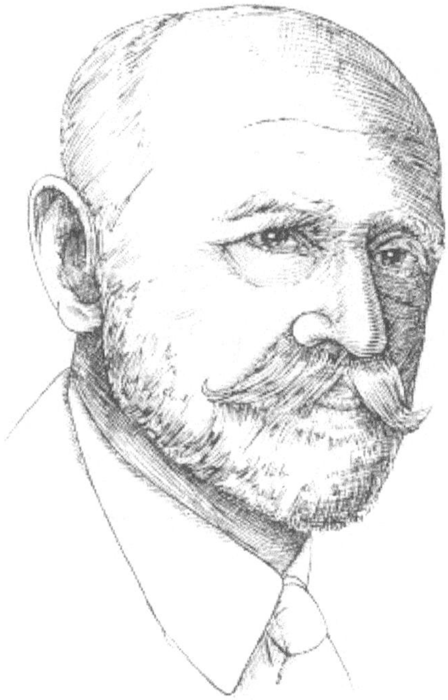

At the 1912 meeting of the Association of American Physicians, James B. Herrick read a paper entitled "Clinical Features of Sudden Obstruction of the Coronary Arteries," which is now considered a classic. For Herrick, however, the event was a disaster:

> In 1912 when I arose to read my paper at the Association, I was elated, for I knew I had a substantial contribution to present. I read it, and it fell flat as a pancake. No one discussed it except Emanuel Libman, and he discussed every paper read there that day. I was sunk in disappointment and despair. (Means, 1961)

It was not until Herrick readdressed the same association in 1919 that his views finally received proper attention.

Born in Oak Park, Illinois, in 1861, Herrick graduated from the University of Michigan in 1882 and taught English, Latin, and Greek for several years in a high school. He graduated from Rush Medical College in 1888 and interned at Cook County Hospital. He entered practice in Chicago in 1890 and was appointed to the staffs of Cook County Hospital and Presbyterian Hospital. His first book, A Manual of Medical Diagnosis, was published in 1895 when he was age 34. In 1900 he decided to engage only in consulting and became widely known as a master clinician and teacher. Aside from his accomplishments in cardiology,

Herrick called attention to anemia secondary to chronic blood loss in 1902, and wrote the first description of sickle cell anemia in 1910.

The prevailing opinion of coronary obstruction in Herrick's early years was that it usually resulted in sudden death because the coronary arteries were believed to be end arteries, lacking sufficient anastomoses. Conheim lent support to this pessimistic view of coronary obstruction; Herrick disagreed, writing:

> Obstruction of a coronary artery or any of its large branches has long been regarded as a serious accident. Several events contributed toward the prevalence of the view that this condition was almost always suddenly fatal ... But there are reasons for believing that even large branches of the coronary arteries may be occluded—at times acutely occluded—without resulting death, at least without death in the immediate future. Even the main trunk may at times be obstructed and the patient live. It is the object of this paper to present a few facts along this line, and particularly to describe some of the clinical manifestations of sudden yet not immediately fatal cases of coronary obstruction. (1912)

Herrick's medical experience at the bedside enabled him to differentiate clinical manifestations of coronary obstruction when no one had before. His classification consisted of the following four events: (1) instantaneous, perhaps painless, death; (2) severe angina followed minutes later by shock and death; (3) mild, nonfatal angina; and (4) severe angina that is usually eventually fatal, but not immediately. Herrick concluded with an insight concerning a therapeutic dilemma that remains today: "The hope for the damaged myocardium lies in the direction of securing a supply of blood through friendly neighboring vessels so as to restore so far as possible its functional integrity". Herrick advocated use of digitalis instead of nitrates in the treatment of sudden coronary obstruction and recommended bed rest for 6 weeks.

In 1930 Herrick received the Kober Medal for distinguished research in medicine conferred by the Association of American Physicians, and in 1939 he received a Distinguished Service Medal from the American Medical Association. His bibliography includes at least 163 medical articles and 9 papers presented to the Chicago Literary Club. Apart from his classical scholarship, Herrick was interested in medical history. In 1942 he published A Short History of Cardiology, which covered the subject from Harvey to Roentgen. In a review of the book, Paul Dudley White wrote:

> The next to the last chapter, devoted to coronary disease, is of particular interest in its attempt to explain the lapse in interest in the subject between 1900 and 1912 ... Sudden deaths and temporary invalidism from heart disease, were occurring commonly throughout that century, pathologists were finding scars in the heart and other evidences of serious coronary disease, but there was no clinician to put all the facts together until Herrick himself analyzed the problem. The occasional references in the literature to which he himself refers, although interesting, and of course accumulative, nevertheless do not take away in my mind at all from the luster of Herrick's own accomplishment in his classic paper in 1912. The only outstanding omission in the book as I see it is the lack of recognition of the importance of his own contribution. It undoubtedly is from sincere modesty. (1942)

Herrick described much of his life in his Memories of Eighty Years, in which he mentions his first encounter with Osler in 1898: "A more inspiring, delightful hour I had never spent. I had fallen victim—a willing one—to the charm of the Osler personality." Herrick died in 1954, having read everything written by Chaucer, his favorite author.

References

1. Herrick JB. Peculiar elongated and sickle-shaped red blood corpuscles in a case of severe anemia. Arch Intern Med. 1910;6:516–21.
2. Herrick JB. Clinical features of sudden obstruction of the coronary arteries. JAMA. 1912;59:2015–20. [PubMed]
3. Means JH. The Association of American Physicians: its first seventy-five years. New York: McGrawHill, 1961:108. [PubMed]
4. White PD. Book review: A short history of cardiology. By Herrick JB. JAMA 1942;202–3.

Roberts CS. Herrick and heart disease. In: Walker HK, Hall WD, Hurst JW, eds. *Clinical Methods: The History, Physical, and Laboratory Examinations.* 3rd ed. Boston: Butterworths; 1990. https://www.ncbi.nlm.nih.gov/books/NBK714/

4

MORPHOLOGIC ASPECTS OF AORTIC DISSECTION

CHARLES ROBERTS, M.D.
WILLIAM ROBERTS, M.D.

Aortic dissection was recognized at necropsy over 200 years ago and clinically over 50 years ago. In a 30-year period, we have studied over 200 necropsy patients with aortic dissection, 95 percent spontaneous and 5 percent iatrogenic.

CHARACTERISTICS

The mean age of death after spontaneous aortic dissection is 59 years (range 17 to 91), and most (62 percent) are men. Aortic dissection is characterized by a longitudinal separation of the media, initiated by a transverse tear of the intima and media. The primary, or entry, tear is located in the ascending aorta in 70 percent of cases, in the descending thoracic aorta in 21 percent, in the arch in 8 percent, and in the abdominal aorta in 1 percent (Table 1). When located in the ascending aorta, the entry tear is usually about 2 cm cephalad to the sinotubular junction, which corresponds to the cephalad extension of the aortic valve cusps. When located in the descending thoracic aorta, the tear is usually near the ligamentum arteriosum. The entry tear usually involved about one-half of the aortic circumference; occasionally much less, and rarely, the entire circumference.

The entry tear nearly always extends through the intima and the inner two-thirds of the media, at which level medial separation occurs, creating a false channel. Thus, aortic dissection results in true and false channels separated by the intima and the inner two-thirds of the media. The outer wall of the false channel consists of the outer one-third of the media and the adventitia. External rupture of the outer wall of the false channel is far more common than internal rupture (re-entry tear) of the inner wall because the outer wall is thinner. The thinner the outer wall of the false channel, the greater the likelihood of fatal rupture (Fig. 1).

Table 1 Sites of Primary Tear in Aortic Dissection

Location of Tear	*Hirst**	*Roberts*
Ascending aorta	62	70
Aortic arch	9	8
Isthmus and descending thoracic aorta	26	21
Abdominal aorta	3	1

*Data from Hirst AE Jr, et al. Dissecting aneurysm of the aorta: A review of 505 cases. Medicine 1958; 37:217–279.

Although dissection represents a longitudinal separation of media, the percentage of aortic circumference involved by the dissection at any particular level of aorta is variable. Most commonly at any level, about one-half of the circumference of the aorta is dissected, and the wall of the other half of aorta is intact. With dissections beginning in the ascending portion, the tear usually involves the right lateral aortic wall, and longitudinal dissection occurs along the greater curvature of the ascending, transverse, and descending thoracic portions of aorta. Extension of the dissection into the innominate, left common carotid, and left subclavian arteries is common.

After a transverse intimal and medial tear, the longitudinal dissection may occur in an antegrade or retrograde direction. The former is far more common. Once blood under pressure enters the media through the tear, the time required thereafter to dissect the media of the entire length of the aorta appears to be only a few seconds. Evidence of the rapidity of the longitudinal dissection once it begins was gained from retrograde aortic dissection observed during attempted cardiopulmonary bypass as well as by the virtually instantaneous deaths of some victims of spontaneous aortic dissection. Presumably, the antegrade aortic dissections occur with similar speed, possibly even more rapidly because, in the natural state, the aorta is exposed to a pulsatile flow rather than entirely to a mean pressure as during cardiopulmonary bypass.

A secondary or re-entry tear allows blood in the false channel to re-enter the true channel, but it is infrequently found (14 percent). A re-entry tear also was identified rarely (10 percent) in the patients collected from previous reports by Hirst et al.[1] The re-entry tear was located in the aorta in about half of the cases, most commonly the abdominal portion, next the descending thoracic portion, and last, the ascending portion. In the other half re-entry was into a peripheral artery, most commonly one or more of the iliac arteries. Rarely, a single tear serves as both the entrance to and the exit from the false channel. In this circumstance, flow within the false channel may be both retrograde and antegrade.

The length of aorta involved by dissection varies. In about half (51 percent) of our necropsy patients, the aorta both proximal and distal to the ligamentum arteriosum (Type I) was dissected. Next most common (29 percent) was involvement proximal to the ligamentum arteriosum (Type II), and least common (20 percent) was involvement only of the aorta located distal to the ligamentum arteriosum (Type III). Thus, the ascending aorta was both the most common portion of aorta involved by dissection and the most common site of an entry tear.

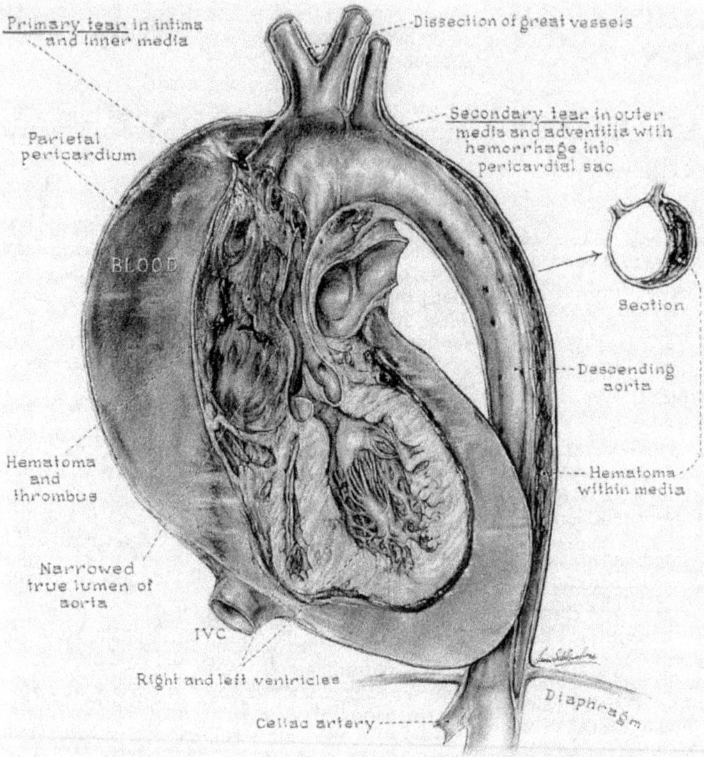

Figure 1 Dissection with initial tear about 8 cm cephalad to the aortic valve and extending to the diaphragm in a 70-year-old man, who died several days after the onset of symptoms resulting from aortic dissection. Thrombus filled the false channel from the tear to the aortic root, causing narrowing of the true channel. The outer wall of the false channel ruptured at the initial tear, causing hemopericardium. The weight of the heart was normal. (Reproduced with permission from Roberts WC. Aortic dissection: Anatomy, consequences and causes. Am Heart J 1981; 101:195–214.)

Entry tears distal to the ligamentum arteriosum cause antegrade dissection and, rarely (1 percent), retrograde dissection.

Why any aortic dissection stops within the aorta, with or without re-entry into the true lumen, is a question that has received little attention. The most common cause of interruption of the longitudinal dissection appears to be extensive atherosclerotic plaque that has caused underlying medial scarring or atrophy, or both, and that prevents further medial separation. A common site of extensive atherosclerotic plaque is the isthmus of the aorta, which is in the vicinity of the ligamentum arteriosum. Extensive atherosclerosis in the abdominal portion of the aorta also may prevent longitudinal dissection. When a fusiform aneurysm of the abdominal aorta is present, distal aortic dissection is nearly always stopped by severe medial atrophy or fibrosis at the site of the aneurysm.

A rare (1 percent) cause of interruption of a dissection involving the ascending and arch portions of the aorta is aortic isthmic coarctation. Aortic rupture, usually with dissection, is a major cause of death in unoperated patients with aortic isthmic coarctation. Because aortic isthmic coarctation represents an invagination of media, longitudinal dissection progressing distally is stopped by a natural coarctation or an aortic coarctation that has been resected and repaired by end-to-end suture anastomosis. Aortic dissection in patients with aortic isthmic coarctation most commonly involves only the portion of aorta proximal to the coarctation, and occasionally the dissection involves only the aorta distal to the coarctation, but never both.

Without extensive aortic atherosclerosis or coarctation, the entire aorta distal to the entrance tear usually dissects. Dissection limited to the ascending and transverse portions of aorta generally indicates the presence of extensive aortic atherosclerotic plaque or coarctation at the aortic isthmus. If aortic isthmic coarctation is absent, aortic dissection in patients younger than 40 years old nearly always involves the entire aorta because atherosclerotic plaquing in them is usually mild. Aortic dissection in patients older than 65 years of age has a greater chance of being localized because of the greater probability of heavy atherosclerotic plaquing, at least among persons residing in the Western world, with or without a fusiform aneurysm.

Recognition of which portion of aorta is involved by dissection has important consequences. Healing or survival beyond 60 days occurs rarely in cases of Type I (3 percent) or Type II (13 percent) spontaneous aortic dissection. Involvement of the ascending aorta, therefore, is an indication for operative intervention. In many patients with an aortic tear distal to the ligamentum arteriosum (Type III), healing occurs, and a re-entry site may be identifiable in them.

In contrast to its inappropriate use in most patients with acute dissection, the term aneurysm is usually appropriate in patients with healed aortic dissection because the false channel usually is large, larger than the true channel, and its wall has focal, frequently multiple, saccular aneurysms, most of which contain thrombi. Occasionally, the false channel is filled completely by thrombus. The lining of the false lumen is usually completely endothelialized and covered by atheroma and thrombi.

The atheromatous plaques in the false channel provide the rare opportunity of studying plaques known to be present for specified periods of time. For example, if the acute dissection occurred 2 years before death, it can be said with certainty that the atheromatous plaque in the false channel had been present no more than 2 years. Most yellow atheromatous plaques in false channels are covered by thrombi, suggesting that the underlying plaques are formed by organization of thrombi. At times, healed aortic dissections are found at necropsy in individuals in whom no earlier clinical event compatible with acute dissection had been apparent, suggesting the existence of clinically silent acute aortic dissections.

Although healing occurs in many patients with Type III aortic dissection, most healed dissections eventually produce significant complications (29 percent nonfatal, 41 percent fatal). External rupture of the false lumen (42 percent) and stenosis of the true lumen from compression by a thrombus-filled false lumen (19 percent) occur with enough frequency to justify early operative therapy in these patients. In general, the rate of healing, or survival, after dissection is proportional to the distance of the intimal and medial tear from the aortic valve. Consequently, few patients with healed aortic dissections have the initial tear in the ascending aorta. Once healing has occurred, however, a longer false channel generally affords longer survival.

COMPLICATIONS

Various complications of aortic dissection are listed in Table 2. Death is most frequent; more than 80 percent of patients die fewer than 60 days after spontaneous acute aortic dissection without operative intervention. External rupture of the false channel is the most common (90 percent) mechanism of death. The site of rupture is usually near the site of the initiating entry tear, which, therefore, often determines the site into which extravasation occurs. The most frequent site of the entry tear is the ascending aorta, which is also the most frequent site of through-and-through rupture (see Fig. 1). Extravasation of blood in this circumstance is nearly always into the pericardial sac (Table 3). Because the parietal pericardium is attached to the ascending aorta just proximal to the origin of the innominate artery, rupture of any portion of the ascending aorta leads to extravasation into the pericardial sac. The usual site of the through-and-through rupture is the right lateral wall, the site of contact of blood ejected from the left ventricle.

Table 2 Complications of Aortic Dissection

Through-and-through rupture of aorta with extravasation of blood into
- Pericardial sac
- Pleural space
- Mediastinum
- Retroperitoneum
- Wall of pulmonary trunk and/or main right and left pulmonary arteries, because of common adventitia with aorta (peripheral pulmonary stenosis)
- Atrial and/or ventricular cardiac septum (atrioventricular conduction defect)
- Lung
- Esophagus

Partial or complete obstruction by medial hematoma of the lumen of an artery arising from aorta
- Cornary (sudden death or acute myocardial infarction)
- Innominate and/or common carotid (syncope, confusion, stroke, coma)
- Innominate and/or subclavian (upper limb gangrene, paralysis)
- Intercostal and/or lumbar (spinal cord ischemia, paraplegia)
- Celiac
- Renal (oliguria)
- Mesenteric (bowel ischemia)
- Common iliac (lower leg gangrene, paralysis)

Separation of branch of aorta from aorta

Aortic regurgitation

Obstruction of aorta itself (true aortic stenosis)
- By compression of true lumen by medial hematoma
- Intussusception of aorta

Table 3 Sites of Hemorrhage in Aortic Dissection

	Incidence (%)	
Site of Hemorrhage	*Hirst**	*Roberts*
Pericardial sac	52	82
Mediastinum	10	2
Pleural space	29	14
Retroperitoneum	6	2
Other	3	0

*Data from Hirst AE Jr et al. Dissecting aneurysm of the aorta: A review of 505 cases. Medicine 1958; 37:217–279.

Before the final external rupture of the ascending aorta and usually rapid death, blood frequently dissects into the adventitia of the wall of the aorta's false channel. Because the ascending aorta and pulmonary trunk have a common adventitia, blood may extend from the adventitia of the aorta into the adventitia of the major pulmonary arteries (Fig. 2). Because the intrapulmonary pressure is low, and because the extravasated aortic blood is forced into the pulmonary arterial adventitia under systemic arterial pressure, the lumens of the major pulmonary arteries may be narrowed by this dissecting adventitial hematoma, leading to a form of peripheral pulmonary stenosis.[2]

Rupture of the aortic arch is most often into the mediastinum; the descending thoracic aorta into the left pleural space; and the abdominal aorta into the retroperitoneum. External rupture of a healed dissection of the descending thoracic aorta may produce massive hemoptysis from an aortopulmonary fistula or hematemesis from an aortoesophageal fistula.

Extension of the medial dissection or hematoma into an artery arising from the aorta may lead to ischemia or necrosis of the organ or tissue normally perfused by that artery. Retrograde longitudinal dissection in the ascending aorta, particularly when it extends into the sinus portion of the aorta, may extend into the media of a major coronary artery, usually the right coronary artery. Medial dissection of an artery the size of a coronary artery commonly leads to luminal narrowing, causing myocardial ischemia, which may be fatal. A second consequence of dissection involving the aortic root is loss of commissural support of one or more aortic valve cusps, with the consequence of aortic regurgitation. A third complication of retrograde aortic dissection is extension of blood into the free walls or septa of the adjacent cardiac atria or ventricles. This may lead to development of an aortico-atrial or aortico-right ventricular fistula or to a high degree of atrioventricular block.

Extension of the longitudinal dissection into the arteries arising from the aortic arch may lead to arm or cerebral ischemia, or both. Extension into one renal artery, usually the left, may produce signs of renal failure and elevation of the systemic blood pressure. Extension into the celiac axis or one or both mesenteric arteries may produce signs of abdominal organ insufficiency. Extension into the common iliac arteries or distally may lead to leg and foot ischemia. On occasion, dissection of the aorta may completely shear off or separate one or more arteries that arise from the aorta. When this situation

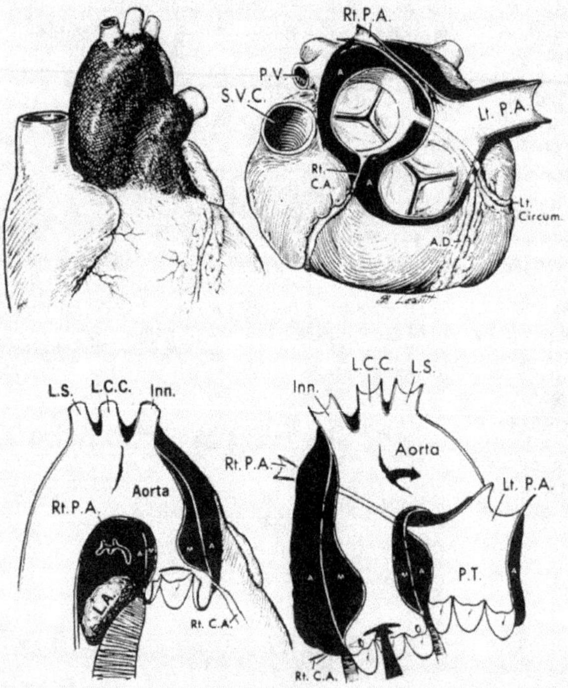

Figure 2 Dissection of the entire aorta with rupture into the pericardial sac in a 57-year-old man who developed chest pain 17 hours before death. He was known to have had systemic hypertension. This patient is described in detail elsewhere. At necropsy, extravasated blood was present in the adventitia (*A*) of both the ascending aorta and the extrapulmonary arteries. Because the ascending aorta and the pulmonary trunk (*PT*) have a common adventitia, dissection of blood into the adventitia of the aorta can extend into the adventitia of the pulmonary arteries and into the main right (*Rt*) and left (*Lt*) pulmonary trunk arteries. This drawing shows how this process leads to severe narrowing of the lumen of the right pulmonary artery. The ascending aorta also was narrowed by blood in the false channel as well as in the adventitia. The entrance site of the dissection was just above the aortic valve, and the exit site was in the arch. The lumen of the right coronary artery (*Rt CA*) also was severely narrowed by the medial (*M*) and adventitial hematoma. PA = Pulmonary artery; PV = portal vein; SVC = superior vena cava; AD = left anterior descending coronary artery; Circum = circumflex coronary artery; LS = left subclavian artery; LCC = left common carotid artery; Inn = innominate artery. (Reproduced with permission from Buja LM, et al. Stenosis of the right main pulmonary artery. A complication of acute dissecting aneurysm of the ascending aorta. Am Heart J 1972; 83:89–98.)

occurs, flow through the branch ceases, but extravasation usually is prevented by drainage into the false channel.

True aortic stenosis, as opposed to aortic valve stenosis, may result when a large hematoma or thrombus fills most or all of the false channel, with resulting compression of the lumen of the true channel. This circumstance is most likely to occur when the dissection occupies a large portion of the circumference of the aorta. Another unappreciated type of true aortic stenosis occurs when the entrance tear into the medial longitudinal dissection involves the entire circumference of the aorta. In this situation, the partition between the true and false channels "rolls up" and is propelled distally into the lumen of the aorta, essentially producing an intussusception.

CAUSES

The cause of spontaneous aortic dissection is usually unknown. An intrinsic abnormality in the wall of the aorta is usually not identified. About 75 percent of patients with aortic dissection have or have had systemic hypertension (Table 4). At necropsy about 90 percent of these patients have left ventricular hypertrophy, with a heart weight of more than 350 g in adult women and more than 400 g in adult men. The most reasonable explanation for this cardiomegaly is systemic hypertension. Aortic dissection often represents the patient's first serious illness, and once the acute dissection has occurred, the blood pressure usually falls. By the time of hospitalization, the systemic hypertension may have vanished. The dissection in some patients causes death so rapidly that the systemic blood pressure may never be obtained. Thus, documentation of systemic hypertension in only 75 percent of these patients is not surprising.

Systemic hypertension appears to be a major risk factor in the development of cardiovascular disease in two ways: by increasing the deposition of atherosclerotic plaque in major arteries, most commonly causing luminal narrowing with resulting organ ischemia, infarction, or both; and by weakening the media of certain arteries, causing aneurysms that may or may not rupture or tears that may or may not dissect. The effect of hypertension on the arterial media is direct, whereas its effect on the arterial intima is indirect. Systemic hypertension is the only known major underlying factor in two conditions: aortic dissection and intracerebral microaneurysm with or without rupture. Better blood pressure control clearly leads to a reduction in the incidence of aortic dissection and of nontraumatic intracerebral hemorrhage.

Thus, aortic dissection may be viewed as representing a therapeutic failure in the management of systemic hypertension. If systemic hypertension were eliminated, spontaneous aortic dissection would virtually disappear. Despite its being the common factor in patients with spontaneous aortic dissection, however, systemic hypertension by itself cannot be viewed as the sole cause of aortic dissection. There are estimated to be 60 million Americans with systemic hypertension, and the frequency of aortic dissection among them is quite low. Furthermore, the pressure in the aorta can be experimentally increased eight times above normal before rupture occurs. Why one hypertensive person has aortic dissection and another of similar age and with similarly elevated pressures does not is unclear. Histologic abnormalities present in the wall of the aorta are infrequent, even at the entrance site into the dissection. Acid mucopolysaccharide material in the aortic media at the site of the aortic tear or in other parts of the aorta in the patients with dissection is usually present in normal amounts.

Other conditions have been associated with aortic dissection, including pregnancy, but the number of reported patients is small. Even among these, little information on the presence or absence of systemic hypertension is available. It is well known that the systemic blood pressure and volume rise during pregnancy, and these increases may lead to an increased frequency of aortic dissection, when compared with similarly aged, nonpregnant women.

Marfan's syndrome and its forme fruste varieties are also often listed as a cause of aortic dissection. This syndrome was rare (3 percent) in our necropsy patients. In patients with both Marfan's syndrome and aortic dissection, the characteristic medial le-

Table 4 Comparison of Clinical and Morphologic Data on Aortic Dissection

Series	Year Published	Mean Age at Death (Years)	Males (%)	Type of Dissection I (%)	II (%)	III (%)	SH (%)	Abnormal Aortic Valve (%)	CoA (%)	Marfan's Syndrome (%)
Wilson[7]	1982	55	65	—60—		40	69	0	0	5
Larson[6]	1984	62	65	54	21	25	58	16	1	4
Roberts	-	59	62	51	29	20	76	8	1	3
Mean		59	64	53	25	23	68	8	1	4

SH = Systemic hypertension; CoA = coarctation of aorta.

sion, namely cystic medial necrosis, is usually absent, and, therefore, the aortic dissection in these patients cannot be attributed to the Marfan-type aorta. Dissection is rare in patients with fusiform aortic root aneurysms.

One type of aortic dissection that may not be associated with systemic hypertension is that occurring in patients with congenitally bicuspid or unicuspid aortic valves, an anomaly present in 8 percent of the necropsy patients. Not only is the frequency of a congenitally bicuspid aortic valve much higher than expected in patients with aortic dissection, but the frequency of aortic dissection is much higher than expected in patients with congenitally bicuspid aortic valves.

Aortic isthmic coarctation clearly is associated with a high frequency of aortic dissection, which is probably two events: systemic hypertension and a common association with congenitally bicuspid aortic valves. The latter, particularly in association with aortic isthmic coarctation, appears to be related in some way to a structurally weaker aorta, compared with patients with three-cuspid aortic valves, with or without associated aortic isthmic coarctation.

Blunt trauma is a well-recognized, but rare, cause of aortic dissection (Fig. 3). The aortic tear usually occurs in the vicinity of the aortic isthmus, where the aorta is tethered by the ligamentum arteriosum.

Iatrogenic, traumatic aortic dissections are primarily of two types: cannulation-induced and aortic incision–induced. The former commonly results from insertion of a cardiopulmonary bypass cannula into the femoral artery, or insertion of an intra-aor-

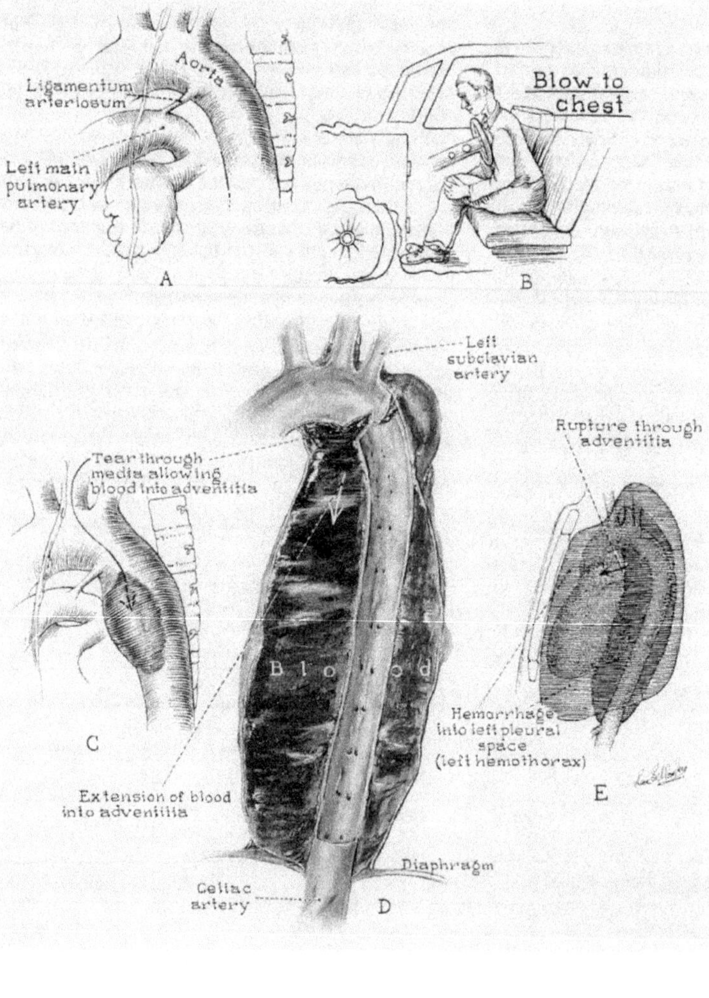

Figure 3 Drawing of the descending thoracic aorta in a 19-year-old man who was in an automobile accident 12 days before death. The aorta was torn (*D*) at the time of the accident but extravasation of blood beyond the media and adventitia did not occur until nearly 2 weeks later. At necropsy, the left pleural space was filled with blood. (Reproduced with permission from Roberts WC. Aortic dissection: Anatomy, consequences, and causes. Am Heart J 1981; 101:195–214.)

tic balloon counterpulsation device. The cannula or catheter tip is inadvertently inserted into the arterial media rather than the lumen. When cardiopulmonary bypass is instituted, arterial blood under pressure causes an immediate retrograde dissection of the aorta by way of the femoral and iliac arteries. Because of these types of accidents, radiographs of the distal aorta and its branches have been recommended before femoral cannulation, particularly in older patients. Cannulation in the proximal aorta has been a safer procedure but has also led to aortic dissection, generally not immediate. Incisions into the ascending aorta for insertion of aortocoronary bypass conduits or for replacement of the aortic valve have been followed, usually late, by aortic dissection initiated at the site of aortic incision.

Atherosclerosis and syphilis also have been listed as causes of aortic dissection, but both appear highly unlikely. Atherosclerosis is, at least initially, an intimal disease. The overlying atherosclerotic plaques may later cause atrophy of the underlying media. Dissection, in contrast, is primarily a medial disease, characterized by medial separation. Rarely are plaques present at the entrance site of the dissection. Although there are many exceptions, the greater the extent of aortic atherosclerosis, the less the likelihood of aortic dissection. Syphilis produces transverse medial scars, which also tend to prevent rather than to initiate aortic dissection.

REFERENCES

1. Hirst AE Jr, Johns VJ Jr, Kine SW Jr. Dissecting aneurysm of the aorta: A review of 505 cases. Medicine 1958; 37:217–279.
2. Roberts WC. Aortic dissection: Anatomy, consequences, and causes. Am Heart J 1981; 101:195–214.
3. Buja LM, Ali N, Fletcher RD, et al. Stenosis of the right main pulmonary artery. A complication of acute dissecting aneurysm of the ascending aorta. Am Heart J 1972; 83:89–98.
4. DeSanctis RW, Doroghazi RM, Austen WG, et al. Aortic dissection. N Engl J Med 1987; 317:1060–1066.
5. DeBakey ME, Henly WS, Cooley DA, et al. Surgical management of dissecting aneurysm of the aorta. J Thorac Cardiovasc Surg 1965; 49:130–149.
6. Larson EW, Edwards WD. Risk factors for aortic dissection: A necropsy study of 161 cases. Am J Cardiol 1984; 53:849–855.
7. Wilson SK, Hutchins GM. Aortic dissecting aneurysms: Causative factors in 204 subjects. Arch Pathol Lab Med 1982; 106:175–180.

Roberts C, Roberts W. Morphologic aspects of aortic dissection. In Ernst CB, Stanley JC, eds. *Current Therapy in Vascular Surgery.* 2nd ed. Philadelphia: B.C. Decker Inc.; 1991: 245–251.

5

Cardiac Surgery in Russia: An Account of a Trip to Sarotov, May 22–29, 1998

At the Raleigh-Durham Airport in the afternoon, I met Gary Boss, Tim Taft, and Paul Tawney. Also in the group was a Russian medical student named Tatiana Kudryashov, from Saratov, Russia. She was just completing three months at the University of North Carolina as part of the exchange program. The plan was for our group to fly to Washington's Dulles Airport, where we would meet Susanne Kirby, and then the six of us would fly directly to Moscow. In Moscow, we would be met by an orthopedic resident trainee from Saratov and also Tatiana's father, Alexander Kudryashov.

Just a brief note about each of the participants from Chapel Hill.

Gary D. Boss is Associate Professor of Surgery (Orthopedics) who specializes in orthopedic oncology. He was born in 1947, participated in the Vietnam War as a navigator on military planes, and then attended the medical school of the University of Chicago, from which he graduated in 1978. He trained at Case Western Reserve in Cleveland, Ohio, and then did a fellowship in orthopedic oncology at the Mayo Clinic. He tells me that every drop of blood in his veins is Dutch. His parents were from western Michigan and Iowa and lived in Dutch communities in those areas. Gary attended seminary briefly before pursuing medicine. He is a member of the Dutch Reform Church which, he relates, is a branch of the Presbyterian Church, just as the French Huguenots were French Calvinists. He is married with two children, one of whom just recently married a Dutch man. He has a gregarious, enthusiastic personality, and he is largely responsible for this entire exchange program.

The other orthopedic surgeon on the trip is Timothy N. Taft, who is Professor of Surgery (Orthopedics) specializing in sports medicine. He is the team doctor for the various athletic teams at UNC. He was originally from St. Louis and received his undergraduate degree from Princeton. He graduated from the School of Medicine at the University of Missouri in 1969 and took his orthopedic training at the University of North Carolina. He reminds me of Uncle Stewart. He is about 6 feet in height and stocky. He is bald on top and wears glasses. His personality is delightful and humorous.

The third man in our group is Paul J. W. Tawney, who happens to live in Southern Village in Chapel Hill. We were born the same year, in 1960, and he is from Albuquerque, New Mexico. He graduated from the University of New Mexico School of Medicine in 1989 and took his training in physical medicine/rehabilitation at the University of Virginia. He is currently Assistant Professor of Physical Medicine and Rehabilitation at UNC, and he specializes in spinal cord injury and back pain. I cross-examined him soon after meeting him on techniques to alleviate back pain. He is slender in appearance, about 5'10" in height. Never having been to Russia, he was surprised to learn that I had packed certain things like antibiotics and tissue paper. He said that he had been so busy right up to this trip that he had prepared little in the way of reading or packing.

We took a United Airlines flight at 4 p.m. to Dulles International Airport. We were delayed leaving Raleigh-Durham and were very concerned that we would miss our transfer to Moscow, but as it happened, when we arrived at the gate in Dulles, no one had boarded yet. We were unclear about whether to stand in front of the empty reception desk at the gate or wait in a long line of Russians to board the plane. Finally, a Delta agent appeared at the desk and we submitted our tickets. To our amazement, there were no more seats in the regular cabin areas, so we were moved to the business class section. We greeted this with contained enthusiasm, as we did not want to somehow sabotage this good fortune. At the airport in Washington, we met Susanne Kirby. At the door to the Aeroflot plane were copies of a small newspaper in English called the *Moscow Times* (since 1992). *Perestroika* occurred in 1991; and since then, Western influence has become apparent in Russia. The flight to Moscow could not have been more relaxing, excepting for the fact that passengers were free to smoke. Two passengers chose to do so in the business class area, and that made things slightly less pleasant. Regrettably, Susanne Kirby remained in the economy class section, because she had met us at the airport and had checked in on time. The stewardesses on the airplane were mostly attractive women who spoke a little English. Our stewardess in the business class was extremely polite and attended well to our needs. I had a Scotch on the rocks to start with, followed by a plateful of appetizers including salmon and bread and cheese and salad. Not knowing that this was the appetizer only, I was surprised when she asked me whether I would like "chicken or meat." I chose meat, and it came with potatoes on the side. All this was followed by coffee and dessert. During most of the trip, I read a book called *Inside Russia Today*, by John Gunther, which was a Penguin paperback appearing in 1964 in that form. The first edition of this book, called *Inside Russia*, was published in 1957 and later revised in 1962. This particular copy cost $6 and was inscribed by the author. I found it in one of the rare book shops in Chapel Hill. It interesting reading primarily because the book was written during the reign of Khrushchev in the middle of the Cold War. Gunther noted that in the mid-1950s, only about 150 Americans were living in the USSR. Our relationship with the USSR he described as "the most important, difficult, and dangerous problem in the world today, on which peace and, no doubt, the future of mankind depend." Some of the basic facts of Russian history are important to note:

600 A.D.	Slavs settle in Russia.
862	Novgorod founded by the Norseman Rurik. Russian history begins.
878	Slavic Kiev is conquered by Norsemen. The two Russias merge.
860-1240	Kiev in Russia. Byzantium brought into Russia.
988	Prince of Kiev baptized into Orthodox Christian Church. Russian conversion to Greek form of Christianity.
1237-1480	Mongolian conquest of Russia (Tatars). Khanate of the Golden Horde. Sarai, near Astrakhan, was the capital. This conquest explains some eastern or Asiatic characteristics of Russians.
1462-1505	Ivan III, the Great. "First national king." Married Sophia, niece of Constantine III. Russia and Byzantium united. Moscow Kremlin built.
1533-1584	Ivan IV, the Terrible. Married a Romanov. Crowned czar. Called "great gatherer of the Russian land." First kazan (1552), then astrakhan (1556).
1613	Mikail Romanov. 300-year throne. Serfdom, the cancer of the old Russia.

1689-1725	Peter the Great ruled. Russian capital moved from Moscow to St. Petersburg. Modern Russian history begins.
1755	Moscow University established, the first in Russia.
1762-1796	Catherine II, the Great. German blood. Hated the French Revolution.
1917	The October Revolution. The Bolshevik Revolution. Organized and led by Lenin. Based in part on the Communist Manifesto (by Marx and Engels, 1948).
1923	Stalin assumes leadership. Union of Soviet Socialist Republics is established (four original republics: Russia proper, the Ukraine, White Russia, and the Transcaucasian Soviet Federated Socialist Republic, composed in turn of Georgia, Armenia, and Azerbaijan).
1936	The new Stalin constitution. There were 11 republics.
1940	The Soviet Union has 15 republics. Area covers 8,602,700 square miles, larger than all Latin America, larger by far than China and India together. Its European section alone is larger than the rest of Europe. It covers almost one-sixth of the total land surface of the globe. More than twice as large as any other country in the world. It spreads 160° of longitude and nearly halfway around the world. (The sun takes 11 hours to cross it.) Moscow to Vladivostok is further than Moscow to New York. No true physical line of demarcation between Europe and Asia. Asia considered to begin not at the Urals, but at the Volga, deep in what we think of as European Russia. Eurasia is a single, indivisible continent. There are three types of land: the tundra, or northern marshland; the taiga, which is wooded area (the largest uninterrupted forest block); and the steppes, or extensive grassland with rich soil. Saratov is located in the "great agricultural triangle" in south-central Russia, where the earth is black and is of unmatched fertility and resource. The rivers were the roads of ancient Russia. Four of the nine longest rivers in the world are Russian: Ob, Amur, Lena, and Yenisei. The Volga, on which Saratov sits, drains an area three times the size of France.
1953	Stalin dies and Khrushchev assumes leadership.
1956	Hungary explodes in a revolution which is suppressed by Marshal Kukov.
1961	Berlin Wall erected. Kennedy and Khrushchev meet.
1985-1991	Mikail Gorbachev assumes leadership. *Perestroika* and *Glasnost* occur.
1991-1998	Boris Yeltsin leads Russia.

May 23,1998

We arrived in Moscow about noon and passed through customs without difficulty. The woman to whom I handed my passport and visa looked at me intensely for a second or two, but said nothing and handed back my documents. Citizens of Russia went down one path, and citizens of all other countries—including citizens from the former USSR—down another. Our bags appeared, and we then filled out a paper to claim what goods we were bringing into Russia. If one claimed more than $3,000, one had to go down a certain path. Tim Taft did so, and this delayed us about 30 minutes as his bags were inspected. The rest of us passed by a bored customs agent about 25 years of age who hardly looked at us. Tim Taft apparently had a screwdriver in his suitcase because he happened to be working on windows of his home when Gary Boss picked him up, and so he simply pocketed the screwdriver. The Russian agent scolded him for having it, but let him pass. Alex, the father of Tatiana, was there to meet us, as well as Victor, the orthopedic trainee. They had come up from Saratov to escort us home. We had several hours to kill, and so we went in a van with all our luggage to see the most conspicuous sights in Moscow: the Kremlin, Red Square, and the Lenin Mausoleum. It could have been any large capital in the world. There were tourists everywhere on the Square, and many groups of teenagers with ribbons around their shoulders, signifying their school. I must add that on the way to Red Square, we saw the Bolshoi Theater from the van. It was an impressive theater on a wide, dusty, unattractive main street. There were very few lines in the road to indicate lanes, and the traffic was bustling, but it did move on. Buildings in general on each side of the main road looked run-down. The major apartment buildings, which are so numerous in Moscow, looked like tenant houses built in the 1960s, except that they are generally white in color, rather than red brick. The Moscow Kremlin was a pleasure to tour. It sits on a hill, and one has to pass through metal detectors to enter. There are at least three churches within the Kremlin, which means "citadel." It was Sophia, the wife of Ivan the Great, who imported from Italy the architects who built the Moscow Kremlin. We entered only one church, which was a small one for the exclusive use of the czar and his family. The religious paintings of Christ and Mary were stunning in their beauty. It was a very cold afternoon, and none of us had brought coats. We had a Russian tour guide whose speech was translated to us by Tatiana. As we began to get colder and colder, one of my Chapel Hill colleagues turned to me and said, "She's telling me more than we want to know right now."

We then went to the Moscow train station, where we sat for two hours or so, waiting for our train to Saratov. The Moscow train station was astonishingly quiet, despite an entire floor full of neatly ordered rows of chairs with families including children. The children seemed to run freely, and several went off to the side to kick a ball around. They couldn't decide whether to bounce it like a basketball or kick it like a soccer ball. I bought a Corona Mexican beer as we waited. We made one excursion to the bathroom, our first in Russia. It was downstairs, and as soon as one hit the floor where the bathrooms were located, the smell pervaded the entire level. We walked past a guard at a desk and then went further into the bathroom area and encountered another desk, where we paid 3 rubles apiece to use the facility. Fortunately, I used only the urinal, but one of my colleagues told me about the condition of the other toilets. He said it was definitely unfavorable. Paul Tawney remarked to me that all the Russians had to do to encourage western tourists was revamp their public bathrooms.

We then boarded a train to Saratov. The train ride would be 16 hours, and we would not arrive until the next day, which would be Sunday. We rode in the first class section, which involved a sleeper car that provided a bed/couch for two people opposite one another. A little table was positioned between the two couches. I was the first on the train, and I entered the first compartment available. As it happened, I was assigned to share this two-person compartment with a Russian stranger. He was not present when I entered the room, but when he appeared, we introduced ourselves. He spoke no English, but I gathered through sign language that he was a urologist in Saratov. He was in his mid-60s, I suspect, and had a terrible case of chronic obstructive pulmonary disease. His breathing was audible at rest, and this was probably a consequence of many years of smoking. As we could not communicate, I spent most of my time lounging in the cabin of Gary Boss and Tim Taft, who kindly allowed me to join them. While it was still light, however, I collapsed in my own bed and was dead to the world for at least six hours. The Russian urologist was awake doing a crossword puzzle when I retired, and when I awoke at 4 a.m., he was asleep.

Sunday, May 24, 1998

I found my dinner, still unopened, in a plastic carton, and took it out into the hall of the moving train. It contained a sealed slab of sausage and another cut of cheese, with a roll of bread. There was also a little container of yogurt. I devoured all this food in the hall and then re-entered the dark cabin. I turned on the little light above my bed and read for two or three hours while the Russian urologist slept. The other seven people in our group going to Saratov slept soundly, they reported. Most of the morning in the train I spent conversing in the cabin with Gary Boss and Tim Taft. Gary Boss was planning out the total knee replacement that he was scheduled to perform in Saratov, and Tim Taft related to me his memories of Cold War America—the bomb shelters, the surveillance of the skies, etc.

We finally arrived in Saratov about noon and were greeted by a contingent of medical people from the University. I was introduced to Constantine, who would be my interpreter and would accompany me while in Saratov. He was a tall (perhaps 6'3"), beefy Russian man about 26 years of age. He told me briefly that he was training in cardiology, "not interventional." We walked out of the Saratov train station, and there was a statue across the way of a man facing away from us. Apparently, the statue is of the founder of the KGB; and in 1991, a crane was ordered to turn the statue so that it did not face people as they exited the railway station. Instead, one saw only the back of his head.

On the way to the hotel, I had a good view of the conditions in Saratov. Once again, I was amazed by the poverty and the decrepit conditions of the citizens. Though the main roads were paved, many of the side roads were unpaved. The sidewalks were generally dirt. I never saw one house that was comparable to any house in Chapel Hill, let alone Southern Village. I saw an endless number of apartment complexes which were about ten stories in height and white in color. Often, laundry hung on lines on each balcony. In some sections of town, there were houses made of wood, but they were generally dirty and boarded up and undesirable dwellings. New Orleans came to mind as I passed through parts of Saratov. I recalled some sections of the poorest parts of New Orleans, where the wooden, single-story homes vaguely resembled these dwellings in Saratov.

We finally made it to our hotel, which was situated on the outskirts of town, enclosed by an iron fence with a guard out front. We were each shown to a room, and mine was satisfactory. The bedding was something one might find in prison. The bathroom was something one might find in the cellar of an unrestored Victorian home built in the 1920s. In fact, I suspect that this building in Russia was built in the 1960s. There was hot water, however, and the toilet was fairly conventional. The bed was not uncomfortable. There was a black and white TV in the room which was unplugged, and there was also an old small refrigerator in the room which was which was unplugged. The television had six channels, and three of them showed "Euro news," which was, for the brief moment I watched it, in Italian.

The five UNC doctors then had lunch in the dining room of this hotel, which was unpopulated except for two women several tables away. We were served by a Russian girl in her 20s who spoke no English and said nothing when she brought each of the three courses: first, a bowl of beets; next, a chicken noodle soup; and finally, some sort of sausage dish. I retired for a nap for two hours and then showered and dressed for dinner.

The five of us were taken to dinner at the home of Tatiana. Her family lived on the sixth floor of a large apartment building similar to the ones I had seen in Moscow and Saratov. It was about ten stores in height, white in color, and each apartment had a balcony. We entered at the ground floor into a dark passageway and rode an elevator to the sixth floor. The entrance could not have been more uninviting to a visitor, but we were greeted by smiling faces at their apartment door. Inside the apartment, they had placed a parquet wood floor in three of the four rooms I saw. Upon entering, there was a kitchen immediately to the left, then a dining room. On the right was their son's bedroom and then, continuing down the hall, was Tatiana's bedroom. The balcony door was through Tatiana's bedroom. The view from the balcony was glorious. The Volga River was very wide, and a bridge connected Saratov to Engels, named after the Communist writer. I should add that Paul Tawney and I were taken to

Tatiana's apartment by her brother, Micha (or Michael), who was 20 years of age and a student in the Academy of Economics in Saratov. He had spent one year in Houston, Texas, in high school and was easy and comfortable in our company. He was driving a Russian-made car about the size of my Volkswagen, and it had 109,000 kilometers on the odometer. None of the cars that I saw on the road were washed, and all were generally in poor condition.

Alec offered me champagne, a gin and tonic, vodka, or red wine, and I chose the last. We sat down to a table full of cold foods first: salami and cheese, crab salad, cold fried fish, and caviar (orange and black) spread lightly over buttered rolls. Once again I was fooled. I thought this was the main event, and so I ate heartily. Then suddenly Galina, Tatiana's mother, came forth with the meat and potatoes and peas. There was enough food for twice the number of guests, and we all ate well. Several Russians made toasts, to which we drank. I was impressed by the Kudryashov family. Alexander and Galina were married in 1969 in Saratov. Their two children, Tatiana and Micha, were attractive and successful. Alexander was a gracious host and told us several times of his own experiences in the United States. He said that first Micha went to Houston for a year; then he (Alexander) went to Columbia, South Carolina, for a year to gain some expertise in his field of electrical appliances; and then finally Tatiana went to Chapel Hill for several months. Alexander's business required him to spend several days every other week in Moscow, and he was apparently very successful. Like many Russian families in Saratov, they had a small cottage 30 kilometers away on the Volga River. At these weekend cottages, they would garden and escape city life. I drank two cups of tea at the end of dinner and enjoyed the cake prepared by Galina. Micha drove Paul and me back to the hotel, where we retired at about 10 p.m.

Monday, May 25, 1998

I rose, wide awake, at about 4:30 a.m. After reading *The New Yorker* cover to cover, I showered and dressed and dictated some notes.

The five American doctors were then taken by car to Saratov Medical University. There we walked briefly through the campus past a fountain in the center of campus which is similar to The Pit at UNC, where many students congregate. We then went to the rector's office (the rector is the Dean of the medical school). The five of us Americans sat in chairs against the wall facing the rector's desk and about fifteen Russian faculty members. The rector gave a formal presentation through an interpreter, then welcomed us.

After that, we each went off with our corresponding faculty member. I was introduced to Vadim A. Prelatov, whose title is Professor and Chief of Surgery and Doctor of Medical Science at the Cardiac Surgery Center. His office was on the fourth floor of the second city hospital. The exterior was run-down, as was most of the interior. Linoleum covered most of the floors. His office had a single plaque over the door, and we entered a large room with a desk and conference table perpendicular to it. Three large bay windows looked out upon the Volga River, which was a block away. He had another smaller room adjacent to his office which was his "break room." It contained a little kitchen table with four chairs, a refrigerator, and a bathroom off to one side. In the bathroom was a toilet, a sink, and a shower. This room also had a large bay window and good light. His office, I should note, also had a ceiling fan and an air conditioner. He had very few things on the wall, but—notably—he had a picture of Leonard Bailey from Loma Linda University standing over a couch full of little children whose hearts he had transplanted. The professor had been to Loma Linda two years ago for three weeks and lived with a friend in Los Angeles during that time. He showed me a brochure of Loma Linda University and was very proud of his brief association with Leonard Bailey. He was slightly embarrassed because his English was not fluent. He told me the story of how he was intently observing Leonard Bailey operating when suddenly Bailey inquired about the health of Yeltsin. Professor Prelatov was speechless because he was concentrating so intently on the operation that he did not understand the quick speech of Bailey. He was embarrassed by his inability to answer. Prelatov also met Gundry and admired both of them.

Prelatov is about 5'9" in height and has a slightly olive complexion. He looks almost Cuban. His hair is white, and he is energetic and slender. He was all movement and enthusiasm. We sat down in his break room, and he served sparkling water and peach juice, and then brought out salami and cheese, which he cut with a large knife.

Constantine (my interpreter) and I got on well throughout the four-day visit. Constantine's father is Chief of Internal Medicine at Saratov State Medical University, and his mother is Greek. Constantine had spent a period of time in Chapel Hill with Wayne Cassio, the cardiologist. He seemed to like the United States, but he told me specifically that he wanted to live in Russia. Later in the week, his father told me that Constantine was about 6'2" in height, and overweight. He smoked intermittently throughout each day and partook in every toast we had. He was ebullient and friendly, and his English was satisfactory. His father asked me specifically about Constantine's level of understanding of English, and I told him that it was 85% complete.

Prelatov then brought some light blue scrubs for me to wear, plus a paper hat and mask. The hat had already been tied in the back and had obviously been worn previously, and so had the mask. I tried to put on the mask, but one of the strings in the back had ripped off, and so Prelatov handed me his mask, which had obviously been previously used. We went downstairs one floor to the operating suites. There appeared to be two or three operating rooms, and Prelatov worked in one specifically. I chose to observe and take pictures the first day. Prelatov had a 9-year-old girl on the table with a ventricular septal defect. When we got to the operating room, the child's chest had been opened and prepared, and the cannulation stitches were in. Prelatov scrubbed in by an elaborate process and then came to the table. He cannulated, went on bypass, cross clamped, and then gave antegrade cardioplegia. He opened the heart through the right atrium and closed a small inlet VSD with a pledgeted Prolene suture. The child came off bypass satisfactorily in sinus rhythm. Prelatov's assistant was a 37-year-old surgeon who was not particularly smooth in technique. The two surgeons as a team, with a female surgical assistant as second assistant, could not be described as "smooth operators." The assistants were constantly petting in Prelatov's way, but they got the job done. There were two operating room nurses scrubbed in and one circulator. The perfusionist was a physician whom they described as a cardio-physiologist. He was a young man, about 30, who was not a surgeon. Their heart-lung machine was basically the same as ours. They used roller pumps. The cardioplegia was delivered by roller pump, as well. I inspected the data sheets of the perfusionist and the anesthesiologist, and both were detailed, with 5-minute recordings on the anesthesiologist's paper. Two female anesthetists worked the ventilator and observed the telemetry unit. The monitoring unit was positioned at about waist level so that the perfusionist and the anesthetist could see it, though the anesthetist had to lean over to look at the numbers. They had blood pressure, heart rate, SVO_2, and SAO_2 on the monitor. I did not have an opportunity to see what sort of lines they placed, however. They had an electrocautery device that was nondisposable and archaic-looking. There may have been a foot pedal, because I did not see an on-off button. When the child was off bypass, Prelatov scrubbed out, and his first and second assistant closed the chest together. I inquired later about his infection rate, and he told me it was about 2%.

After the operation, we went back to the break room adjacent to his office, where we were visited by several of the hospital administrators. It was then decided that there would be a picnic in the forest that afternoon. We left in three or four cars and went off into the countryside. I really had no idea where we were going, and we landed on a horse farm about 30 miles outside of Saratov. I must add that we went through a village associated with a collective farm. My hosts were particularly proud of this village and the collective farm, and I was told that it was very productive. The horse farm was associated with this collective farm, and I was told that their best horses were kept here and that some champion race horses trained here. I think we were taken to the horse farm because it was their impression that Americans love horses. I inspected all the horses, and then we went on a buggy ride around the horse track. The trainer was a 16-year-old boy who seemed very competent with the horses. They brought out their prize horse for me to inspect, and pictures were taken of us standing in front of the horse.

We then piled back into cars and drove back down the highway, then into the woods. In this pine forest there suddenly appeared two picnic benches and several people congregated around an open fire. The hospital ambulance was parked between trees nearby, so it was obvious that the hospital ambulance doubled as the catering truck today. With us at the table sat Professor Prelatov; myself; Constantine, the translator; Sergei Dodiu, who was "the chief of the Second City Hospital"; Oleg Kostin, who was the main health care administrator of Kirov's district of Saratov; Kostin's wife, who was an attorney and much younger than he; and Mr. Feldman, who was the chief of all hospitals in the largest district of the Saratov region. To be an administrator in the hospital system in Russia appears to be prestigious, and doctors seem to jump at administrative posts whenever the opportunity arises.

Roberts CS. Cardiac surgery in Russia: An account of a trip to Sarotov, May 22-29, 1998. Address at Grand Rounds, Department of Surgery, University of North Carolina School of Medicine, Chapel Hill, North Carolina, August 26, 1998 (previously unpublished).

6

A Note on Mr. Christopher Lincoln as Teacher, on the Occasion of His Retirement

Albert Schweitzer once wrote that EXAMPLE is not the *main* thing in influencing others; it is the *only* thing. Having spent one year recently with Mr. Lincoln at the Royal Brompton Hospital, what I learned more than anything else were professional habits to carry one through 25 years in the field of cardiac surgery. I observed these habits very carefully with the hope that I could adopt most of them and by doing so, conduct a successful practice—not just where to put in the stitch, but also how to conduct a practice.

Mr. Lincoln rounded every Monday and Thursday with the team, and these rounds were a model of efficiency. We reviewed the angiogram. Televisions were turned off. Risks were described carefully to each patient. Mr. Lincoln did not think aloud. The patient was entitled to his conclusions, not his mental mechanisms.

Most Monday afternoons, he brought back a cake from a bakery near the Wellington Hospital. We ate it in his office while strategizing for the week: who would do which case, what operative approach to take, etc. Mr. Lincoln, of course, never ate. Like Samuel Johnson, he drank tea all day. Every Thursday, he instructed the members of his team to "improve your mind," and he meant just that. On Tuesday, Wednesday, and Friday, Mr. Lincoln operated at the Brompton and during the year performed 476 operations. As his fellow, I participated in 300. During the first 5 months, I assisted almost exclusively; and during the latter 7 months, I performed certain operations independently.

Mr. Lincoln's method of teaching was unlike any method I had experienced in my 10 years of training in the States. First of all, he never assisted me on an operation, except one, in the entire year. He either performed the operation himself or he turned it over to a trainee and did not scrub in. He told me to perform a mitral valve replacement early after my arrival; and upon opening the left atrium, I accidentally entered the right atrium. He was leaning over the ether screen and said, "Stop! Do not move. This will not do." He scrubbed in. I walked to the other side of the table, humiliated, and for the rest of the year we called it "The Roberts maneuver." But I must tell you, I have never made that mistake again.

However harsh his teaching methods were on occasion, they were—in my case—effective. You had to learn his technique exactly. That was the criterion to operate independently under his supervision. I memorized his technique of coarctation repair precisely, knowing that if I neglected a step in the operative set-up, he would take the case. More importantly, if I followed exactly his technique, the case would go easily and the patient was assured of a good result.

The surgery of Mr. Lincoln was simple, straightforward, and safe. He liked to quote Lord Moynihan, who said, "When I need an operation, oh Lord, save me from the gifted surgeon." To emphasize a pearl, he would say, "I want this tattooed across my chest: close my aortotomy in two layers" or "Use interrupted suture inside my heart." He believed in efficiency in theatre and used to say "every extra unnecessary minute in theatre leads to 10 extra minutes in the ICU." He liked quiet in his operating room and used to repeat the sign in the red buses: "Do not speak to or distract the driver when the bus is in motion."

Working with Mr. Lincoln was to work in a larger world. In my first operation assisting him, there was a second assistant from Cuba, a scrub nurse from Vietnam, a German cardiologist, and a South African anesthetist in the room. He exclaimed, "This is a world event." My grandfather once wrote that "no provincialist can be a great teacher of medicine," and Mr. Lincoln was certainly no provincialist. I asked once about the European Community, and he said, "I am not a European. I am a citizen of the world."

Frequently, blending the old with the new, the past with the present, Mr. Lincoln quoted Panneth, Tubbs, Ross, Aberdeen, Waterston, Kirklin, Shumway, and most of all Lord Brock. He frequently gave credit to his teachers by saying, "Ross taught me this" or "Senning showed me this" or "My mother taught me that." When I say it was a larger world working for Mr. Lincoln, I also mean that my education was not confined to the operating room and wards. One learned many of his views on the world.

Mr. Lincoln also included me in six social occasions at his home on Pembroke Square, which was a treat. This privileged interaction was extremely rare in my experience in the States. Dr. John Simpson, the anesthetist, remarked to me, shortly after I arrived, "If you ever get an invitation to dine at Christopher Lincoln's home, cancel your invitation to the American Embassy and go. It will be well worth it."

One Saturday, Mr. Lincoln took me and my fellow American trainee Francis Ferdinand to Harvey and Hudson on Jermyn Street, where he had his shirts made, and introduced us to Mr. Harvey. He would frequently leave articles from the *Financial Times*, his favorite newspaper, in my mailbox.

One final important aspect of his teaching is that he occasionally described to me clinical mistakes that he had made in his own career, with the obvious purpose that I would avoid them in my career. No other surgeon in my experience of ten years in training had been so candid; and to me, it was an admirable expression of humility. "You take these complications with you to the grave," he would say.

Shortly after I had arrived in London in 1996, he said to me, "Charles, this will be the greatest year of your life," and as a mentor, Mr. Lincoln made every effort to make it so. I feel privileged to have been one of his 27 foreign fellows. He has been the wise friend of my clinical life in Chapel Hill, and the unseen consultant with my patients. His words and manner still ring in my ears on the wards in Chapel Hill, and I am certain that the memories will linger for a lifetime.

Roberts WC. A note on Mr. Christopher Lincoln as teacher, on the occasion of his retirement, 1999. Address at Advances in Paediatric Cardiac Surgery, 1973-1999. A Festschrift for Christopher Lincoln, Royal Brompton Hospital, London, United Kingdom, June 4, 1999 (previously unpublished).

7

EDITORIALS

Postoperative Drug Therapy To Extend Survival After Coronary Artery Bypass Grafting

Charles S. Roberts, MD

Division of Cardiothoracic Surgery, University of North Carolina School of Medicine, Chapel Hill, North Carolina

The debate on the best form of therapy for coronary artery disease has been framed historically in terms of medicine versus surgery. Physicians and surgeons engaged in this debate often have failed to avail their patients of the potential benefit of multimodality therapy. Several modes of therapy extend survival in patients with coronary artery disease (Table 1), and they can be combined to achieve maximal benefit.

In a metaanalysis by Yusuf and associates [1], coronary artery bypass grafting (CABG) was shown to lower the 5-year mortality rate by 39% compared with medical therapy in the era before statin drugs. In the trials that form the basis of the metaanalysis, patients were enrolled between 1972 and 1984, and only 10% of the CABG patients had an internal mammary arterial conduit. Because CABG with one or both internal mammary arterial conduits confers a survival benefit superior to that with only vein conduits [2, 3], one can project an even better effect on survival than that reported in the metaanalysis.

Three major secondary preventive trials support the use of statin drugs in patients with coronary artery disease [4–6]. In the Scandinavian Simvastatin Survival Study, the simvastatin group had a 42% reduction in coronary deaths at 5.4 years compared with the placebo group [4]. In the Cholesterol and Recurrent Events (CARE) study, in which about one fourth of the patients had a previous CABG, a 24% reduction in fatal coronary events or nonfatal myocardial infarction occurred over 5 years with pravastatin compared with placebo [5]. Specifically, the survival benefit of the CABG patients taking pravastatin versus placebo was 38% [7]. In the Long-term Intervention with Pravastatin in Ischaemic Disease (LIPID) study, in which about one fourth of the patients also had had CABG, a relative risk reduction of 24% in mortality rate from coronary artery disease occurred over 6 years with pravastatin [6]. Although this editorial concerns the survival benefit of statin drugs, the positive effect of lowering lipid levels on graft patency after CABG has been well demonstrated [8].

In a metaanalysis of 145 trials of antiplatelet drugs (mainly aspirin), involving about 70,000 high-risk patients with atherothrombotic diseases of various kinds, the incidence of myocardial infarction was reduced by 30% and vascular death by 17% after 2 years [9]. For patients with either acute or healed myocardial infarcts, aspirin prevented about 40 vascular events per 1,000 patients treated for 1 month or 2 years, respectively [9].

Trials of inhibitors of angiotensin-converting-enzymes have shown improved symptoms and reduced mortality rates in patients with congestive heart failure [10, 11]. More recently, the Heart Outcomes Prevention Evaluation (HOPE) study showed that ramipril (10 mg daily) reduced cardiovascular deaths by 25% and nonfatal myocardial infarction by 20% in high-risk patients, compared with matching placebo over 5 years [12]. The average blood pressure reduction was only 3/2 mm Hg, and the benefit of ramipril was independent of ejection fraction. Like the statin drugs, angiotensin-converting-enzyme inhibitors might accomplish their beneficial effect by improving systemic endothelial function [13].

Two major metaanalyses of beta-blockade after myocardial infarction have shown conclusively a reduction in cardiovascular mortality rate of approximately 23% at 5 years [14, 15]. The benefit of beta-blockade applies to patients with acute or healed myocardial infarcts, which is nearly half of all CABG patients [16].

In summary, virtually all CABG patients should probably be started on a statin drug with the goal of maintaining a low-density lipoprotein-cholesterol level of 100 mg/dL or less. Contraindications would be active liver disease or women of child-bearing age. Postoperatively aspirin should be prescribed routinely except in patients with an allergy or gastric intolerance, in which case clopidogrel can be substituted. An angiotensin-converting-enzyme inhibitor appears warranted in CABG patients with an abnormal ejection fraction and perhaps in all CABG patients, as data from the HOPE study suggests. Beta-blockers should be restricted to patients who have had a myocardial infarction and should be avoided in patients with overt congestive heart failure, heart block, or bradycardia.

Each of those five forms of therapy confers a survival benefit in patients with coronary artery disease. Although CABG is beneficial in selected patients with coronary artery disease compared with historical medical therapy, it is not the only form of therapy that can extend life. A surgeon who treats a patient with CABG has the responsibility to initiate or continue multimodality therapy while that patient is under his or her care. Incorporating risk reduction drug therapy into routine postoperative and discharge orders may reduce the frequency of reintervention and, more importantly, extend survival after CABG.

Address reprint requests to Dr Roberts, Division of Cardiothoracic Surgery, University of North Carolina School of Medicine, 108 Burnett-Womack Building, CB 7065, Chapel Hill, NC 27599-7065; e-mail: charless@med.unc.edu.

Published by Elsevier Science Inc

Ann Thorac Surg 2000;69:1315–6 • 0003-4975/00/$20.00
PII S0003-4975(00)01216-9

Table 1. Approximate Cardiovascular Mortality Rate Reduction by Various Interventions

Intervention	Approximate Cardiovascular Mortality Reduction at 5 Years (%)	Reference
CABG	39	1[a]
Statin drug	30	4–7[b]
Aspirin	17	9[c]
ACE inhibitor	25	12
Beta-blocker	23	14, 15[d]

[a] Risk reduction was 68% if left main artery and 42% if three-vessel disease. [b] Risk reductions in the 4S, CARE, and LIPID studies were 42%, 24%, and 24%, respectively. [c] The average duration of these trials was 2 years. [d] In patients who had a myocardial infarction.

ACE = angiotensin converting enzyme; CABG = coronary artery bypass grafting.

References

1. Yusuf S, Zucker D, Peduzzi P, et al. Effect of coronary artery bypass graft surgery on survival: overview of 10-year results from randomised trials by the Coronary Artery Bypass Graft Surgery Trialists Collaboration. Lancet 1994;344:563–70.
2. Loop FD, Lytle BW, Cosgrove DM, et al. Influence of the internal-mammary-artery graft on 10-year survival and other cardiac events. N Engl J Med 1986;314:1–6.
3. Lytle BW, Blackstone EH, Loop FD, et al. Two internal thoracic artery grafts are better than one. J Thorac Cardiovasc Surg 1999;117:855–72.
4. Scandinavian Simvastatin Survival Study Group. Randomised trial of cholesterol lowering in 4444 patients with coronary heart disease: the Scandinavian Simvastatin Survival Study (4S). Lancet 1994;344:1383–9.
5. Sacks FM, Pfeffer MA, Moye LA, et al. The effect of pravastatin on coronary events after myocardial infarction in patients with average cholesterol levels. N Engl J Med 1996; 335:1001–9.
6. The Long-term Intervention with Pravastatin in Ischaemic Disease (LIPID) Study Group. Prevention of cardiovascular events and death with pravastatin in patients with coronary heart disease and a broad range of initial cholesterol levels. N Engl J Med 1998;339:1349–57.
7. Flaker GC, Warnica JW, Sacks FM, et al. Pravastatin prevents clinical events in revascularized patients with average cholesterol concentrations. J Am Coll Cardiol 1999;34:106–12.
8. The Post Coronary Artery Bypass Graft Trial Investigators. The effect of aggressive lowering of low-density lipoprotein cholesterol levels and low-dose anticoagulation on obstructive changes in saphenous-vein coronary-artery bypass grafts. N Engl J Med 1997;336:153–62.
9. Antiplatelet Trialists' Collaboration. Collaborative overview of randomised trials of antiplatelet therapy—I: prevention of death, myocardial infarction, and stroke by prolonged antiplatelet therapy in various categories of patients. BMJ 1994; 308:81–106.
10. The CONSENSUS Trial Study Group. Effects of enalapril on mortality in severe congestive heart failure: results of the Cooperative North Scandinavian Enalapril Survival Study (CONSENSUS). N Engl J Med 1987;316:1429–35.
11. The SOLVD Investigators. Effect of enalapril on survival in patients with reduced left ventricular ejection fractions and congestive heart failure. N Engl J Med 1991;325:293–302.
12. The Heart Outcomes Prevention Evaluation Study Investigators. Effects of an angiotensin-converting-enzyme inhibitor, ramipril, on cardiovascular events in high-risk patients. N Engl J Med 2000;342:145–53.
13. Oosterga M, Voors AA, Buikema H, et al. Functional effects of ACE-inhibitors on angiotensin I conversion in human vasculature. J Am Coll Cardiol 1998;31(suppl A):239A–40A.
14. Yusuf S, Peto R, Lewis J, Collins R, Sleight P. Beta blockade during and after myocardial infarction: overview of the randomized trials. Prog Cardiovasc Dis 1985;27:335–71.
15. Teo KK, Yusuf S, Furberg CD. Effects of prophylactic antiarrhythmic drug therapy in acute myocardial infarction: an overview of results from randomized controlled trials. JAMA 1993;270:1589–95.
16. Edwards FH, Carey JS, Grover FL, Bero JW, Hartz RS. Impact of gender on coronary bypass operative mortality. Ann Thorac Surg 1998;66:125–31.

Roberts CS. Postoperative drug therapy to extend survival after coronary artery bypass grafting. *Ann Thorac Surg*. 2000;69(5):1315-1316. doi:10.1016/s0003-4975(00)01216-9

8

Death and the Research Imperative

To the Editor: Callahan's belief that 65 years is a sufficient life span to experience "the typical range of human possibilities and aspirations" brings to mind Sir William Osler's "two fixed ideas": that one's best work is done by the age of 40, and that one should retire at the age of 60. Osler humorously referred to Anthony Trollope's novel *The Fixed Period,* in which "the plot hinges upon the admirable scheme of a college into which at sixty men retired for a year of contemplation before a peaceful departure by chloroform."[1] These remarks drew such criticism that Osler tendered his "heartfelt regrets" in the preface to the second edition of *Aequanimitas.* Osler repeated, however, his original belief that "the real work of life is done before the fortieth year and after the sixtieth year it would be best for the world and best for themselves if men rested from their labours."[1]

Of course, healthy human longevity has increased since Osler's day. However, Callahan correctly suggests that the current research imperative to eradicate death at all ages should refocus on the promotion of health and the prevention of disease. For no disease is this strategy more appropriate than it is for atherosclerosis.

The "bright line" between the living and the dying is not bright too often in my practice; nearly half of my patients who have undergone coronary bypass are at least 65 years of age. My colleagues and I fight death to the end, even in elderly patients with severe atherosclerosis. But I also agree with Callahan that these patients should be allowed to consider carefully, and without reproach, a peaceful death with noninvasive care.

CHARLES S. ROBERTS, M.D.
University of North Carolina
Chapel Hill, NC 27599-7065

1. Osler W. Aequanimitas: with other addresses to medical students, nurses and practitioners of medicine. 2nd ed. Philadelphia: Blakiston, 1906.

Roberts CS. Death and the research imperative. *N Engl J Med.* 2000;343(3):224-225.

9

DISEASE MANAGEMENT

10 Questions—and 10 Answers—About the Role of "Statin" Therapy after Coronary Artery Bypass Grafting

Charles S. Roberts, MD, Kimberly D. Donovan, MS, ANP

Over the past 30 years, coronary artery bypass grafting (CABG) has become commonplace. About a million CABG procedures are now done every year in the United States. This means that several million individuals are eligible for secondary preventive measures, the goal being to avoid future cardiovascular events. In this article we answer ten questions pertinent to the use of 3-hydroxy-3-methylgluraryl-coenzyme A inhibitors ("statin" therapy) to lower cholesterol synthesis and thereby improve blood lipids after CABG.

(1) What percentage of CABG patients have had a cardiovascular event? Nearly all. The CABG database of the Society of Thoracic Surgeons indicates that at the time of CABG surgery, 59% of patients have unstable angina pectoris, 47% have had a myocardial infarction, 12% have congestive heart failure, and 2% are in cardiogenic shock.[1] Atherosclerosis is clinically demonstrable in cerebral or peripheral vessels in 20% of CABG patients.[1]

(2) How extensive is the coronary atherosclerosis in CABG patients? Based on angiograms (which generally underestimate the extent of coronary atherosclerosis compared to autopsy studies[2]), most patients have "three-vessel disease"; the database of the Society of Thoracic Surgeons indicates that 73% have atherosclerotic narrowing of all three major epicardial coronary arteries, 21% have narrowing of two, and 6% have narrowing of one.[1] About 20% have significant narrowing of the left main coronary artery.[1] It seems clear that CABG patients carry a heavy burden of atherosclerosis.

Dr. Roberts is Assistant Professor of Surgery, University of North Carolina School of Medicine at Chapel Hill. Ms. Donovan is an Adult Nurse Practitioner in the Lipid Clinic of the University of North Carolina Health Care System. Contact Dr. Roberts at 919/966-3381 or charless@med.unc.edu

(3) What drugs are usually prescribed after CABG? Shortly after surgery, most CABG patients need analgesics and diuretics. Over the long term, most are told to take an aspirin tablet every day. If they have had a myocardial infarction in the past, a beta-adrenergic blocking drug is usually prescribed. But it is not likely that a CABG patient will get a prescription for a statin drug. It is also not likely that patients will have taken a statin before surgery. Cardiac surgeons tend to continue preoperative medications after surgery, except for nitrates, which are routinely discontinued.

(4) Has CABG been compared to statin therapy in a clinical trial? No. Randomized trials comparing CABG to medical therapy were carried out before statin drugs were available. A 1992 meta-analysis by Yusuf and associates concluded that CABG improved 5-year survival by an average of 39% compared to medical therapy.[3] But only 10% of the CABG patients in the trials had an internal mammary arterial conduit, which is standard today. Thus, neither the surgical nor the medical treatments used in the randomized studies of coronary artery disease is comparable to today's approaches, when internal mammary arteries are used routinely and statin drugs are part of standard medical therapy.

(5) Does statin therapy improve conduit patency after CABG? Yes. The Post Coronary Artery Bypass Graft Trial[4] studied whether aggressively lowering low-density lipoprotein (LDL) cholesterol levels affected saphenous vein conduits. Reducing the LDL-cholesterol level to below 100 mg/dL significantly reduced angiographically evident atherosclerosis in saphenous vein conduits, which are already less disposed to atherosclerosis than arterial conduits.

(6) Does statin therapy reduce the need for a second CABG? Probably. The Post Coronary Artery Bypass Graft Trial found that those whose LDL-cholesterol levels were aggressively lowered to below 100 mg/dL had a 29% lower rate of revascularization over four years compared to those receiving moderate treatment (p=0.03).[4] Analysis of a subset of 1091 CABG patients in the CARE study found that revascularization was 14% less likely in patients treated with pravastatin compared to placebo, but the difference was not statistically significant.[5]

(7) Why is it important to avoid a second CABG? The early mortality rate for a second CABG is about 5-10%, roughly twice that for a first operation.[6,7] Risks unique to the second CABG include catastrophic hemorrhage during sternal reopening; injury to patent conduits (particularly the left internal mammary artery); embolism during manipulation of old conduits; greater requirement for an intra-aortic balloon pump; greater incidence of low cardiac output syndrome; greater frequency of perioperative myocardial infarction; and greater likelihood of continuing angina pectoris.[8-10]

(8) Does statin therapy reduce the frequency of cardiovascular events after CABG? Yes. Two of the three major secondary prevention trials[11-13] included patients who had already undergone CABG. In the CARE study,[11] 1091 patients (about 27%) had prior CABG; separate examination of the results in these patients showed a 33% risk reduction in coronary death or nonfatal myocardial infarction in those receiving pravastatin compared to placebo.[5] Similarly, 27% of subjects in the LIPID study had had CABG; the incidence of adverse cardiovascular events in this subpopulation was consistently lower among patients receiving pravastatin, but these patients have not been examined as a separate group.[12]

(9) Does statin therapy prolong survival after CABG? Yes. In the CARE study, CABG patients given pravastatin had a 38% survival benefit at 5 years and 44% fewer deaths from coronary artery disease compared to those given placebo.[5] The LIPID study showed a 24% relative reduction in risk of death from coronary artery disease, and overall mortality was reduced by 22% in the pravastatin group.[12] The third secondary prevention trial (the 4S study[13]) excluded patients who had already had CABG, but who did have angina pectoris or myocardial infarction, just as do most CABG patients. The group given simvastatin had a survival benefit at 5.4 years of 30% compared to the placebo group.[13]

(10) What should we routinely do after CABG? Recognizing that all therapy must be individualized, we have some general recommendations. With few exceptions, a statin drug and an aspirin should be prescribed after CABG.[14] Patients with systemic hypertension or abnormal left ventricular ejection fraction should be given an angiotensin converting enzyme inhibitor.[15] Patients who have already had a myocardial infarction should be on a beta blocker, unless there is overt congestive heart failure or bradycardia.[16] We recommend follow-up of CABG patients three and six months after surgery to adjust the statin dose (to achieve an LDL cholesterol level under 100 mg/dL[15]) and to modify other cardiovascular risk factors such as smoking and obesity.

References

1 Edwards FH, Carey JS, Grover FL, et al. Impact of gender on coronary bypass operative mortality. Ann Thorac Surg 1998;66:125-31.

2 Roberts, WC. Qualitative and quantitative comparison of amounts of narrowing by atherosclerotic plaques in the major epicardial coronary arteries at necropsy in sudden coronary death, transmural acute myocardial infarction, transmural healed myocardial infarction and unstable angina pectoris. Am J Cardiol 1989;64:324-8.

3 Yusuf S, Zucker D, Peduzzi P, et al. Effect of coronary artery bypass graft surgery on survival: overview of 10-year results from randomised trials by the Coronary Artery Bypass Graft Surgery Trialists Collaboration. Lancet 1994;344:563-70.

4 The Post Coronary Artery Bypass Graft Trial Investigators. The effect of aggressive lowering of low-density lipoprotein cholesterol levels and low-dose anticoagulation on obstructive changes in saphenous-vein coronary-artery bypass grafts. N Engl J Med 1997;336:153-62.

5 Flaker GC, Warnica JW, Sacks FM, et al. Pravastatin prevents clinical events in revascularized patients with average cholesterol concentrations. J Am Coll Cardiol 1999;34:106-12.

6 He G-W, Acuff TE, Ryan WH, et al. Determinants of operative mortality in reoperative coronary artery bypass grafting. J Thorac Cardiovasc Surg 1995;110:971-8.

7 Weintraub WS, Jones EL, Craver JM, et al. In-hospital and long-term outcome after reoperative coronary artery bypass graft surgery. Circulation 1995;92(suppl II):II50-7.

8 Dobell ARC, Jain AK. Catastrophic hemorrhage during redo sternotomy. Ann Thorac Surg 1984;37:273-8.

9 Gillinov AM, Casselman FP, Lytle BW, et al. Injury to a patent left internal thoracic artery graft at coronary reoperation. Ann Thorac Surg 1999:67:382-6.

10 Lytle BW. Coronary reoperations. Coronary Artery Dis 1993;4:703-6.

11 Sacks FM, Pfeffer MA, Moye LA, et al. The effect of pravastatin on coronary events after myocardial infarction in patients with average cholesterol levels. N Engl J Med 1996;335:1001-9.

12 The Long-Term Intervention with Pravastatin in Ischaemic Disease (LIPID) Study Group. Prevention of cardiovascular events and death with pravastatin in patients with coronary heart disease and a broad range of initial cholesterol levels. N Engl J Med 1998;339:1349-57.

13 Scandinavian Simvastatin Survival Study Group. Randomised trial of cholesterol lowering in 4444 patients with coronary heart disease: the Scandinavian Simvastatin Survival Study (4S). Lancet 1994;344:1383-9.

14 Antiplatelet Trialists' Collaboration. Collaborative overview of randomised trials of antiplatelet therapy-I. Prevention of death, myocardial infarction, and stroke by prolonged antiplatelet

therapy in various categories of patients. Br Med J 1994:308:81-106.

15 The Heart Outcomes Prevention Evaluation Study Investigators. Effects of an angiotensin-converting-enzyme inhibitor, ramipril, on cardiovascular events in high-risk patients. N Engl J Med 2000;342:145-53.

16 Yusuf S, Peto R, Lewis J, et al. Beta blockade during and after myocardial infarction: an overview of the randomized trials. Prog Cardiovasc Dis 1985;27:335-71.

17 Grundy SM, Balady GJ, Criqui MH, et al. When to start cholesterol-lowering therapy in patients with coronary heart disease: a statement for healthcare professionals from the American Heart Association Task Force on Risk Reduction. Circulation 1997;95:1683-5.

Roberts S, Donovan KD. 10 questions—and 10 answers—about the role of "statin" therapy after coronary artery bypass grafting. *N Carolina Med J.* 2000 July/August;61(4):220-222.

10

Harvey's Experiment on Occlusion of the Vena Cava
To the Editor:

To relieve acute pulmonary hypertension during beating heart operations, Drs Dagenais and Cartier [1] recommend placing a snare to occlude the inferior vena cava, partially or totally, in patients with low-to-moderate mitral regurgitation or severe left ventricular dysfunction. In his book *The Motion of the Heart and Blood*, published in 1628, Dr William Harvey [2] describes a similar technique applied to the heart of a live snake, presumably without valvar regurgitation or ventricular dysfunction: "Now, pinching off the vena cava with a forceps or between finger and thumb, the course of blood being intercepted some distance below the heart, you will see that the space between the finger and the heart is drained at once, the blood being emptied by the heart beat. At the same time, the heart becomes much paler even in distention, smaller from lack of blood, and beats more slowly, so that it seems to be dying. Immediately on releasing the vein, the color and size of the heart return to normal."

After numerous observations and experiments in various species, Dr Harvey demonstrated, for the first time in human history, that the heart pumped all the blood from veins to arteries in a circular system. Producing bradycardia by interrupting venous return to the heart was indirect evidence of the pumping function of the heart.

Charles S. Roberts, MD

Division of Cardiothoracic Surgery
University of North Carolina at Chapel Hill
CB 7065, 108 Burnett-Womack Bldg
Chapel Hill, NC 27599
e-mail: charless@med.unc.edu.

References

1. Dagenais F, Cartier R. Pulmonary hypertension during beating heart coronary surgery: intermittent inferior vena cava snaring. Ann Thorac Surg 1999;68:1094–5.
2. Harvey W. Exercitatio anatomica de motu cordis et sanguinis in animalibus, 4th ed. Springfield: Charles C Thomas, 1958:84.

Reply
To the Editor:

Of course, we are all grateful to William Harvey (1578–1657), whose concept of continuous blood circulation in a contained system has been one of the most contributory accomplishments in physiology in the 17th century. Nevertheless, Harvey had precursors [1] such as Michael Servetous (1511–1553), Matteo Realdo Colombo (1516–1559), and Andrea Cesalpino (1519–1603), who proposed the concept of separated pulmonary transit of the blood. Cesalpino was the first to propose the term "circulation" and to put together the knowledge of greater (systemic) and lesser (pulmonary) circulation. But more interesting is the fact that Harvey's work was poorly received by his peers. Even 20 years after his publication *Exercitatio Anatomica de Motu Cordis et Sanguinis in Animalibus* (1615) his work was ignored by the medical community. For these men of "Science," who adhered to Galenism Theory (blood arising from the liver, transiting from the right heart to the left heart by "septal pores" before vanishing in the peripheral tissues), the granting of a "respectable status" in the community was more important than the virtuous principles of experimental science.

So far we have been proud to apply Harvey's experimental observations to beating heart surgical procedures. We have shared our technique with other surgeons who are quite pleased with the results.

Raymond Cartier, MD

Department of Surgery
Montreal Heart Institute
5000 Belanger St E
Montreal, PQ, Canada H1T 1C8

Reference

1. Lyons AS, Petrucelli RJ. Medicine, an illustrated history. New York: Harry N. Abrams, 1978.

Patient-Prosthesis Mismatch Is Not Negligible
To the Editor:

We read with interest the article by Izzat and associates [1] on the impact of patient-prosthesis mismatch in modern cardiac prostheses. Physiologically, it must be remembered that transvalvular gradients are essentially determined by two factors (see Gorlin equation): the effective orifice area of the valve and transvalvular flow. In turn, transvalvular flow is related to cardiac output, which at rest is largely determined by body surface area. Accordingly, we have repeatedly demonstrated that the parameter that best correlates ($r > 0.80$) with postoperative resting and exercise gradients is the indexed valve area, that is, the effective orifice area of the prosthetic valve divided by body surface area (see reference and bibliography) [2]. Hence, it is surprising that Izzat and associates have omitted in their statistical analysis the most important factor associated with mismatch (ie, the indexed valve area). Also, they used a multivariate linear analysis, whereas the relationship between transvalvular gradients and body surface area or valve area is nonlinear [2]. Finally, the study included a cohort of patients with a narrow range of body surface areas and indexed valve areas, and two groups (St. Jude bileaflet 21 mm and Carbomedics 21 mm) had markedly lower average cardiac indices (1.56 L/min/m^2) compared with the four other groups (2.5 to 3.2 L/min/m^2), thus suggesting the inclusion of patients with significant left ventricular dysfunction, which per se would tend to decrease gradients. All these important biases thus compromise the reliability of the multivariate analysis and the conclusions of the study. Furthermore, when the average values of the resting and stress mean gradients reported by Izzat and associates are plotted as a function of the average indexed valve areas (see Fig 1), a strong curvilinear relationship is found, similar to those that we previously reported [2]. The only exceptions are the two groups with abnormally low cardiac output, which is not surprising given that the decrease in transvalvular flow will result in lower gradients than expected. The conclusion that "these prostheses can be used without concern" also implies that resting gradients of 19, 22, and 30 mm Hg and stress gradients of 33, 42, and 49 mm Hg, corresponding to indexed valve areas of 0.56, 0.58, and 0.65 cm^2/m^2, are acceptable without any other form of discussion. In this context, it should be remembered that previous studies have demonstrated that patients with evidence of mismatch as defined by an indexed valve area <0.85 cm^2/m^2 have less symptomatic improvement, worse hemodynamics, and less regression of left ventricular hypertrophy after operation [2, 3]. Furthermore, Rao and associates have recently reported in a study of 2,516 patients that the indexed valve area but not the

Ann Thorac Surg 2000;69:1983–96 • 0003-4975/00/$20.00
PII S0003-4975(00)01121-8

Roberts CS. Harvey's experiment on occlusion of the vena cava. *Ann Thorac Surg.* 2000;69(6):1983. doi:10.1016/s0003-4975(00)01121-8

11

The Scholarship of *De Motu Cordis*: Whom Did Harvey Reference?

> In discussing the movements and functions of the heart and arteries, we should first consider what others have said on these matters and what the common and traditional viewpoint is. —William Harvey, *De Motu Cordis*, 1628

Most medical or scientific publications contain references to previous work in the field, and the author's choice of references is often a clue to the author's scholarship. In his *De Motu Cordis*, William Harvey refers to 17 persons, all but 2 of whom were physicians. The references span 20 centuries, from Hippocrates to Riolan, with Galen and Aristotle mentioned most often.

Harvey was 50 years of age in 1628 when his book on the circulation appeared. It was 5 years after Shakespeare's First Folio appeared and 3 years after Charles I was crowned. Harvey was a first-born, a Loyalist, a conservative, married and childless, and a somewhat reluctant author—his lecture notes indicate knowledge of the circulation some 8 years before the book was published. His choice of references in *De Motu Cordis* indicates that he did not work in a vacuum, but rather had a keen knowledge of medical history.

My reprinted copy of *De Motu Cordis* has 165 pages in 13 chapters. Chapter 8 is the critical chapter in which Harvey first uses the word circle to describe the flow of blood in the human body.

Harvey mentions 17 persons in De Motu, in chronological order in history (not in chronological order in the book). Galen is mentioned 31 times and several persons are mentioned only once. Of the 17 persons mentioned, only Hoffman and Riolan were alive in 1628, the year of publication. Each person mentioned has a unique reason for being referenced by Harvey.

Hippocrates of Cos (460-370 BC)

Hippocrates is only mentioned once by Harvey. The Hippocratic corpus is a compilation of about 80 anonymous medical works that became a part of the library of Alexandria about 250 BC. Hippocrates is especially known for the concept of the 4 humours, but of particular interest to Harvey must have been "De Corde," a brief essay on the heart in the Hippocratic collection. The heart is considered the central organ of life, with a respiratory function. The left ventricle was noted to be thicker than the right...to protect the soul.

Aristotle of Macedonia (324-322 BC)

Harvey claimed to have two guiding lights—Fabricius, his mentor in Padua, and Aristotle. Although his teacher, Plato, distrusted the senses, Aristotle began the scientific principle of systematic observation. For almost 2,000 years, Aristotle's ideas on scientific investigation formed the basis for experimentation, and he was the first scientist to apply findings in anatomical dissection to biomedical theories. Harvey is the first real disciple of Aristotle.

Aristotle also regarded the heart as the most important organ in the body, and as the seat of the soul. Developing embryos were not considered alive until a heartbeat was distinguished. The heart was seen as the source of innate heat within the body. All sensory systems were assumed to link back to the heart. The brain and lungs were merely devices for cooling down the innate heat. Aristotle described a "pneuma," which was akin to innate heat, and which was unrelated to the outside air. This pneuma, along with innate heat, was used to describe a myriad of physiological mysteries, including the connection between the body and the soul.

Aristotle was a comparative biologist who dissected innumerable animals. Harvey describes cardiovascular anatomy in 45 animals in *De Motu Cordis*. Aristotle is responsible for the idea that a rational relationship exists between the structure and function of an organ. He wrote 4 main biological works: *History of Animals, Parts of Animals, Generation,* and *Movement of Animals*. Harvey's other major medical treatise was called *Generation.*

Terrance of Rome

Terrance is not referred to by name, but is simply called "the old man." Harvey quotes a passage from *Adelphi*, a comedy written by Terrance.

Erasistratus of Alexandria (310-250 BC)

Considered to be the Father of Physiology, Erasistratus is a controversial figure in medical history. After training in Athens, he supposedly worked in Alexandria, experimenting on living animals and, some speculate, even on humans. Erasistratus believed that arteries carried "pneuma" and veins carried blood, supplied by the liver. He believed that arteries showed blood when cut, only because nature abhorred a vacuum—the outward flow of pneuma was matched by an inward flow of blood. Erasistratus believed that food was necessary for the production of blood and, like Aristotle, that pneuma was integral to the body.

Galen of Pergamos (131-201)

Galen wrote a myriad of medical texts, including 16 books on the pulse. His system of medicine established on the minutiae of pulse variations persisted into the 18th century. Galen's observation that arteries contain blood, not air, was crucial in Harvey's work on the circulation. Galen also showed that practically all the blood can be withdrawn by an arteriotomy, proving a connection between veins and arteries.

Harvey disputed Galen on several points: (1) that the function of the heart and lung movements were identical; (2) that the ventricles and large arteries simultaneously expand; (3) that the function of the right and left ventricles was different; (4) that the cardiac valves were incompetent; and (5) that pores existed in the interventricular septum.

Galen's legacy has been the longest in medical history, lasting some 15 centuries. He was finally superseded in anatomy by Vesalius, in physiology by Harvey, and in pathology by Boerhaave.

Avicenna of Persia (980-1037)

The Latin translation of Avicenna's *Cannon of Medicine* was the second most published book in the world for a time, after the Bible. Avicenna was a supporter of Aristotle and continued to maintain that the heart had 3 ventricles and was the central organ in the body. He never performed dissections but rather engaged in "speculative anatomy." Though Avicenna drew criticism for rejecting Galenic views, he performed the Galenic role of philosopher-physician and linked the medical traditions of the East and West.

Sylvius of Paris (1478-1555)

Jacobus Sylvius, a Parisian medical humanist, contributed to medicine by his vehement support of Galen and in his role as teacher of Vesalius. His two books, *Introduction to Anatomy* (1555) and *Order and Way of Reading Hippocrates and Galen* (1539), served to renew the Galenic tradition. In fact, Sylvius was so deeply rooted in that tradition that if any anatomical discrepancies were found during dissection, the fault was attributed to the corpse rather than Galen. Sylvius described tuberculosis as a disease of the lungs and recorded that tubercules softened and suppurated to form cavities.

Fracastoro of Verona (1478-1553)

Giroloamo Fracastoro is considered to be the Father of Epidemiology. His main contributions to medicine were his two major publications—one on syphilis and the other on contagion. The first work is a poetic description of the symptoms and signs and treatment of syphilis. The second elaborates on the ideas of Epicurus and Lucretius in explaining contagious disease through "seeds," or seminaria, that infected from a distance, or through "fomites," that harbored these seeds and transmitted them directly. This book formed a crude beginning to the germ theory. Harvey's single reference to Fracastoro concerns the motion of the heart, which the Verona physician thought was something "to be understood by God alone."

Hollerius (1498-1562)

There is a single reference to this person, whose identity in history remains unknown to me.

Vesalius of Padua (1514-1564)

Although taught by Sylvius, a supporter of Galen, Vesalius had no compunction about exposing Galen's errors. His book, *De Humani Corporis Fabrica* (On the Structure of the Human Body, 1543), corrected Galen's errors with information gathered from frequent human dissections. For example, Vesalius described the sternum as composed of 3 bones instead of the 7 proposed by Galen. The liver no longer contained 5 lobes, but still was thought to produce blood.

Perhaps the most important correction involved the heart and was introduced in the second edition of the *Fabrica* (1555). Vesalius denied the tenet that the ventricular septum was permeable—he saw no pores, indicating that a pulmonary circulation did exist. Harvey took note of this. Although many observations by Vesalius were soon corrected as well, his daringness to oppose Galen led to the acceptance of anatomy based on dissection, and thus, his title as the Father of Anatomy.

Columbo of Rome (1515-1559)

Although a lesser known anatomist, Realdo Columbo was one of the most influential for Harvey. His *De Re Anatomica* was published in 1559 in the style of Galen and as a succession to the work of Vesalius. Columbo accused Vesalius of passing animal anatomy off as human, exactly the same charge that Vesalius had put against Galen.

Columbo's description of the pulmonary circulation was monumental, though he may have read the account of Servetus which was published 6 years earlier. Columbo proved that the pulmonary vasculature took blood to the lungs to mix with air, rather than air passing to the heart to mix with blood. He also showed that the interventricular septum was impermeable to blood.

Columbo also described the heartbeat and broke tradition in theorizing that (1) the heart worked with greater force during systole than during diastole, and (2) the heart discharged blood into the arteries. These two ideas were crucial for Harvey as well. Columbo also gave a clear description of the mode of action of the cardiac valves.

Botallus of France (1530-)

Though born in Italy, Leonardo Botallo (Botallus) spent most of his life working as prebendary of the Abbye of Saint Marie de Chelles near Meux. Probably his most important contribution was a description of the ductus arteriosus. He was also physician to French royalty, including Charles IX and William, Duke of Brabont. In *De lue veneria* (1563), he advocated the use of mercury to combat syphilis.

Fabricius of Padua (1537-1619)

From his home in Padua, Fabrizzi (Hieronymus Fabricius of Aquapendente) aspired to produce Totius Animalis Fabricate Theatrum (The Theatre of the Entire Animal Structure), but only parts were published. He was less concerned with anatomy than with function. Although he was not the first to discover the venous valves, he published *De Venarum Ostiolis* (On the Valves of the Veins) in 1603, the year Harvey returned to London. It describes the venous valves at length. Fabricius believed the purpose of the valves was merely to delay the flow of blood. Harvey's experiments established their true purpose—to keep blood from pooling in the extremities, establishing equal systemic flow. This idea was crucial for Harvey's discovery of circulation.

Fabricius also thought that the pulmonary vein was the most important structure of the lungs and that they were designed to house that one vessel. He described systole and diastole, as well as the separate purpose of the lungs in providing air for the heart. The writings of Fabricius include the anatomy of almost all parts of the body except the heart.

Laurens of Paris (1558-1609)

Andre du Laurens was physician to Henri IV and Professor at Montpellier. He published a *Discourse of the Preservation of the Sight; of Melancholic Diseases; of Rheumes and of Old Age* in 1597. Laurens maintained that the causes of aging were mental as well as physical. "Nothing hastens old age more that idleness," he wrote. Laurens also wrote *Historia Anatomica Humani Corporis* in 1602. He believed that the heart was "as perplexing as the flux and reflux of Euripus was to Aristotle," which is the quote included by Harvey.

Bauhin of Basle (1560-1624)

Caspar Bauhin was Professor of Anatomy, Botany, Greek, and Medicine, as well as rector of the University at Basle. He produced *Pinax Theatric Botanici* (A Catalogue of Botanical Theatre) in 1627, a year before Harvey's *De Motu* appeared. It included over 6,000 specimens and was the most up to date botanical synthesis.

In Harvey's book, he is credited with noting the 4 distinct motions of the heart in time and space. Harvey refutes this, describing 4 motions in space (of the 4 chambers), and only 2 in time (the two atria and the two ventricles each contract "simultaneously").

Hofmann of Altdorf (1572-1648)

As professor of medicine at Nuremberg, Friedrich Hofmann was the most important of the "Iatromechanists." He wrote about an ether that flowed through the nervous system, producing muscle tone. Harvey's description of the circulation made no positive impression on Hofmann (or Riolan), who continued to preach the Galenic doctrine. Hofmann, Riolan, and Harvey were each former students of Fabricius.

Riolan of Paris (1580-1657)

Jean Riolan the Younger was the most fierce opponent of Harvey. In *Encheiridium Anatomicum* (1648) and in *Opuscula Anatomica Nova* (1649), Riolan vehemently upheld the physiology and anatomy of Galen, some 20 years after Harvey's book appeared. Riolan still believed that blood, for the most part, remained stationary in the body. Like Bauhin, Riolan also believed that there were 4 movements of the heart in time and space. Harvey, of course, disproved both of these theories.

The criticism by Riolan was the only criticism to which Harvey ever chose to reply, in the form of two published letters in 1649, just after the publication of Riolan's books.

Previous Works Not Cited by Harvey

Several authors of important cardiovascular contributions go unmentioned by Harvey.

Conclusion

Harvey had a keen knowledge of medical history, which helped him formulate his case for the concept of a complete circulation of blood. While he made reference to Galen most frequently, Harvey seems to have admired Aristotle the most and gained much from his Padua mentor, Fabricius. Harvey "discovered" the circulation about 4 centuries ago. His brief book of 1628, *De Motu Cordis*, remains exciting to read, not only as a report of a new idea, but also as an example of scholarship.

Roberts CS. The scholarship of *De Motu Cordis*: Whom did Harvey reference? Presented in abstract form at the American Osler Society annual meeting in Houston, Texas, April 23, 2004.

12

Oversupply of Cardiothoracic Surgeons: Its Consequences and Correction

While the number of operations performed by our specialty in the USA is diminishing, the number of residents being trained for our specialty remains fairly constant. The supply of cardiothoracic surgeons, in my view, needs to be brought into balance with the demand for our services. In brief, too many cardiothoracic residents are being trained to do too few operations in practice, which is detrimental to all parties—the patients, the practitioners, and the residents.

Diminishing operations. The most common procedure performed by cardiothoracic surgeons as a group is coronary artery bypass grafting (CABG). The number of patients referred by cardiologists for CABG has declined at virtually all institutions, translating into fewer cardiac operations, overall, per surgeon. The obvious reason for the decrease in CABG referrals is the increase in percutaneous interventions to treat atherosclerosis. Vascular surgeons have experienced this phenomenon in nearly all operations for atherosclerosis. Open procedures are in decline. Closed procedures are on the rise.

Will the trend continue? Probably yes. Percutaneous interventions and medicines will improve and continue to dominant therapy for atherosclerosis. CABG will be applied more and more selectively in the future, for patients with advanced disease—probably after all percutaneous options have been exhausted.

Effect on patients. The diminishing number of operations in our specialty will impact our care of patients. The relation of surgeon volume and patient outcome was recently studied in a large sample of Medicare patients who underwent one of four cardiothoracic operations—CABG, aortic valve replacement, pulmonary resection, or esophagectomy (1). For each operation, higher surgeon volume was associated with lower operative mortality. For CABG, the mortality was 4.0% when the annual surgeon volume was >162 cases, and 5.4% when it was <101 cases.

A survey of cardiothoracic surgeons in 1999 showed that among adult cardiac surgeons also performing general thoracic surgery, the median number of cardiac cases was 174 per year (2). If the average adult cardiac surgeon performed, let's say, 150 cardiac operations last year, 125 this year, 100 next year, and so on as the CABG numbers diminish, patients face the probability of a higher operative risk, because of the surgeon's lower annual volume.

Effect on practitioners. While CABG numbers have declined, outcome expectations for all cardiothoracic operations have risen. Our surgical outcomes, especially for CABG, are feverishly analyzed, perhaps more so than any results in the history of surgery. To exceed national benchmarks in any complication category alarms our local critics. Red flags are raised. In this milieu, one year with a high complication numerator and a low volume denominator may be ruinous for a young surgeon, or even a seasoned one.

The decline in CABG numbers will affect all cardiothoracic surgeons, not just those whose practice is dominated by CABG procedures. The competition for valve referrals will increase, as will competition for general thoracic referrals. Vascular surgeons will also be impacted, as many cardiothoracic surgeons train their eyes on other vascular beds. The loss of concentration of valve, general thoracic, and vascular cases among subspecializing surgeons will ultimately mean higher rates of adverse outcomes.

Effect on residents. To train many residents for a specialty that has few openings in practice is unfair to trainees. Two "Situations Available" appeared in the January issue of the Annals of Thoracic Surgery this year, compared with 21 listings ten years ago; and yet, about 140 cardiothoracic residency positions remain available each year.

Medical students and general surgery residents have sensed the imbalance in our specialty and fewer apply each year for cardiothoracic positions. Fewer than 10% of applicants who attended American medical schools are rejected from cardiothoracic training (3), and this loss of competition to enter our specialty does not bode well for patients in the future.

The solution. The number of cardiothoracic training positions in the USA should be significantly decreased. Whether to decrease the number by a fourth, by a third, or by half, is debatable. The process of eliminating training positions is also debatable. Perhaps small training programs doing fewer than 400 adult cardiac operations per year, or some reasonable number, should phase out their programs. Perhaps large training programs with multiple slots should decrease the number of those slots by half. In the face of an unrelenting decline in CABG numbers, prompt correction of the oversupply of cardiothoracic surgeons is in the best interest of patients.

References

1. Birkmeyer JD, Stukel TA, Siewers AE, Goodney PP, Wennberg DE, Lucas FL. Surgeon volume and operative mortality in the United States. *N Engl J Med* 2003; 349: 2117-27
2. Shemin RJ, Dziuban SW, Kaiser LR, Lowe JE, Nugent WC, Oz MC, Turney DA, Wallace JK. Thoracic surgery workforce: snapshot at the end of the twentieth century and its implications for the new millennium. *Ann Thorac Surg* 2002; 73:2014-32
3. Orringer MB. Unity and participation: embracing counterintuitive survival skills. *Ann Thorac Surg* 2002; 74:3-12

Roberts CS. Oversupply of Cardiothoracic Surgeons: Its Consequences and Correction. *CTSNet,* September 3, 2004. https://www.ctsnet.org/article/oversupply-cardiothoracic-surgeons-its-consequences- and-correction

13

READERS' COMMENTS

Another View of Dr. Perloff's Personal Coronary Bypass Experience

"The most tragic thing in the world is a sick doctor."

George Bernard Shaw
The Doctor's Dilemma, Act I

"As to how I am, well, a respectable doctor is never sick. If ever anything happens to him, he dies at once, and that is all."

Ivan Turgenev
A Month in the Country, Act I

The practice of surgery is often misunderstood to mean "cutting and sewing" in the operating room, and little else. It is similar to believing that the practice of medicine means prescribing pills, and little else. Properly understood, surgery involves the preoperative consultation with all its nuances, the operation itself, and postoperative care for a minimum of 1 month and usually 2. Surgeons are *required* to focus on all 3 phases of surgical care, and neglect of any phase can jeopardize patients.

The recent article in this *Journal* by the Doctors Perloff, "Coronary Artery Bypass: A User's Manual,"[1] makes uncomfortable reading for a cardiac surgeon, because it exposes shortcomings in the postoperative care of a certain patient, Dr. Joseph E. Perloff, the distinguished cardiologist and author of 3 books with many editions. The patient's wife, Dr. Marjorie Perloff, happens to be a distinguished literary critic and author of 12 books. When the Doctors Perloff combined forces, a case report was produced, which describes the saga of the medical Dr. Perloff as patient.

Their case report is presented by the cardiologist and his literary wife, in their words, as "a user's manual" for coronary artery bypass. This is unfair, I believe, because their postoperative experience represents the exception, not the rule. "Coronary Artery Bypass: A Cautionary Tale" might be a more appropriate title.

Their article was not accompanied in this *Journal* by an independent commentary, but one is warranted. The physicians and surgeons at UCLA involved in the care of Dr. Perloff are unlikely to respond publicly to the many criticisms made in the article. I offer the following observations, therefore, based on a decade of evaluating patients for coronary artery bypass grafting (CABG), performing the operation, and caring for the patients postoperatively in both a university and a private practice setting.

The case summarized: A 78-year-old active cardiologist had "inappropriate fatigue" for 2 years. One night he had an ischemic event. He was taken to his own university hospital where an emergency cardiac catherization was performed followed immediately by CABG. The patient survived without stroke or reoperation for bleeding or mediastinitis. On postoperative day 6 he was discharged. He had a miserable first postoperative month, requiring frequent office visits, medication changes, repeated thoracentesis, and house calls by physicians.

His care inconvenienced a number of people, including his wife and daughter. By 2 months, the patient was able to function independently. A retrospective piece was published by the patient and his wife, who reported that "To me, Joe seems to be reborn, his walking is better than before surgery, his color is good, his spirit is improving."

The ischemic event: Because his myocardial ischemia went unrecognized until his nocturnal ischemic event, Dr. Perloff and his wife disparage the physicians who, they believe, missed the opportunity to diagnose it when he complained of fatigue. Dr. Perloff had been dismissive of the usefulness of an exercise test, he admits. "Because I did not personally believe that an exercise stress test was necessary," he writes, "my general physician did not bring up the subject in deference to my opinion."

Perhaps half of the patients I evaluate in consultation for CABG had no knowledge of their severe coronary atherosclerosis until coronary angiography. President Clinton, who recently had CABG, had no knowledge of his severe coronary atherosclerosis before his first ischemic event, despite the attention of numerous physicians for years.

Dr. Perloff seems amazed at the timing of his first ischemic event—that it did not happen during his world travels, but rather happened at home. Many of my patients express amazement at the timing of their first atherosclerotic event; some are reluctant to believe that they have severe coronary atherosclerosis, and a few, like Dr. Perloff, are critical of their general physicians for not diagnosing it earlier.

The operation: The CABG operation that Dr. Perloff underwent at UCLA took 6.5 hours, he states, which is 3 to 4 hours longer than a standard CABG procedure takes, if measured by skin-to-skin time. The duration of the operation, if accurately reported by the patient, suggests that this CABG procedure was not straightforward—perhaps the anastomoses were difficult, the weaning from cardiopulmonary bypass was slow, or some other difficulty was encountered. We are given no information except the operative time.

A longer operation, unfortunately, *often* means a slower recovery. The combination of advanced patient age and long operation time *usually* means a slower recovery.

The discharge: The patient was discharged too soon for reasons unclear to me. I do not recall sending home a CABG patient in an ambulance, or requiring stretcher-bearers to raise him to the second floor of his home. Dr. Perloff

Letters (from the United States) concerning a particular article in *The American Journal of Cardiology®* must be received within 2 months of the article's publication, and should be limited (with rare exceptions) to 2 double-spaced typewritten pages. Two copies must be submitted.

0002-9149/05/$–see front matter

states, "During the first week, I could not move in bed. . . ." His fecal incontinence, his apparent inability to ambulate, and the late hour of the day all suggest that discharge home on day 6 was too early. Furthermore, the necessity of a devoted wife and daughter, a housekeeper, and a private duty nurse to manage a CABG patient full time at home postoperatively is highly irregular. Nineteen medicines prescribed at discharge is clearly unusual.

Notwithstanding the concerns of the Doctors Perloff, I believe that his postoperative situation is atypical for UCLA and elsewhere. To justify discharging a patient, our group generally requires that patient to ambulate, to eat and drink, to move bowels appropriately, to weigh near the usual body weight, and to appear comfortable. The UCLA surgeons undoubtedly have similar criteria, which were put aside in the care of Dr. Perloff.

An assessment of the home situation by the surgeon is mandatory. Virtually all single patients, without family to live with, go to "rehab." Most patients >75 years of age, like Dr. Perloff, are also encouraged to transfer to an inpatient rehabilitation unit before going home. The attending cardiologist "suggested" this transfer, but it was not to be. The patient apparently "insisted that (he) could not tolerate another night in the hospital," and his wife admits that he was "so adamant about going home."

The literary Dr. Perloff concluded that postoperative care "lag(s) way behind" operative advances in the treatment of cardiovascular disease, a conclusion that must be based on her husband's singular experience. In fact, good postoperative care at UCLA is one reason why the medical Dr. Perloff is alive today. Excellent intensive care is now taken for granted. Despite the advancing age of patients having CABG, major complication rates in CABG continue to decline worldwide.

The lessons: The main lesson in this case report, in my judgment, is that postoperative patients must meet certain criteria to be discharged home, without exception. Unfortunately, every surgeon in every specialty has a nightmare tale of a patient going home too soon, and this report is one. Although the Doctors Perloff express concern that their personal experience is shared by many, I believe their experience is shared by very few indeed.

Discharging a patient home too soon postoperatively means more work for all concerned—multiple phone calls, frequent office visits, etc.—and so it is never in anyone's best interest to create the situation in which the Perloffs found themselves the first postoperative month. The safest path for the patient is usually also the most efficient path for the surgeon. In Dr. Perloff's particular case, his early discharge created more work for everyone, especially the family.

This case report is also a reminder of the principle that a physician should avoid being his or her own doctor. When the patient influences practice decisions too much, such as whether to get a stress test or when to go home postoperatively, clinical routines are disrupted. Had the patient not been a prominent cardiologist, he would have probably undergone a routine stress test to sort out the cause of his fatigue. After CABG, he would have probably stayed longer in the hospital and then gone to "rehab," which would have been routine postoperative care.

Charles Stewart Roberts, MD
Winchester Virginia
4 October 2004

1. Perloff JE, Perloff M. Coronary artery bypass: a user's manual. *Am J Cardiol* 2004;94:172–177.

doi:10.1016/j.amjcard.2004.11.016

Roberts CS. Another view of Dr. Perloff's personal coronary bypass experience. *Am J Cardiol.* 2005;95(5):705-706. doi:10.1016/j.amjcard.2004.11.016

14

Am Heart Hosp J. 2007;5:107–109

Commentary

Counsel for the Coronary Surgeon

Charles Stewart Roberts, MD

Young coronary surgeons fresh out of training face challenging circumstances: fewer operations, sicker patients, and greater scrutiny. With this milieu in mind, the author offers 28 suggestions for the inexperienced surgeon performing coronary artery bypass grafting. ©2007 Le Jacq

The best surgeon, like the best general, is he who makes the fewest mistakes. —Sir Astley Cooper, Lectures on Surgery

The young coronary surgeon faces challenging circumstances: fewer operations, sicker patients, and greater scrutiny. First, the number of coronary artery bypass grafting (CABG) procedures has fallen with the rise in percutaneous coronary interventions. Thoracic surgeons now do fewer operations in training and in practice. The relation of surgical volume to adverse outcome in CABG is controversial. The concern is that a fall in the number of cases per surgeon or per institution may lead to a rise in the number of complications.

Second, the current CABG patient is less healthy than in years past. Coronary stents have lengthened the interval from the first presentation of coronary atherosclerosis to the referral for CABG. The CABG patient now is older, the burden of atherosclerosis is greater, and concomitant diseases such as obesity and diabetes mellitus are more frequent.

Third, the oversight of CABG outcomes is increasingly intense. Perhaps no other operation in the history of surgery has been so analyzed, particularly with respect to early outcomes. In some states, the CABG results of individual surgeons are published. Referring cardiologists and hospital administrators are keenly aware of complication rates above the benchmarks.

With this milieu in mind, I offer to the inexperienced coronary surgeon some personal lessons learned, invariably, the hard way. Perhaps the young coronary surgeon, with less quantitative experience, may find the following qualitative advice useful.

- *Spend at least 30 minutes with every preoperative CABG candidate (excepting emergencies).* Even if you learn all you think you need to know in 20 minutes, spend another 10 in the patient's room. The mind requires time to process the many variables involved in a cardiac operation. Thirty minutes is minimal consideration to give a patient whose life will be significantly altered by your operation.
- *Describe potential complications slowly and clearly.* Let there be no doubt in the mind of the patient and his or her family members in the room that death and stroke are possibilities. I usually initiate the discussion by pointing out that driving on Interstate 81 has risks—and so does the operation. Give your best estimate. I usually say the risks of death, stroke, and infection are 3%, 2%, and 1%, respectively—easy to remember. The leery patient may be reminded that there are risks in not doing CABG as well. Handing the patient the consent form and pen, I usually say, "By signing this you are acknowledging that I have described the risks to you." This is not litigation phobia. It is common sense.
- *Be courteous at all times to patients and their families.* Go out of your way to be polite. Discourtesy

• From The Heart and Vascular Center, Winchester Medical Center, Valley Health System, Winchester, VA

• Address for correspondence: Charles Stewart Roberts, MD, Suite 2A, Medical Office Building I, 1870 Amherst Street, Winchester, VA 22601; e-mail: csrwinchester@hotmail.com

www.lejacq.com ID: 5793

toward patients or colleagues is unbecoming of a physician. If you are impatient with an impatient family member, you will regret it later when you find yourself having to discuss a complication that occurred in a loved one. When entering a new patient's room, identify yourself, greet everyone, and then politely ask the patient if you may sit down and ask him or her a few questions. Courtesy is disarming.

- *Turn down certain patients for CABG.* This is the hardest lesson to learn. In some patients, the risk of a bad outcome is simply too high to justify the operation. Performing CABG in a 79-year-old morbidly obese and diabetic woman who is oxygen-dependent and has a creatinine of 2.7 mg/dL is simply unwise. Your reputation will suffer more for a failed operation, however difficult, than by declining to operate. Your reputation may, indeed, rise when your thoughtful assessment leads you to advocate nonoperative therapy. At the end of the year, if your mortality rate exceeds the benchmark, no explanation to your peers, or referring cardiologists, or hospital administrators will matter.
- *Decline to operate on coronary patients in cardiogenic shock.* Evidence indicates that CABG is not superior to medical therapy in these patients. The circumstance will usually be an emergency consultation in the cardiac catheterization laboratory for a patient in the throes of a myocardial infarction (MI). Delay is appropriate. Emergencies (and reoperations) are invariably associated with higher early mortality in CABG. The iatrogenic catheter-related catastrophe and the mechanical complication from an acute MI are different scenarios that may indeed require emergency operation.
- *Avoid operating within 48 hours of an acute MI if feasible.* The longer CABG is delayed after an acute MI, the lower the early mortality. CABG in the face of a fresh anterior-wall MI can be disastrous. An intra-aortic balloon pump (IABP) is usually better than a CABG in the first 48 hours.
- *Beware of patients with a body mass index of 40 kg/m^2 or higher.* The morbidly obese patient is a physical challenge for the entire heart team. A complication of some kind is inevitable.
- *Adopt a stroke prevention protocol and follow it.* Ours includes preoperative carotid duplex scanning, intraoperative epiaortic ultrasound, selective aortic cannula filtration, high mean arterial pressures during cardiopulmonary bypass (CPB), an arterial line filter, avoidance of cardiotomy suction, the single aortic cross-clamp, full-dose aprotinin, and maintenance of strict euglycemia. This author avoids the prophylactic or combined carotid endarterectomy in the symptomatic coronary patient. If a stroke prevention protocol is not in place, one will be foisted on you before long. Patients fear stroke more than death.
- *Prepare for the calcified aorta.* Routine, intraoperative epiaortic ultrasound does prompt one to give attention to the ascending aorta in a deliberate, habitual way. Calcific deposits can be identified and the operation altered if clamping the aorta appears too dangerous.
- *Keep the operating room quiet and peaceful.* Some surgeons play loud music, but this author believes that the team generally prefers efficiency to entertainment. This author focuses best when the operating room is like a library.
- *Place a right subclavian central venous catheter in all patients before incision.* This is in addition to the usual Swan-Ganz catheter in the right jugular vein, which is soon removed. Venous access problems during the hospital stay are eliminated.
- *Add a femoral arterial line before incision in all reoperative patients and all primary patients with an ejection fraction of 0.30 or less.* It allows easy access for an IABP, should that be necessary to wean from CPB. Trying to place a femoral arterial line during the weaning process with nonpulsatile flow is sometimes difficult and introduces a technical distraction from the weaning process.
- *Pause before a repeat sternotomy.* Make sure that every precaution is in place—CPB lines divided, femoral cannulas in the room, a Foley catheter on the table, heparin drawn up, blood products available, and have the team ready in the event of bleeding.
- *Decompress, decompress, decompress.* Have a low threshold to place a left ventricular vent through the right superior pulmonary vein. A distended heart at any point in the operation threatens future contractility. Prolonged distention dooms the heart. In addition, for exposure purposes when sewing distal anastomoses, a decompressed heart is ideal. One never regrets decompressing the heart.
- *Avoid the trap of the extremely difficult distal anastomosis.* Fewer grafts are sometimes safer for the patient than many grafts with a long aortic cross-clamp period. The considerations include the quality of the conduit, coronary target, myocardial protection, and exposure. Sewing a small vein graft to a small ramus in its proximal portion in the setting of cardiomegaly can be harrowing.

The 30-minute anastomosis is rarely worthwhile. Think through the bypass plan before applying the aortic cross-clamp.

- *Wean from CPB slowly.* I call for "half-flows," then wait. Chest tubes can be placed while the anesthesiologist and perfusionist prepare. The triad—surgeon, anesthesiologist, and perfusionist—need to be of the same mind when separating the patient from CPB. Too many times I have weaned too quickly, and recovery is sometimes difficult.
- *Take time for hemostasis before closing.* Have a deliberate process (same way every time) to achieve hemostasis—and be patient. Excessive bleeding and take-backs are dangerous for the patient and time consuming for the surgeon. A bedside vigil over a bleeding patient takes a month off the surgeon's life. Complete hemostasis the first time keeps your evenings undisturbed.
- *Cover the heart with a pleuropericardial flap.* Bring the left pleural edge (the left pleural space is opened when taking down the left internal mammary artery) to the right pericardial edge over the aorta with 2 stitches to cover the grafts. It will make reoperation safer and mediastinitis less dangerous.
- *Use double wires to close the sternum.* Most Americans are overweight or obese, but sternal dehiscence from mechanical stress is preventable. Double wires around the body of the sternum add security. Using the hook to cinch down the wires is foolproof.
- *Dictate immediately after degowning in the operating room.* Describe all usual and unusual aspects of the case. Remember that the opportunity to examine the heart in situ is a privilege—a careful description of operative findings is an obligation. This is also your best chance to tell the world what you did and why. All later explanations will be discredited. Undictated recollections are illegitimate in the eyes of attorneys, administrators, and even your peers who may be asked to review a case. As Osler wrote, "The further away from the mountain, the hazier it is. Memory plays strange pranks." Consider the dictation part of the operation.
- *Call the referring cardiologist as soon as the patient arrives in the intensive care unit.* This simple habit took me too many years to adopt. We've heard of the fury of the woman scorned; there is also the fury of the cardiologist uninformed. Cardiologists appreciate communication, however brief, and these calls are brief. The call acknowledges the cardiologist's status as referring physician, your status as consulting surgeon, and a transfer of information occurs. More communication between the subspecialties will result in greater mutual understanding.
- *Delay removing the IABP and endotracheal tube in the marginal patient.* Though the patient with an ejection fraction of 0.20 may appear to be recovering brilliantly on day 1, don't be fooled into withdrawing hemodynamic and ventilatory support promptly and simultaneously. Go slowly. Reinsertion of the IABP and reintubation are setbacks that are sometimes hard to overcome.
- *Take back bleeding patients promptly.* Excessive transfusions are harmful. Persistent bleeding puts the patient, the patient's family, and the surgeon through a nightmare. On my first encounter with the patient's family in the waiting room after CABG, I always inform them of the possibility of a reoperation for bleeding, though the likelihood is very low. This makes it easier to address later, if necessary.
- *Leave pleural drains in for 2 or 3 days.* An extra day with a chest tube saves having to perform thoracentesis later in the office. This extra procedure is sometimes painful for the patient and always a nuisance for the surgeon.
- *Transfer the sick patient back to the intensive care unit sooner rather than later.* No one regrets moving an unstable patient back to the intensive care unit, but we all regret allowing one to linger on the ward. When in doubt, transfer the patient to where the patient/nurse ratio is 1:1.
- *Review your outcome data yearly.* Contribute to the database of the Society of Thoracic Surgeons, and compare your individual data to its benchmarks. Analyses more frequent than yearly are usually inappropriate because the denominator is too small, but a careful yearly review is mandatory.
- *Go regularly to surgical meetings—at least twice a year.* It clears the mind of clinical burdens and allows one to ponder opportunities for quality improvement. Compare your protocols and practices regularly with those of other coronary surgeons.
- *Leave your work behind on holiday.* Clear up your practice to the best of your ability, then depart and do not call. Checking in with your partners about your patients during vacation rarely brings contentment. Cultivate the peace of mind that comes from knowing that you have done your best at work, and that your rest from work is well deserved.

Roberts CS. Counsel for the coronary surgeon. *Am Heart Hosp J.* 2007;5(2):107-109. doi:10.1111/j.1541-9215.2007.05793.x

15

Cusp Configuration in Aortic Stenosis

Charles Stewart Roberts, MD
From the Section of Thoracic and Cardiovascular Surgery, The Heart and Vascular Center, Winchester Medical Center, Valley Health, Winchester, VA
Address for correspondence: Charles Stewart Roberts, MD, 1870 Amherst Street, Suite 2A, Winchester, VA, 22601
E-mail: croberts@valleyhealthlink.com

Aortic valve replacement is the standard therapy for severe stenosis of the aortic valve (AV), irrespective of age. An echocardiogram is requisite in the preoperative evaluation; the AV gradient and area are always determined.[1] In addition, the configuration of the cusps of the stenotic AV is often determined preoperatively by echocardiography. Sometimes that specific anatomical information is unknown, however; either it is not determined or not recorded. Therefore, whether the patient has a unicuspid or bicuspid or tricuspid AV is sometimes determined for the first time at operation by direct visual examination. A careful examination is critical because of certain intraoperative and postoperative implications.

A unicuspid AV (Figure 1) has 1 leaflet and 1 commissure. A bicuspid AV (Figure 2) has 2 leaflets and 1 commissure. The 2 leaflets can be either in an anterior-posterior orientation, with both coronary ostia arising above the anterior leaflet, or in a left-right orientation, with the right coronary artery arising above the right leaflet and the left main coronary artery arising above the left leaflet. If a raphe is present, it is always in the anterior leaflet in the anterior-posterior cases and in the right leaflet in the right-left cases. A tricuspid AV (Figure 3) has 3 leaflets and 3 commissures.

Why is this specific "operative finding" important? For 3 main reasons. First, from the standpoint of intraoperative management, the patient with a congenitally malformed AV (unicuspid or bicuspid) may have, in association, a dilated ascending aorta that requires repair during AV replacement. The ascending aorta in patients with a congenitally malformed valve is morphologically abnormal.[2] The frequency of a hypoplastic aorta, coarctation of the aorta, aortic aneurysm, and aortic dissection are all higher in patients with a unicuspid or bicuspid AV. The ascending aorta dilates with age in these patients, beginning in childhood.

As a general guideline in the management of ascending aortic aneurysm, patients with an ascending aortic diameter >5.5 cm should undergo operative repair. Patients with the Marfan syndrome or with a congenitally malformed AV, however, should be considered for repair of the ascending aorta when the diameter is >4.5 cm, with or without AV replacement, because the risk of dissection is comparatively high.[3]

Geriatric patients with a unicuspid or bicuspid AV who undergo AV replacement should be examined for ascending aortic dilation. If the diameter exceeds 4 cm, then reduction aortoplasty is indicated.[4] The aortotomy used to perform AV replacement is simply extended distally in the ascending aorta and a linear strip of aorta is

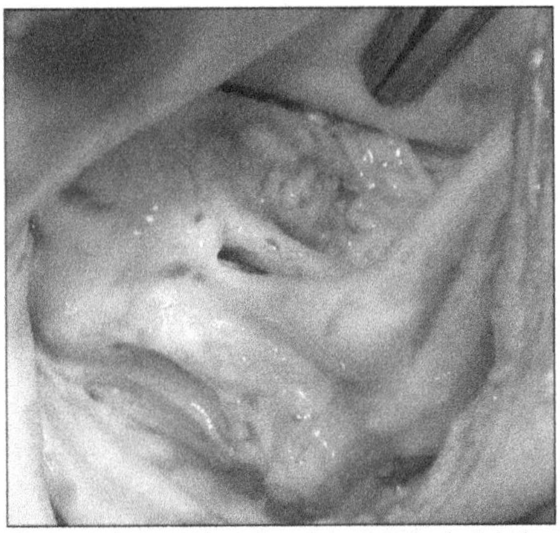

Figure 1. Unicuspid aortic valve photographed before replacement.

www.lejacq.com ID: 6468

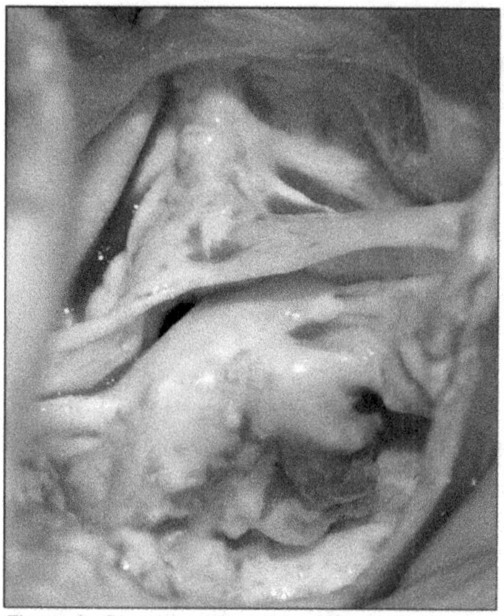

Figure 2. Bicuspid aortic valve photographed before replacement.

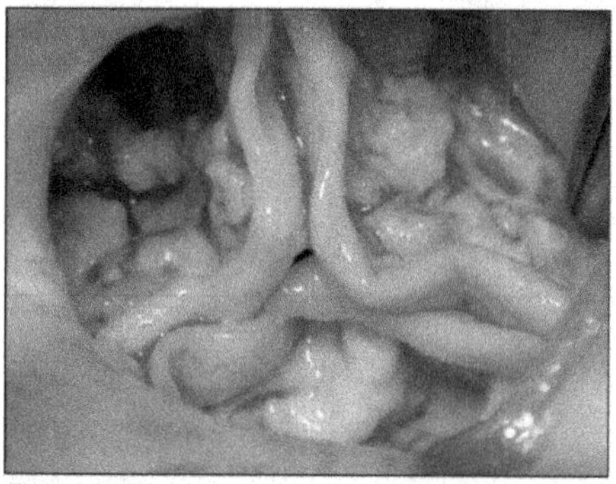

Figure 3. Tricuspid aortic valve photographed before replacement.

excised, reducing the aortic diameter to <3.5 cm. Reduction aortoplasty is a simple addition to standard AV replacement. It preserves the patient's own aortic endothelium and creates a fibrous scar along the aortotomy in the anterolateral zone of the ascending aorta where an entry tear in aortic dissection is most common.

Second, the determination of cusp configuration is important because postoperative surveillance of the ascending aorta, repaired or not repaired, is warranted. Echocardiography or computed tomography is indicated yearly. The ascending aorta enlarges in patients with a congenitally malformed AV, whether the AV functions well or poorly and whether the native AV remains undisturbed or is replaced. Aortic dissection remains a risk in postoperative patients who were born with a malformed AV.[5]

A third reason to determine cusp configuration is that the cause of a congenital malformation of the AV appears to be a genetic mutation with hereditary implications.[6] Children or siblings of a geriatric patient with a congenitally malformed AV may, therefore, be at risk for this condition. Sir William Osler first observed the predisposition of congenitally malformed valves to infective endocarditis. At the very least, a child or sibling who shares the inheritance of a unicuspid or bicuspid AV would benefit from antibiotic prophylaxis before dental or gastrointestinal procedures. A congenital malformation of the AV (unicuspid or bicuspid AV) is a class I (level of evidence: C) indication for endocarditis prophylaxis.[1]

Furthermore, the fibrous thickening and calcium deposition that occurs prematurely on the malformed AV may be related to hypercholesterolemia as well as genetic factors.[7] Cholesterol-lowering therapy may be warranted in the younger genetic relative who has a unicuspid or bicuspid AV, to avoid the same fate as the geriatric patient who required AV replacement. No trials have been undertaken, however, to justify a formal recommendation for statin therapy in congenital malformation of the AV.[1]

References

1 Bonow RO, Carabello BA, Chatterjee K, et al, for the American College of Cardiology, American Heart Association Task Force on Practice Guidelines, Society of Cardiovascular Anesthesiologists, Society for Cardiovascular Angiography and Interventions, and Society of Thoracic Surgeons. ACC/AHA 2006 guidelines for the management of patients with valvular heart disease: a report of the American College of Cardiology/American Heart Association Task Force on Practice Guidelines (writing Committee to Revise the 1998 guidelines for the management of patients with Valvular Heart Disease) developed in collaboration with the Society of Cardiovascular Anesthesiologists Endorsed by the Society of Cardiovascular Angiography and Interventions and the Society of Thoracic Surgeons. *J Am Coll Cardiol*. 2006;48:1–148.

2 Bauer M, Pasic M, Meyer R, et al. Morphometric analysis of aortic media in patients with bicuspid and tricuspid aortic valve. *Ann Thorac Surg*. 2002;74:58–62.

3 Borger MA, Preston M, Ivanov J, et al. Should the ascending aorta be replaced more frequently in patients with bicuspid aortic valve disease? *J Thorac Cardiovasc Surg*. 2004;128:677–683.

4 Bauer M, Pasic M, Schaffarzyk R, et al. Reduction aortoplasty for dilatation of the ascending aorta in patients with bicuspid aortic valve. *Ann Thorac Surg*. 2002;73:720–723.

5 Russo CF, Mazzetti S, Garatti A, et al. Aortic complications

after bicuspid aortic valve replacement: long-term results. *Ann Thorac Surg.* 2002;74:S1773–S1776.

6 Garg V, Muth AN, Ransom JF, et al. Mutations in NOTCH1 cause aortic valve disease. *Nature.* 2005;437:270–274.

7 Chui MC, Newby DE, Panarelli M, et al. Association between calcific aortic stenosis and hypercholesterolemia: is there a need for a randomized controlled trial of cholesterol-lowering therapy? *Clin Cardiol.* 2001;24:52–55.

Roberts CS. Cusp configuration in aortic stenosis. *Am J Geriatr Cardiol.* 2007;16(3):197-199. doi:10.1111/j.1076-7460.2007.06468.x

16

Endarterectomy for Carotid Atherosclerosis

Charles Stewart Roberts, MD
From the Section of Thoracic and Cardiovascular Surgery, The Heart and Vascular Center, Winchester Medical Center, Valley Health, Winchester, VA
Address for correspondence: Charles Stewart Roberts, MD, 1870 Campus Boulevard, Suite 2A, Winchester, VA 22601
E-mail: csrwinchester@hotmail.com

After coronary artery bypass grafting, the most common surgical operation for atherosclerosis is carotid endarterectomy (CEA). Indeed, in 2006, the author performed 153 coronary artery bypass grafting procedures and 37 CEA procedures. Though the disease is the same, the anatomic location and the surgical techniques are different. Atherosclerotic obstructions in coronary arteries, in general, are bypassed. Carotid arterial stenoses, in general, are removed—hence the term endarterectomy.

Indications for CEA depend on whether the patient is symptomatic or asymptomatic. Symptoms of carotid atherosclerosis are neurologic: ischemic stroke or transient ischemic attack (TIA). Stroke indicates that a brain infarct is present. TIA indicates brain ischemia, but not infarction. Historically, a time criteria has been applied to the definition of TIA (an ischemic event beginning and ending within 24 hours), but use of the time period to diagnose TIA is controversial.[1] Transient monocular blindness (amaurosis fugax) is a TIA resulting from embolism from a carotid atherosclerotic plaque. Carotid atherosclerosis in geriatric patients with TIA or stroke is probably underdiagnosed and undertreated.[2]

The purpose of CEA is to reduce the risk of stroke.[3] For a symptomatic patient, CEA is appropriate if the internal carotid narrowing is >50% of the luminal diameter (hemodynamically significant).[4] The benefit of CEA is greatest in those with greater stenoses, those aged 75 years or older, men, those with recent stroke rather than TIA, and those with hemispheric symptoms instead of amaurosis fugax.[4] For an asymptomatic patient, CEA is considered appropriate if the stenosis is >70% (critical), and the majority of patients who undergo CEA are asymptomatic.[5] When the degree of carotid stenosis is <50%, CEA is not indicated.[4,5] Of course, these clinical decisions also depend on the complication rate of the surgeon or institution. A high complication rate negates the benefit of CEA.[4,5]

www.lejacq.com ID: 6224

A carotid duplex scan is useful in the screening and surveillance of carotid atherosclerosis. Before a CEA, however, an angiogram obtained by magnetic resonance imaging, computed tomography, or direct arterial contrast injection is usually required for operative planning. Most patients with carotid atherosclerosis have coronary atherosclerosis as well, and a preoperative screening study for myocardial ischemia is appropriate. In the geriatric population, roughly half of patients with ischemic stroke have coronary artery disease.[6]

At operation, the anesthesia can be general or regional/local—I prefer general. Because it is necessary to clamp the carotid arteries (common, internal, and external) to remove the atherosclerotic plaque, consideration must be given to brain protection during the period of clamping.[3] Some surgeons routinely place a small shunt from the common carotid artery to the internal carotid artery during the clamp period. Others surgeons shunt selectively, an approach which I prefer, based on objective criteria. All patients in my practice are subjected to intraoperative electroencephalography. If a change occurs on the electroencephalogram when the clamps are placed, a shunt is inserted. Some surgeons measure the "stump pressure" above the clamp in the internal carotid artery to determine whether a shunt is necessary—if the stump pressure is low (<50 mm Hg), then a shunt is inserted.

The endarterectomy is usually done through an arteriotomy extending from the common carotid artery across the bifurcation into the internal

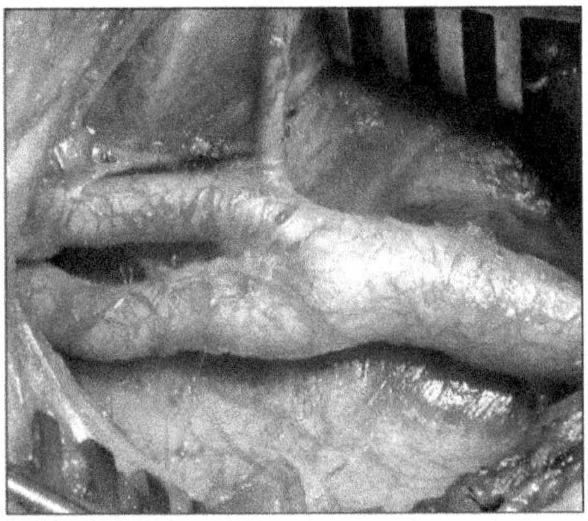

Figure 1. An operative photograph showing the right carotid bifurcation.

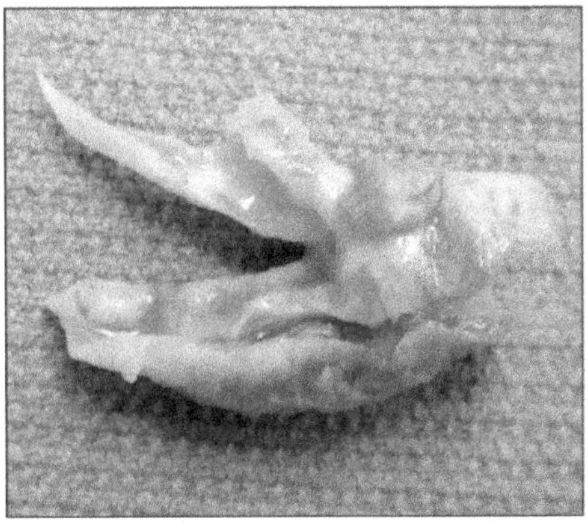

Figure 2. A photograph of an atherosclerotic plaque removed from the carotid bifurcation.

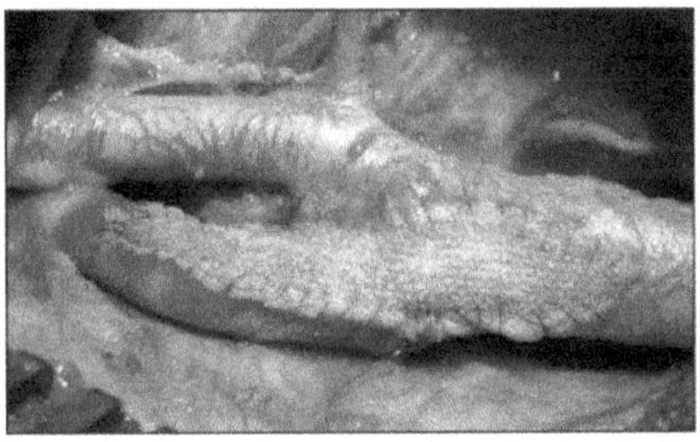

Figure 3. An operative photograph showing a polyester patch extending from the right common carotid artery across the bifurcation onto the right internal carotid artery.

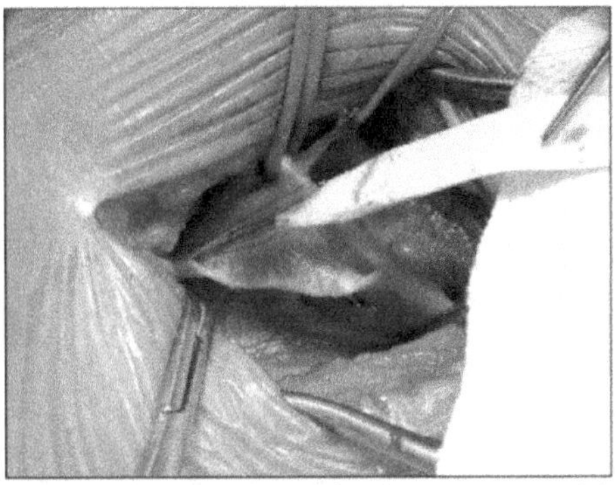

Figure 4. In the typical carotid endarterectomy, a patch angioplasty is done, which involves sewing a synthetic patch across the bifurcation to close the arteriotomy, after the plaque has been removed.

carotid artery (Figure 1, Figure 2, and Figure 3). If the appropriate plane in the media of the artery is found, the plaque usually comes away cleanly in one piece. The so-called end point of the plaque in the internal carotid artery is critical; the transition must be smooth to avoid a dissection plane when the clamps are removed. Sometimes several fine tacking sutures are placed to make certain the end point is smooth. Plaque in the external carotid artery is usually easily removed by everting that artery and pulling out the plaque with forceps. The subject of whether to patch the artery has been debated for years. Primary closure (without a patch) is quicker and avoids foreign material; however, poorer outcomes are associated with this technique.[7] In my practice, a polyester patch is routinely used (Figure 4).

After CEA, patients are awakened and extubated in the operating room and then cared for overnight in our step-down unit, in which the care is below intensive but above that in the regular ward. The majority of patients are discharged on the first postoperative day with a mild analgesic and their usual medicines, which should include an aspirin and a statin if not contraindicated.

Early outcomes after CEA are usually expressed as the combined stroke and mortality rate in the first 30 postoperative days. A rate of <1% is desirable. A rate >3% negates the preventive benefit of CEA.[5] A surgeon who performs CEA should probably perform 12 a year at a minimum, or none at all.[8] I avoid simultaneous CEA and coronary artery bypass grafting, which may be associated with a higher risk of stroke and death than are staged procedures.[9]

Carotid stenting is being performed more frequently. No level I evidence supports the position, however, that carotid stenting is superior to CEA or even better than the best medical therapy. It seems appropriate to consider stenting in the symptomatic patient who is simply unfit for surgery, including those who have comorbidities that are too severe or too numerous.[4] Symptomatic patients with restenosis after CEA or with a "hostile" neck (history of neck radiation or surgery) may be better served by stent therapy as well.[4] Carotid stenting in the asymptomatic patient is currently unsupported by randomized trials. CEA and carotid stenting should be viewed as complimentary, not competing, forms of therapy.

References

1 Albers GW, Caplan LR, Easton JD, et al, for the TIA Working Group. Transient ischemic attack—a proposal for a new definition. *N Engl J Med.* 2002;347:1713–1716.

2 Fairhead JF, Rothwell PM. Underinvestigation and undertreatment of carotid disease in elderly patients with transient ischaemic attack and stroke: comparative population based study. *BMJ.* 2006;333:525–527.

3 Pruitt JC. *A Crusade for Stroke Prevention: A Program for Immediate, Aggressive Utilization of New Knowledge and Technology That Could Reduce Strokes by 90 Percent.* Tampa, FL: University of Tampa Press; 2000.

4 Sacco RL, Adams R, Albers G, et al. Guidelines for prevention of stroke in patients with ischemic stroke or transient ischemic attack. A statement for healthcare professionals from the American Heart Association/American Stroke Association Council on Stroke: co-sponsored by the Council on Cardiovascular Radiology and Intervention: the Academy of Neurology affirms the value of this guideline. *Stroke.* 2006;37:577–617.

5 Sacco RL. Extracranial carotid stenosis. *N Engl J Med.* 2001;345:1113–1118.

6 Ness J, Aronow WS. Prevalence of coexistence of coronary artery disease, ischemic stroke, and peripheral arterial disease in older persons, mean age 80 years, in an academic hospital-based geriatrics practice. *J Am Geriatr Soc.* 1999;47:1255–1256.

7 Rockman CB, Halm EA, Wang JJ, et al. Primary closure of the carotid artery is associated with poorer outcomes during carotid endarterectomy. *J Vasc Surg.* 2005;42:870–877.

8 Cowan JA Jr, Dimick JB, Thompson G, et al. Surgeon volume as an indicator of outcomes after carotid endarterectomy: an effect independent of specialty practice and hospital volume. *J Am Coll Surg.* 2002;195:814–821.

9 Borger MA, Fremes SE, Weisel RD, et al. Coronary bypass and carotid endarterectomy: does a combined approach increase risk? A metaanalysis. *Ann Thorac Surg.* 1999;68:14–21.

Roberts CS. Endarterectomy for carotid atherosclerosis. *Am J Geriatr Cardiol.* 2007;16(4):259-261. doi:10.1111/j.1076-7460.2007.06224.x

17

Cardiovascular Surgery for the Cardiologist

Charles Stewart Roberts, MD, Section Editor
Winchester Medical Center, Winchester, VA

Coronary Artery Bypass Grafting After 40 Years (1967–2007)

Charles Stewart Roberts, MD
From the Section of Thoracic and Cardiovascular Surgery, The Heart and Vascular Center, Winchester Medical Center, Valley Health, Winchester, VA
Address for correspondence: Charles Stewart Roberts, MD, 1870 Campus Boulevard, Suite 2A, Winchester, VA 22601
E-mail: csrwinchester@hotmail.com

Four decades have passed since the introduction of coronary artery bypass grafting (CABG) into the clinical arena, which was arguably in 1967. Before that year, sporadic procedures involving a single bypass to a coronary artery had been performed, but usually as an unplanned consequence of a surgical misadventure during coronary endarterectomy.[1] These isolated procedures were not reproduced, and sometimes not even reported until years later. In 1967, however, Kolessov[2] of Lenningrad described 6 patients in whom the left internal mammary artery was sewn to a left coronary artery without using the heart-lung machine, through a left thoracotomy approach, without preoperative angiography. In the same year, Favaloro,[3] an Argentine surgeon at the Cleveland Clinic, began a series of single aortocoronary bypass procedures using autologous saphenous vein; 15 patients were reported the following year, with an appendum adding 53 more patients. Surgeons began performing the procedure at other institutions in 1967, and soon thereafter, CABG became the most commonly performed cardiovascular procedure.

In 1993, the Society of Thoracic Surgeons (STS) established the National Adult Cardiac Database, which is now the largest registry of any subspecialty in the country. It includes nearly 800 participating sites and more than 3 million patient records.[4] Because of its size, the STS database provides the most stable benchmarks for results in clinical cardiac surgery. This piece is intended to profile the CABG procedure in brief terms, based on the STS database: who has the procedure, how it is performed, and what are the early results.

www.lejacq.com ID: 6225

The mean age of patients at surgery is 65 years; half of CABG patients are 65 years or older. Only 1 of 5 patients is at ideal body weight today, and about one third have diabetes mellitus. Almost half (47%) have had a myocardial infarction at some point, and most (83%) have angina pectoris. Nearly all CABG patients have 3-vessel disease (77%), left main disease (31%), or both, and 1 of 5 has an ejection fraction <0.40. Twenty-two percent of CABG patients had a previous percutaneous coronary intervention.

Four of 5 patients receive at least 3 bypass grafts, and an internal mammary artery is used in >90% of CABG procedures (Figure 1). The creation of that anastomosis in millions of patients, I believe, has been the greatest contribution by cardiac surgeons to mankind. Loop and associates[5] at the Cleveland Clinic deserve primary credit for having demonstrated the clinical superiority of the internal mammary artery over the greater saphenous vein as a conduit.

The heart-lung machine is still used in 4 of 5 CABG procedures. No significant differences in major morbidity or mortality between on-pump and off-pump techniques (Figure 2) have emerged,[6] although the clinical trials and the debate continue. Off-pump CABG may offer slightly lower in-hospital mortality, but long-term outcomes are similar, and revascularization rates may be lower with on-pump CABG.[7] In the geriatric population, off-pump CABG may have a slight advantage in early mortality.[8]

Operative mortality after CABG has continued to decline, and is now at 2.1% (the unadjusted rate in the STS database). Five major complications are routinely scrutinized: ventilation >48 hours (8.9%), any reoperation (5.1%), acute renal failure

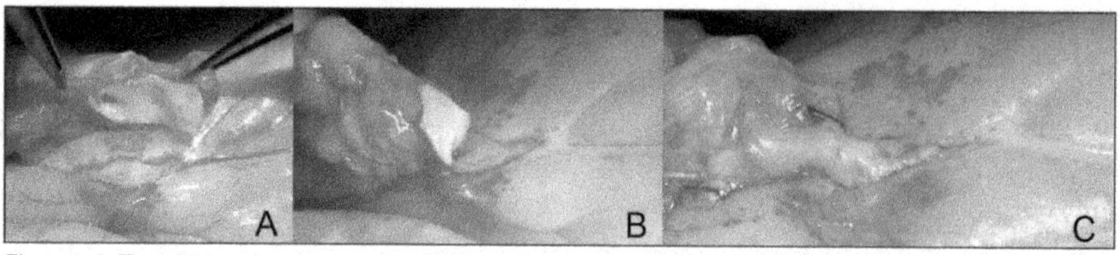

Figure 1. A, The left internal mammary artery (LIMA) positioned alongside the opened left anterior descending (LAD) coronary artery in an on-pump coronary artery bypass graft procedure. B, The LIMA-LAD anastomosis in progress. C, The completed LIMA-LAD anastamosis.

(3.6%), permanent stroke (1.2%), and deep sternal wound infection (0.4%). Eighty-five percent of patients survive 30 days, are discharged, and experience none of the 5 major complications.

The STS presented a comprehensive rating system for cardiac surgical programs for the first time in its spring report of 2007. A composite score was developed based on 11 CABG measures of quality (not only operative mortality), endorsed by the National Quality Forum.[9] Provider institutions are rated according to a 3-tier system: 1 star, 2 stars, or 3 stars (approximately 15% of hospitals receive 3 stars). For example, based on 2006 data, Winchester Medical Center was in the highest quality tier, thereby receiving an STS 3-star rating.

In the next 40 years (2007–2047), CABG as a palliative therapy for severe coronary atherosclerosis may decrease; however, I predict that it will still be a common procedure in 2047. Preventive therapy for atherosclerosis remains inadequate, obesity is on the rise worldwide, and the benefits of percutaneous coronary interventions have been limited. The mammary-coronary anastomosis, in particular, is likely to remain an excellent treatment option for myocardial ischemia.

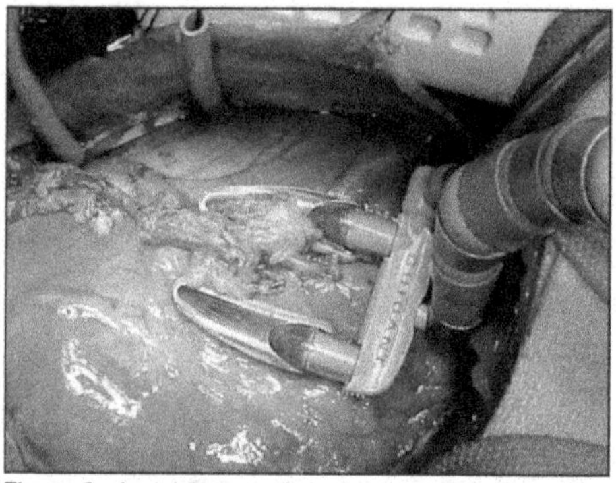

Figure 2. A stablizer positioned on the anterior surface of the heart (the left internal mammary artery-left anterior descending anastomosis is completed) in an off-pump coronary artery bypass graft procedure. Courtesy of Dr Denton Stam.

References

1 Shumaker HB Jr. *The Evolution of Cardiac Surgery.* Indianapolis, IN: Indiana University Press, 1992.

2 Kolessov VI. Mammary artery-coronary artery anastomosis as method of treatment for angina pectoris. *J Thorac Cardiovasc Surg.* 1967;54:535–544.

3 Favaloro RG. Saphenous vein autograft replacement of severe segmental coronary artery occlusion: operative technique. *Ann Thorac Surg.* 1968;5:334–339.

4 Duke Clinical Research Institute. *Data Analysis of The Society of Thoracic Surgeons National Adult Cardiac Surgery Database.* Chicago, IL: The Society of Thoracic Surgeons; 2007.

5 Loop FD, Lytle BW, Cosgrove DM, et al. Influence of the internal-mammary-artery graft on 10-year survival and other cardiac events. *N Engl J Med.* 1986;314:1–6.

6 Parolari A, alamanni F, Cannata A, et al. Off-pump versus on-pump coronary artery bypass: meta-analysis of currently available randomized trials. *Ann Thorac Surg.* 2003;76:37–40.

7 Hannan EL, Wu C, Smith CR, et al. Off-pump versus on-pump coronary artery bypass graft surgery. Differences in short-term outcomes and in long-term mortality and need for subsequent revascularization. [published online ahead of print August 20, 2007] *Circulation.* 2007;116:1145–1152.

8 Panesar SS, Athanasiou T, Nair S, et al. Early outcomes in the elderly: a meta-analysis of 4921 patients undergoing coronary artery bypass grafting—comparison between off-pump and on-pump techniques. *Heart.* 2006;92:1808–1816.

9 Shahian DM, Edwards FH, Ferraris VA, et al. Quality measurement in adult cardiac surgery: part 1—conceptual framework and measure selection. *Ann Thorac Surg.* 2007;83:S3–S12.

Roberts CS. Coronary artery bypass grafting after 40 years (1967-2007). *Am J Geriatr Cardiol.* 2007;16(6):384-385. doi:10.1111/j.1076-7460.2007.06225.x

18

Editorials

EDITORIAL

Cardiovascular surgery as a single specialty: The case to unify cardiac and vascular surgery

Charles Stewart Roberts, MD

Cardiovascular surgery came of age in the 20th century. Carrel,[1,2] in the first decade, described an end-to-end suture technique to connect blood vessels, which launched vascular surgery. Gibbon[3] in 1953 first used a heart–lung machine clinically, which launched cardiac surgery. Cardiovascular deaths in the United States have led all others every year of the 20th century except 1918, the year of the influenza epidemic.

By the end of the 20th century, cardiovascular surgery was formally separated into two different disciplines, *cardiac surgery* and *vascular surgery*. Cardiac surgery is paired with general thoracic surgery as part of the specialty, *thoracic surgery*, which became a primary board specialty in 1971. Vascular surgery more recently emerged as a surgical specialty, first by establishing its own residency programs and later by gaining approval for a primary certificate in vascular surgery by the American Board of Surgery.[4] Both cardiac and vascular surgery address disorders of the circulation. In my opinion, they are unnaturally separated and should be unified into one specialty. Here's why:

The organ system is the best determinant of a surgical specialty, not a region of the body such as the thorax or the abdomen. William Harvey, in his 1628 book on the movement of the heart and blood, described arteries, veins, and the heart as a system.[5] Harvey used the term *circle* and it variants (circulation, circulate, circular, circuit) 27 times in the last 10 chapters (none in the first 7). It seems incongruous today to partition the circle, to have one specialty treat one part of the circulation and another specialty treat another part of the circulation, depending on its position in relation to the diaphragm or clavicle or whether the heart lung machine is necessary.

Cardiovascular is a better term to describe a surgical specialty than *cardiothoracic*. Whereas the term cardiovascular defines an organ system, the term cardiothoracic describes a single organ *and* a region of the body. A parallel term, *esophagothoracic*, for example, is not used. The confusion is heightened because *cardiothoracic surgery*, although it conveniently describes many surgical units in the United States, is not the formal term used to describe the current specialty, which is *thoracic surgery*.

A lifelong study of the circulation is required in both cardiac and vascular surgery. MedicineWorld.Org provides a list of 125 journals under the heading of "cardiology". It lists 187 under the heading of "cancer." No single surgeon can stay current in both cardiovascular disease and neoplastic disease. A cardiovascular surgeon, in contrast to a thoracic surgeon, would be able to focus on the circulatory system and its diseases, which is sufficient for one career.

The dominant disease treated by cardiac and vascular surgeons is the same, namely, atherosclerosis. It is the same disease, of course, in the coronary, carotid, and femoral arteries.[6] Although operative treatment of a single arterial bed may vary in technical ways, systemic treatment of atherosclerosis is virtually identical for coronary artery disease and peripheral arterial disease.

A surgeon familiar with coronary atherosclerosis is well suited to treat carotid or femoral atherosclerosis. Performance of a coronary artery bypass grafting (CABG)

From the Section of Thoracic and Cardiovascular Surgery, The Heart and Vascular Center, Winchester Medical Center, Valley Health System, Winchester, Va.

Received for publication Feb 29, 2008; accepted for publication April 17, 2008.

Address for reprints: Charles Stewart Roberts, MD, 190 Campus Blvd, Suite 410, Winchester, VA 22601 (E-mail: croberts@valleyhealthlink.com).

J Thorac Cardiovasc Surg 2008;136:267-70

0022-5223/$34.00

doi:10.1016/j.jtcvs.2008.04.010

Abbreviations and Acronyms
AATS = American Association for Thoracic Surgery
STS = Society of Thoracic Surgeons
CABG = coronary artery bypass grafting

procedure in the morning and a lobectomy in the afternoon is certainly an everyday occurrence in the United States, but a far more natural sequence is to follow the CABG with a carotid endarterectomy or a femoropopliteal bypass or repair of an abdominal aortic aneurysm.

The same surgeon can treat the single patient with atherosclerosis in different arterial beds. Many of my patients who have undergone CABG have required carotid endarterectomy or femoropopliteal bypass and vice versa. Knowledge of the consequences of atherosclerosis in one arterial bed is useful in the treatment of atherosclerosis in another arterial bed. For example, an expertise in carotid atherosclerosis is useful in the evaluation of a patient with concomitant coronary atherosclerosis and vice versa. Whereas operations to treat aneurysms tend to be curative, operations to treat blockages are palliative. Atherosclerotic patients keep coming back, some presenting first with coronary artery disease, others presenting with peripheral arterial disease, and many presenting with both.

Aneurysms and dissections of the aorta and its branches, no matter what location, can be treated by the same surgeon. Endovascular repair of aortic aneurysms has been developed by vascular surgeons and many now treat thoracic aortic aneurysms. Thoracic surgeons also perform this procedure now, however, and the overlap is obviously unnecessary. The marriage of cardiac and vascular surgeons would eliminate overlap or barriers in the treatment of aortic disease by open or closed techniques. Hybrid procedures, involving combined endovascular and open techniques, inside or outside of the chest, become less complicated when the treating surgeon is not limited to an anatomic region.

The surgical techniques necessary in both coronary and noncoronary arterial surgery are similar. Operating on arteries inside and outside the thoracic cage involves similar techniques—proximal and distal control, use of autologous and nonautologous conduits, vascular anastomoses, patch or primary closures, antegrade and retrograde flushing, avoidance of end-organ ischemia and embolization, anticoagulation and its reversal, and so on. These standard vascular methods are currently learned by both vascular and thoracic surgeons but are intended to be applied only outside the chest by vascular surgeons and inside the chest by thoracic surgeons.

Cardiovascular surgeons may benefit from the combination of open cardiac and vascular cases. The rise of closed procedures on the aorta and all of its branches has meant fewer open procedures. The number of CABG procedures, in particular, has declined in recent years. The same is true for open revascularization procedures for the lower extremities.

The implications for cardiac and vascular surgeons and patients are profound if one considers the inverse relation of surgical volume and adverse outcome. Performing fewer CABG procedures yearly, for example, may be concerning if the other operations in one's case mix are video-assisted thoracic surgery, mediastinoscopy, lobectomy, decortication, and esophagectomy. However, if the other operations are open vascular procedures, such as carotid endarterectomy, and various peripheral arterial operations, then the technical requirements overlap with CABG—fewer CABG procedures annually may not spell disaster.

Vascular surgeons, perhaps more so than cardiac surgeons, feel the pull of the angiography suite and endovascular therapy. This evolution, however, diminishes considerably the vascular surgeon's experience in open procedures. For the vascular surgeon whose bent is open procedures, adding CABG procedures to the practice may enhance his or her skill in open operations.

A cardiovascular surgery specialty is historically fitting. One of the first monograms on this subject, *Surgery of the Vascular System,* was published in 1913 by Bertram M. Bernheim[7] of Baltimore, who was first in the United States (1915) to interpose an autologous vein graft after resecting a popliteal aneurysm.[8] The book contains chapters on general technique, transfusion, end-to-end suture, lateral anastomosis, transplantation of a segment of vein or artery, arteriovenous anastomosis (reversal of the circulation), varicose veins, and aneurysms, with exquisite illustrations. Chapter 13 is called "Surgery of the Heart," the point being that cardiac surgery was originally considered to be within the field of vascular surgery. It was part of "the field of blood-vessel surgery."

Early pediatric cardiovascular operations were purely vascular. In 1938 Gross ligated a patent ductus arteriosus,[9] and in 1944, Blalock constructed a subclavian–pulmonary anastomosis for a patient with the tetralogy of Fallot.[10] Other common pediatric cardiovascular operations are purely vascular, including repair of coarctation of the aorta.

Many early cardiac surgeons began as general surgeons, thoracic surgeons, and vascular surgeons, and many became cardiovascular surgeons, contributing in both cardiac and vascular arenas. Michael E. DeBakey was the founding editor of the *Journal of Vascular Surgery.* His original contributions to the surgical treatment of aneurysms and atherosclerosis in multiple arterial beds were numerous.[11,12] His surgical creativity was not limited by the diaphragm or the clavicle or the heart–lung machine. In an interview in 1997, he remarked: "The cardiac and vascular services are separated in many places. I object to that for the simple reason that I consider the cardiovascular system a unified system."[13]

Denton A. Cooley, known for his numerous contributions to the treatment of congenital and acquired cardiovascular disease, performed the first successful carotid endarterectomy in 1956.[14] His book with Wukasch, *Techniques in Vascular Surgery,* was my guide when developing a practice of vascular surgery.[15] His namesake society is called the Denton A. Cooley Cardiovascular Surgical Society. The term used is *cardiovascular*—not cardiac or vascular or thoracic or cardiothoracic.

The specialty of thoracic surgery was founded on general thoracic surgery, not cardiovascular disease. The focus early in the 20th century was on the operative treatment of pulmonary infections, particularly tuberculosis. Lung cancer before 1930 was infrequent, and cardiovascular operations inside the chest were virtually nonexistent.

In his 1953 book, *A Practice of Thoracic Surgery*, A. L. d'Abreu[16] of Birmingham, England, wrote, "In 1934, largely through the kind encouragement of the late Professor Lyle Cummins, the Professor of Tuberculosis in the University of Wales, I started the study and practice of thoracic surgery." One did not enter thoracic surgery at that time to treat cardiovascular disease. His book contains 27 chapters, only 5 of which pertain to the cardiovascular system (2 diagnostic and 3 surgical), representing 18% of the book by pages. General thoracic surgery dominates, with sections on bronchopulmonary anatomy, pyogenic infection, pulmonary tuberculosis, diseases of the esophagus, and diaphragmatic problems. D'Abreu's book appeared the year the heart–lung machine was first introduced clinically.

Also in 1953, Lindskog and Liebow[17] published *Thoracic Surgery and Related Pathology*, another book dominated by infectious and neoplastic diseases. The follow-up book appeared in 1962 with a title change, now called *Thoracic and Cardiovascular Surgery with Related Pathology*, with the contribution of the cardiovascular surgeon, William Glenn.[18] This new version had two parts: thoracic surgery, which contained 28 chapters (580 pages), and cardiovascular surgery, which contained 21 chapters (444 pages)—two completely different fields of study. This was the beginning of the complicated marriage of cardiovascular surgery and general surgery inside the chest.

The major surgical societies currently do not completely serve the many surgeons who practice cardiovascular surgery. The dominant societies segregate cardiac and vascular surgeons. In the annual meetings of The American Association for Thoracic Surgery (AATS) and The Society of Thoracic Surgeons (STS), peripheral vascular surgery is not part of the program, and a significant portion of both meetings is devoted to general thoracic surgery. The Society for Vascular Surgery does not address the surgical treatment of the first branches of the aorta (coronary arteries) and gives probably inadequate attention to intrathoracic vascular surgery.

The AATS was founded in 1917 on general thoracic surgery, before the advent of antimicrobial therapy. *The Journal of Thoracic Surgery*, the official journal of the AATS, was first published in 1931, and none of the 6 original articles in the first issue concerned cardiovascular surgery. By 1959, the Association was faced with the rapid progress of cardiovascular surgery, and it changed the name of its publication to *The Journal of Thoracic and Cardiovascular Surgery*.[19] It currently divides its subject matter between intrathoracic cardiovascular surgery and general thoracic surgery, having abandoned peripheral vascular surgery altogether. In the February 2008 issue of *The Journal of Thoracic and Cardiovascular Surgery*, the 41 articles included 33 on intrathoracic cardiovascular conditions (1 on thoracoabdominal aortic aneurysm) and 8 on general thoracic conditions.

The STS was founded in 1963. On its emblem, adopted in 1965, there were four drawings—a heart, an esophagus, the lungs, and the abdominal aorta. The emblem was changed in 1994 to reflect the abandonment of extrathoracic vascular surgery. Now there appear four drawings—the heart, the lungs, three structures together (the thoracic aorta, the trachea, and the esophagus), and the thoracic cage. This change is certainly understandable, given the Society's focus on thoracic surgery, but it clearly partitions the cardiovascular system. Sidney Levitsky,[20] in his presidential address to the STS in 2006, reflected on the change: "The peripheral vascular portion of the STS logo, exemplified by the abdominal aortic aneurysm, was changed in 1994 to the thoracic aorta as cardiac surgeons turned away from peripheral vascular surgery and focused their attention on coronary artery surgery...Both specialties and our patients would benefit, if reunification occurred."

The official journal of the STS, *The Annals of Thoracic Surgery*, first published in 1964, also has a division in its subject matter across four organ systems—the cardiovascular system, the respiratory system, the alimentary tract, and the musculoskeletal system. In simplistic terms, of course, it has two subjects, cardiovascular surgery within the chest and general thoracic surgery. In the February 2008 issue, the 40 "original articles" are neatly separated under two different headings: 10 articles appeared under "general thoracic" and 30 under "cardiovascular." No article addressed extrathoracic vascular surgery.

The Society for Vascular Surgery was founded in 1947. In the February 2008 issue of its *Journal of Vascular Surgery*, 3 of the 25 articles under the first section, "Clinical Research," addressed intrathoracic vascular conditions. The lead article was on thoracic endovascular aneurysm repair, and the published presidential address was on carotid stenting, which reflect the clinical range encompassed now by the specialty.

In my own practice, which consisted of 340 operations in 2007, the two most common operations are CABG and carotid endarterectomy, which are the two most common operations in thoracic and vascular surgery, respectively. This cardiovascular surgical practice, however, requires two different national society meetings, two different specialty journals, and two different Web sites (CTSNet and VascularWeb) to keep abreast.

The concept of the "Heart and Vascular Center" or "Cardiovascular Institute" makes sense and fits well with a "cardiovascular" surgical specialty and service line. One does not see the "Heart and Esophageal Center" or the "Lung and Vascular Center." Cardiac and vascular surgeons are already co-located in these cardiovascular centers. A cardiovascular surgeon would be well suited to provide all surgical services in a "Heart and Vascular Center."

A single cardiovascular surgical specialty may enhance relations with other specialties. Cardiologists have no self-imposed barriers, such as the diaphragm and the clavicle. Their realm now is the entire circulatory system. A cardiovascular surgeon may be of the same mind. The referring cardiologist or primary care physician need not inquire whether the thoracic surgeon or the vascular surgeon does this or that operation.

Vascular surgeons attract a considerable number of referrals directly from internists, family practitioners, podiatrists, and others. This position of actually evaluating and treating patients with atherosclerosis or aneurysms is different from the usual position of the thoracic surgeon, who is referred a patient for an operation after a rather thorough evaluation by a cardiologist. After performing a cardiovascular operation in the chest, such as CABG, the thoracic surgeon usually relinquishes the patient by 2 months postoperatively. Vascular surgeons, in contrast, make most clinical decisions about the treatment of noncoronary arterial disease in their patients. As a cardiovascular surgeon, I refer numerous patients with atherosclerosis to cardiologists for cardiac studies, particularly in preparation for noncoronary arterial operations. The relationship with cardiologists, therefore, achieves better balance.

A unification of cardiac and vascular surgery would bring all open and closed cardiovascular operations to bear in a single specialty. Vascular surgeons already are comfortable in the angiographic suite. Cardiac surgeons are slowly adopting more closed procedures. Expertise in closed and hybrid procedures may be a requirement for a viable cardiovascular surgical practice in the future. A merger of cardiac and vascular surgery may facilitate the free flow of ideas and techniques. Numerous closed cardiac procedures such as percutaneous aortic valve insertion and percutaneous mitral valve repair are gaining a foothold, and the combined expertise of cardiac and vascular surgeons might bring more progress.

Cardiac surgeons who are part-time cancer surgeons may serve the cancer patients less well than full-time general thoracic surgeons. Cardiovascular and cancer conferences are entirely different. Cardiovascular conferences involve cardiologists and interventional radiologists, all discussing diseases of the circulatory system, usually atherosclerosis. Cancer conferences involve medical oncologists, surgical oncologists, radiation oncologists, and specialty radiologists (eg, mammogram experts), all discussing tumors. Virtually no overlap of participation occurs in cancer and cardiovascular conferences, except by thoracic surgeons. This duality seems out of step with postmillenium health care delivery.

A cardiovascular surgical residency may attract top trainees. In the 2008 match for thoracic surgery, 96 residents applied for 130 positions and some 81 (67%) positions were filled.[21] For vascular surgery, 139 residents applied for 119 positions and some 115 (97%) positions were filled.[22] One may conclude that medical students and residents have minimal interest now in both thoracic surgery and vascular surgery as separate surgical specialties. Furthermore, the training positions are secured with minimal competition—91% of thoracic surgery applicants matched and 83% of vascular surgery applicants matched.[21,22]

The unification of cardiac and vascular surgery into one residency training program, in my opinion, would be a win–win proposition. A unified cardiovascular surgical training program not only would attract more applicants but also would promote more keen competition for positions, and the final product would be more valuable.

References

1. Carrel A. Surgical technique for vascular anastomoses and organ transplants [French]. *Lyon Med.* 1902;98:859-63.
2. Carrel A. The surgery of blood vessels. *Johns Hopkins Hosp Bull.* 1907;18:18.
3. Gibbon JH Jr. Application of a mechanical heart and lung apparatus to cardiac surgery. *Minn Med.* 1954;37:171-80.
4. Cronenwett JL, Liapis CD. Vascular surgery training and certification: an international perspective. *J Vasc Surg.* 2007;46:621-9.
5. Harvey W. Exercitatio anatomica de motu cordis et sanquinis in animalibus. 4th ed. (Translated by Chauncey D. Leake.) Springfield [IL]: Charles C Thomas Publisher; 1958.
6. Roberts WC. Atherosclerosis: its cause and its prevention. *Am J Cardiol.* 2006;98:1550-5.
7. Bernheim BM. Surgery of the vascular system. Philadelphia: J.B. Lippincott; 1913.
8. Bernheim BM. The ideal operation for aneurysms of the extremity: report of a case. *Johns Hopkins Hosp Bull.* 1916;27:1.
9. Gross RE, Hubbard JP. Surgical ligation of patent ductus arteriosus. *JAMA.* 1939;112:729-31.
10. Blalock A, Taussig HB. The surgical treatment of malformations of the heart in which there is pulmonary stenosis or pulmonary atresia. *JAMA.* 1945;128:189-202.
11. DeBakey ME. The development of vascular surgery. *Am J Surg.* 1979;137:697-738.
12. DeBakey ME, Lawrie GM, Glaeser DH. Patterns of atherosclerosis and their surgical significance. *Ann Surg.* 1985;201:115-31.
13. DeBakey MD, Roberts WC. Michael Ellis DeBakey: a conversation with the editor. *Am J Cardiol.* 1997;79:929-50.
14. Al-Naaman YD, Carton CA, Cooley DA. Surgical treatment of arteriosclerotic occlusion of common carotid artery. *J Neurosurg.* 1956;13:500-6.
15. Cooley DA, Wukasch DC. Techniques in vascular surgery. Philadelphia: W.B. Saunders; 1979.
16. D'Abreu AL. A practice of thoracic surgery. London: Edward Arnold & Co; 1953.
17. Lindskog GE, Liebow AA. Thoracic surgery and related pathology. New York: Appleton-Century-Crofts; 1953.
18. Lindskog GE, Liebow AA, Glenn WWL. Thoracic and cardiovascular surgery with related pathology. New York: Appleton-Century-Crofts; 1962.
19. Ferguson TB. The Journal of Thoracic and Cardiovascular Surgery diamond jubilee—a reflection. *J Thorac Cardiovasc Surg.* 2006;132:451-2.
20. Levitsky S. Navigating the new "flat world" of cardiothoracic surgery. *Ann Thorac Surg.* 2007;83:361-9.
21. Vital Signs. Thoracic surgery fellowship 2008 matches. *Thoracic Surgery News.* 2007;3(5):1.
22. Vital Signs. Vascular surgery fellowship 2008 matches. *Vascular Specialist.* 2007;3(5):1.

Roberts CS. Cardiovascular surgery as a single specialty: the case to unify cardiac and vascular surgery. *J Thorac Cardiovasc Surg.* 2008;136(2):267-270. doi:10.1016/j.jtcvs.2008.04.010

19

Priorities in Polyvascular Disease

Charles Stewart Roberts, MD
From the Section of Thoracic and Cardiovascular Surgery, The Heart and Vascular Center, Winchester Medical Center, Valley Health, Winchester, VA
Address for correspondence: Charles Stewart Roberts, MD, 1870 Campus Boulevard, Suite 2A, Winchester, VA 22601
E-mail: csrwinchester@hotmail.com

Clinicians are occasionally presented with patients who have active problems in multiple arterial beds. Among patients with symptomatic atherothrombosis in a contemporary registry, 16% had symptomatic polyvascular disease.[1] Sometimes this requires prioritizing the problems if they cannot be simultaneously treated. While the care of each patient must be individualized, the following principles may be useful to consider in the staged treatment of multiple arterial conditions.

LIFE-THREATENING BEFORE LIMB-THREATENING

This principle is obvious and illustrated in the case of R.W., a 72-year-old man who presented with thromboembolism in his left foot. Imaging studies disclosed a 9-cm abdominal aortic aneurysm (AAA) (Figure 1) and a 5-cm left popliteal aneurysm (Figure 2). Rupture of the AAA would likely be fatal, while embolism from or rupture of the popliteal aneurysm may result in gangrene and require limb amputation. Therefore, the AAA was treated first by endovascular repair. A month later, the left popliteal aneurysm was treated by ligation (proximally and distally) of the aneurysm and a bypass graft (autologous saphenous vein) from the superficial femoral artery to the infrageniculate popliteal artery. The patient recovered well from these staged procedures.

HEART BEFORE AORTA

Problems in both locations can be life-threatening. If open operations to treat both conditions are required, then the heart is usually addressed first. An open aortic operation in the setting of myocardial ischemia is dangerous.[2] J.M., a 71-year-old man, presented with such a dilemma. He had previous coronary artery bypass grafting surgery (CABG) at 46 years of age. He presented with atrial fibrillation. Catheterization disclosed multivessel coronary atherosclerosis (Figure 3), with an ejection fraction of 15%. Both old vein grafts were occluded. Imaging studies also revealed a 7-cm AAA (Figure 4), which was not amenable to endovascular repair.

A redo-CABG procedure was carried out first, followed 1 month later by open repair of the AAA. The patient recovered well from both procedures. It should be noted that the patient also had asymptomatic, bilateral carotid stenosis (an occluded right internal carotid artery and a 70% narrowing of his left internal carotid artery), which will be addressed later.

SYMPTOMATIC BEFORE ASYMPTOMATIC

When a patient has a severe carotid stenosis and severe multivessel coronary arterial stenoses, the question occasionally arises: which should be done first, carotid endarterectomy (CEA) or CABG? At some institutions, these procedures are simultaneously performed,[3] but most surgeons prefer a staged approach, which has been associated with a lower complication rate.[4] In general, the symptomatic arterial bed is treated first.

J.P., a 68-year-old man, had unstable angina pectoris and also complained of near-syncope, which was probably cardiogenic. Five years before, he had a left CEA for an asymptomatic carotid stenosis. Cardiac catheterization disclosed 3-vessel coronary arterial disease, and findings from magnetic resonance angiography disclosed a significant narrowing in his right internal carotid artery. CABG was carried out first, followed 6 months later by CEA. He recovered well after both procedures.

www.lejacq.com ID: 7706

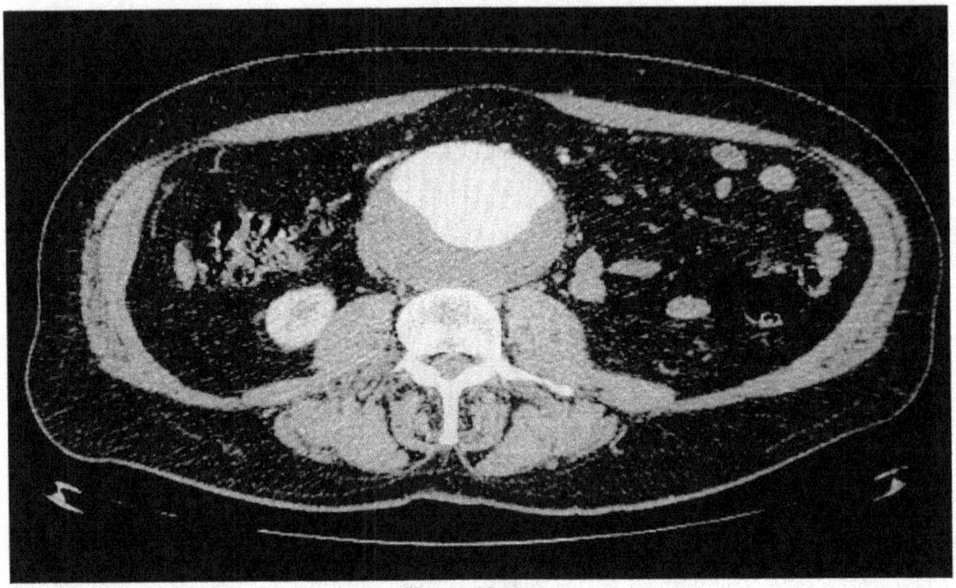

Figure 1. A 9-cm abdominal aortic aneurysm in a 72-year-old man.

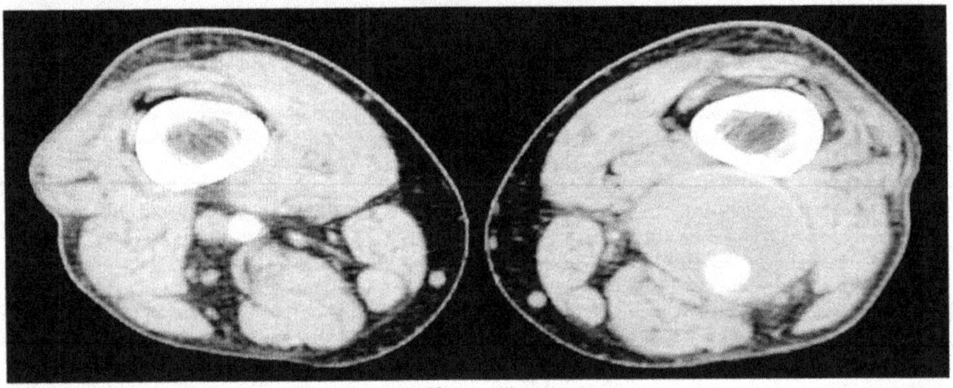

Figure 2. A 5-cm left popliteal aneurysm in the same 72-year-old man.

CLOSED PROCEDURE BEFORE OPEN PROCEDURE

This principle is often appropriate. For example, a patient with concomitant AAA and multivessel coronary artery disease may be best served by endovascular repair of the AAA before CABG—a minimally invasive procedure followed by a maximally invasive procedure. Another example to illustrate this principle is the case of a patient with a critical stenosis in both the aortoiliac system and in the femoropopliteal system. Stent implant in a common iliac artery first, followed later by open bypass grafting of an occluded superficial femoral artery, for example, would also conform to the principle of treating *inflow before outflow* narrowings from atherosclerosis.

References

1 Bhatt DL, Steg PG, Ohman EM, et al: REACH Registry Investigators. International prevalence, recognition, and treatment of cardiovascular risk factors in outpatients with atherothrombosis. *JAMA*. 2006;295:180–189.

2 Golden MA, Whittemore AD, Donaldson MC, et al. Selective evaluation and management of coronary artery disease in patients undergoing repair of abdominal aortic aneurysm.

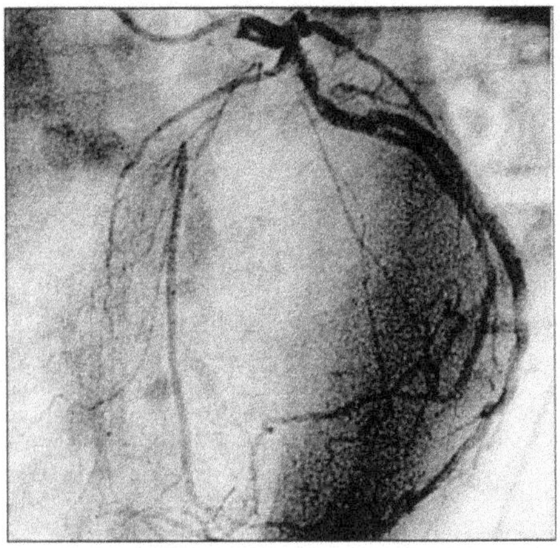

Figure 3. A totally occluded left anterior descending coronary artery with reconstituted flow in a 71-year-old man.

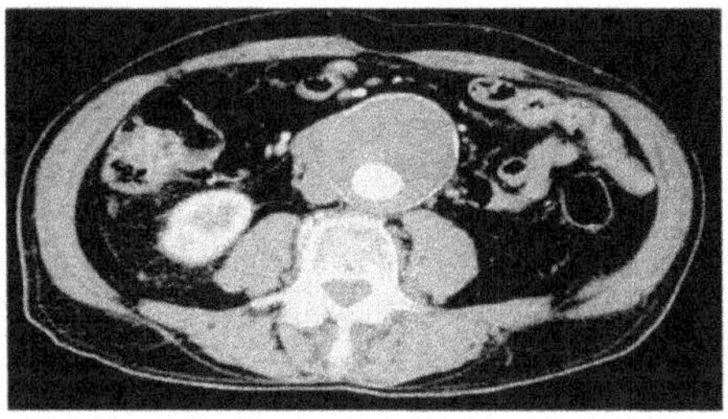

Figure 4. A 7-cm abdominal aortic aneurysm in the same 71-year-old man.

A 16-year experience. *Ann Surg.* 1990;212:415–420.

3 Akins CW, Hilgenberg AD, Vlahakes GJ, et al. Late results of combined carotid and coronary surgery using actual versus actuarial methodology. *Ann Thorac Surg.* 2005;80:2091–2097.

4 Borger MA, Fremes SE, Weisel RD, et al. Coronary bypass and carotid endarterectomy: does a combined approach increase risk? A metaanalysis. *Ann Thorac Surg.* 1999;68:14–21.

Roberts CS. Priorities in polyvascular disease. *Am J Geriatr Cardiol.* 2008;17(2):125-127.

20

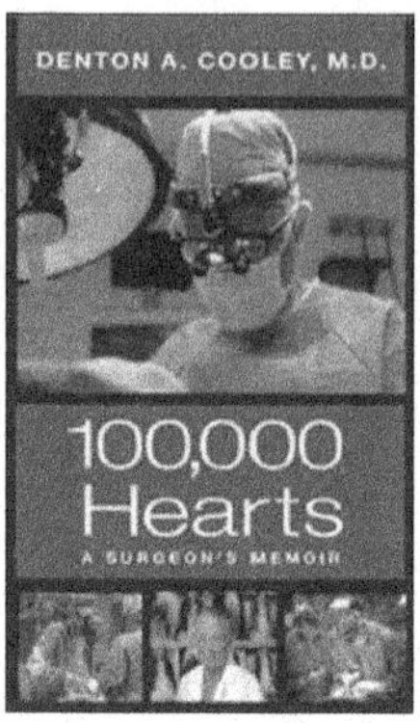

100,000 Hearts: A Surgeon's Memoir by Denton A. Cooley, MD

Austin, TX: Briscoe Center of American History, 2012.
Hardcover, 323 pp., $29.95.

Reviewed by Charles Stewart Roberts, MD

Each time I opened Denton Cooley's memoir, intending to breeze through a couple of chapters, I could not close it without advancing 100 pages. Some chapters, such as the "Reconciliation with Mike," I read twice. No cardiac surgeon could be indifferent to this book. It is a superb memoir of a gifted human being who rose to the peak of his profession. As an intern at Hopkins in 1944, Cooley found cardiovascular surgery a paltry field; he is leaving it a blooming one.

The first thing that strikes me about the book is its thoroughness. Cooley seems to cover life from early to late, including the highs and the lows, with a full range of telling photographs. In the appendices, we find diagrams, a glossary, various lists (personal contributions to cardiovascular surgery, inventions and products, and selected publications), and a curriculum vitae. The beauty of the book, however, is in the story, told as if he is there in the room.

A cardiac surgeon, Dr. Michael D. Crittenden, with whom I worked at the National Institutes of Health some 25 years ago, used to say, "Cardiac surgery is a brutal business." For a long, successful career in cardiac surgery, physical stamina is necessary, as well as a kind of emotional resilience, both of which Cooley clearly had. He was a gifted athlete who worked as a surgeon from 6:00 AM to 8:30 PM daily for decades—one of the few who were able to continue operating beyond the age of three score and ten. He appears to have lived by the dictum *Labor omnia vincit*, which means "Labor conquers all."

Along with endurance, Cooley had that human quality that allowed him to take in stride the brutal lows in cardiac surgery, along with the wonderful highs. Osler called that quality *aequanimitas*, or equanimity (1). The old television show, *Wide World of Sports*, used to open with the phrase, "The thrill of victory . . . and the agony of defeat." I knew one surgeon who would cry in his office after a patient died. Another would hardly speak for a week. Another would take it out on subordinates. Cooley shares with us that a round of golf in the open air helped him move forward.

Thomas Jefferson founded a university; Cooley founded an institute. One expects that the Texas Heart Institute will endure. As a natural leader, Cooley also seems to have lived by the Jeffersonian recommendation to "take things by the smooth handle." In his autobiography, Dr. Christiaan Barnard, the South African who later performed the first heart transplant, made these observations of Cooley during a visit to the Texas Heart Institute as a young surgeon:

> It was the most beautiful surgery I had ever seen in my life. Every movement had a purpose and achieved its aim. Where most surgeons would take three hours, he could do the same operation in one hour. It went forward like a broad river—never fast, never in obvious haste, yet never going back. . . . Dr. Cooley's skill was matched by his grace and kindness toward me. He invited me into his theater, showed me everything, and politely answered all questions (2).

Nearly every cardiac surgeon in North America whose surgical career overlapped that of Denton Cooley can find some connection to him. I am no different. Cooley's book on *Techniques in Vascular Surgery*, coauthored with Dr. Don C. Wukasch, was my go-to book in vascular surgery (3). Published in 1979, the prose is simple and clear and the illustrations are superb. And yet it is surely one of Cooley's minor publications.

Another connection was more personal. As an Emory medical student, I spent a month as an extern at Duke in 1985 and happened to board in the same home in Durham in which one of Cooley's daughters lived while receiving treatment at Duke. The homeowners, who had no children, were very fond of her and lamented her early death, which Cooley described poignantly in his memoir, some 30 years later, as the greatest tragedy of his life.

Cooley spent a year at the Royal Brompton Hospital in London, and his description of that year is delightful. I too spent a year there (1997–98), and my mentor, Mr. Christopher Lincoln, occasionally spoke of Cooley—how he became a "locum consultant" during the medical leave of the thoracic surgeon Oswald Sydney Tubbs, how he had a full operative "list," and how he wrote in a large handwriting. The impression Cooley made at the Brompton had lasted decades.

In 1999, my chief at the University of North Carolina, Dr. Benson R. Wilcox, handed me a letter that he received from Cooley concerning a book I wrote (4). The letter, handwritten by Cooley, reads:

> Dear Ben,
>
> Not knowing Charles Roberts personally, I am writing you to express my enjoyment of reading his book, *Stoking the Fire*. Of course my appreciation comes from having spent a similar year in London with Russell Brock and the other surgical dignitaries at the Brompton and the U.K. Dr. Roberts' observation and descriptions brought back vivid memories which I hold. As an author he has a real talent and may consider a future as a John

Grisham! Please extend my congratulations and encouragement to him. I wish that I had kept a full diary of my year. I can still quote sayings from Brock, Tubbs, Barrett, and Price Thomas.

I hope the summer is going well—

Sincerely yours,
Denton

The passages in Cooley's memoir concerning Dr. Michael E. DeBakey ("Mike" as he is called in the book) are interesting to many of us who have observed this rivalry in Houston from afar. Of course, the Cooley memoir represents one perspective. We will have no perspective from DeBakey, though I suspect he would disagree on many points, including various firsts in cardiovascular surgery. Nevertheless, their reconciliation, in the end, was good for the field of medicine. The photograph of the two surgeons together, shaking hands, late in life, is framed in my office, as a kind of inspiration. Both men are founding fathers of cardiovascular surgery in the 20th century.

1. Osler W. *Aequanimitas with Other Addresses to Medical Students, Nurses and Practitioners of Medicine.* New York: Blakiston Company, 1904.
2. Barnard C, Pepper CB. *Christiaan Barnard. One Life.* New York: MacMillan, 1969:242–243.
3. Cooley DA, Wukasch DC. *Techniques in Vascular Surgery.* Philadelphia: W. B. Saunders, 1979.
4. Roberts CS. *Stoking the Fire. A Surgical Memoir of London.* Armonk, NY: Futura, 1999.

The reviewer, **Charles Stewart Roberts, MD,** is a cardiothoracic surgeon at Winchester Medical Center in Winchester, Virginia.

Roberts CS. Book review: *100,000 Hearts: A Surgeon's Memoir* by Denton A. Cooley. *Proc (Bayl Univ Med Cent).* 2012;25(3):296-297.

21

The Honey Metaphor to Explain the Contribution of William Harvey

The bees steal from this flower and that, but afterward turn their pilferings into honey, which is their own.
—Michel de Montaigne

In 1628 at fifty years of age, William Harvey of England published a book which made the case that blood flows in a circle, pumped by the heart. His book is commonly referred to as *De Motu Cordis*, short for *Exercitatio Anatomica De Motu Cordis et Sanguinis in Animalibus* (Anatomical Exercises on the Movement of the Heart and Blood in Animals). Not until Chapter VIII does Harvey bring forward the argument: "…I began to think there was a sort of motion as in a circle." Indeed the word "Circular" appears in the title of Chapter VIII, and the word "Circulation" appears in the title of eight of the last nine chapters. The origin of the word "circle" meant flow in one direction. No one before him had made such an argument.

The author of Genesis had God create Earth from nothing. For mere mortals, however, nothing comes from nothing, which is to say, being creative requires a treasury of knowledge, a sort of scaffolding for further inquiry. Harvey's vast inventory of knowledge is apparent, not only in De Motu Cordis, but also in his earlier anatomical lectures under the title Prelectiones Anatomiae Universalis, which cover a period from 1616 to 1619. Both of these Latin books in English translation leave a reader with the unmistakable impression that Harvey was a scholar, thoroughly versed in the "ancients" and the "moderns."

Put another way, Harvey's creative contribution to science and to medicine did not arise in a vacuum. It was from slow, deliberate study. Montaigne described the honey metaphor above, and added, "…So the pupil will transform and fuse together the passages that he borrows from others, to make of them something entirely his own; that is to say, his own judgement. His education, his labor, and his study have no other aim but to form this."

The top ten physicians or scientists that Harvey cites both in his Lectures and in De Motu Cordis are listed in Table 1. Anyone interested in medical history may find this list to be a useful starting place to understand what came before in the study of the cardiovascular system. Aristotle and Galen were Harvey's two clear intellectual mentors, with Vesalius and Hippocrates, next among the "ancients." Columbo, Bauhin, Fallopius, and DuLaurens were cited most frequently among the "moderns."

Shakespeare died 400 years ago in 1616, the year Harvey was appointed Professor of Anatomy at the Royal College of Physicians, and the year his lecture notes appear to have begun. The honey metaphor can be applied similarly to Shakespeare. His sources of nectar were numerous—Ovid, Seneca, Lucretius. The honey he made was his own. Like Harvey, his inventory of knowledge was vast.

The example of Harvey may be useful to current students of cardiovascular surgery, particularly those striving to make an historical contribution. In his essay, "How to Think Like Shakespeare," Scott L. Newstok of Rhodes College wrote that "You cannot simply transform tradition (a creative ideal) without first knowing it (a conserving ideal)." Adding cardiovascular and thoracic surgical history to the inventory of knowledge of our trainees may prove to be worthwhile for our specialty.

Roberts CS. The honey metaphor to explain the contribution of William Harvey. Address at annual meeting of the American Osler Society, Atlanta, Georgia, April 12, 2017 (previously unpublished).

22

Charles L. McIntosh, MD, PhD (1938 to 2017): NIH Surgeon and Industry Executive

Achieving distinction in one domain is usually enough for one lifetime. Charles L. McIntosh, MD, PhD (hereafter CLM) had a bipartite career in which he rose to eminence in two fields, first in clinical cardiac surgery at the National Institutes of Health (NIH) in Bethesda, Maryland, and then in the medical device industry with Cook Group of Bloomington, Indiana. His success was understandable. His operative skill and standards were of the first order, his connection to patients was warm and often lifelong, his mastery of the English language was pleasing to the ear and to the eye, and his professional personality was unfailingly collegial, including to those of us who came under his mentorship during surgical training.

NIH Surgeon

After 3 years of general surgical training under Dr. Warren Cole at the University of Illinois in Chicago, CLM went to the National Heart Institute of NIH in Bethesda for the 2-year Clinical Associate program under Dr. Andrew Glenn Morrow. Dr. Morrow had been appointed the first Chief of the Clinic of Surgery of the National Heart Institute in 1953 and remained in that position until his death in 1982. He had 138 Clinical Associates during this 30-year period. Among his many accomplishments, Dr. Morrow was especially known for the "Morrow Procedure," a left ventricular myotomy/myectomy operation to treat the obstructive form of hypertrophic cardiomyopathy, then called idiopathic hypertrophic subaortic stenosis.

During this 2-year NIH fellowship, CLM favorably impressed Dr. Morrow, who invited and encouraged CLM to skip the 2 remaining years of general surgical residency in Illinois and instead remain at NIH and complete his cardiac surgical training under him (the only clinical associate so invited). CLM agreed and was soon thereafter appointed staff surgeon in the National Heart Institute, where he remained for the next 20 years. He also joined the Public Health Service and attained the rank of Captain.

During these 2 decades (1970 to 1990), CLM authored or co-authored 86 articles on cardiovascular disease, primarily on valvular heart disease and on hypertrophic cardiomyopathy. His operative techniques in valvular heart procedures were safe and precise and methodical, acquired in an era before the domination of coronary artery bypass surgery. Double and even triple valve replacements were routine for CLM. Long-term follow-up studies were published on these patients. In 1975, CLM was first author of an article on their initial 5 year clinical experience with replacement of the mitral and/or tricuspid valve with a Hancock porcine xenograft, concluding that it was the "prosthesis of choice."[1]

Unlike most cardiac surgeons then or now, CLM, along with all cardiac surgeons at NIH, was subjected to an intense degree of clinical review at NIH, owing to research protocols in place which required all postoperative patients to undergo a thorough reevaluation at 6 months, including repeat cardiac catheterization and echocardiogram. Indeed once a week at NIH there was a combined conference of cardiology and cardiac surgery, in which all surgical patients were discussed. In an NIH file of mine, I found a 6-page document addressed to "Dr. McIntosh," written by a peer Clinical Associate, detailing the clinical course of 1 patient who died postoperatively. No complications went unexamined.

During my 2 years as a Clinical Associate, 1988 to 1990, CLM held the title of Director of the Clinical Service of the Surgery Branch of the National Heart, Lung, and Blood Institute. When one entered his office, with its bookcases and oriental rug, classical music was always in the background. His knowledge of his patients before and after the operation was thorough. His missing out on the final 2 years of general surgical residency had no bearing on his overall clinical acumen, which was superb.

It seems meaningful to point out that CLM maintained decade-long excellent relationships with his colleagues at NIH. In cardiology, there was particular collaboration with Dr. Robert O. Bonow, now an international expert on valvular heart disease (presently at Northwestern University) and Dr. Barry J. Maron, surely the world's present authority on hypertrophic cardiomyopathy (now at Tufts Medical Center).

With Dr. William C. Roberts, his colleague in cardiovascular pathology (presently at Baylor University Medical Center in Dallas), CLM enjoyed a positive relationship and co-authorship of numerous articles. CLM later wrote in a personal letter to me, "If I became a good cardiac surgeon it was in part based on your father's teaching in his laboratory and conferences. He was not always correct but he always made one think and without question altered the way I did certain operations. He was the only individual with enough conviction and courage to speak out when [Claude] Lenfant closed the Surgery Branch. . ."

CLM cherished his relationships with many clinical associates, cultivating friendships that continued even as he went into medical industry. In 1991, when my parents separated, CLM sent me a 4-page hand-written letter. Among several pearls of wisdom, he shared the view that to achieve balance, it was important to develop interests outside of medicine, which he undertook, regretfully, only later in his surgical career.

CLM had suggested at one time that I undertake a biography of Dr. Warren Cole, his general surgical mentor at Illinois, who had retired to Ashville, North Carolina. During a brief vacation I stopped in to meet Dr. Cole and took many notes which I shared with CLM. Although I declined to undertake the project, a good book was finally written by another author. CLM wrote, "Your idea of a format for his biography I believe would have provided a more appropriate tribute. You know my feelings that what people write about you is not as important as what the individuals you train accomplish in their careers. That really casts a legacy."

0002-9149/
https://doi.org/10.1016/j.amjcard.2018.06.020

It was also during this 20-year period at NIH that CLM met his wife Dr. Deborah Barbour, most recently a distinguished cardiologist in Chevy Chase, Maryland, and Chief of Cardiology in the Bureau of Medical Services of the U.S. Department of State. She had trained at Georgetown University and was a senior fellow first in cardiac pathology and then cardiology at NIH during the same years. They were married for 32 years and maintained 2 gracious homes in Maryland, one in Silver Spring and another in their beloved Oxford on the Tred Avon River on the Eastern Shore. In Oxford they enjoyed a beautiful antebellum home, the Bratt Mansion (Academy House), which had served as quarters for the officers of the Maryland Military Academy. They shared a love of entertaining, of dogs and of antiques, and oriental rugs and found well-being in their wide circle of friends in Silver Spring, Oxford and Bloomington, Indiana.

With the death of Dr. Morrow in 1982, CLM became the premier surgeon for hypertrophic cardiomyopathy in North America. He wrote several articles on the subject as first author, the first with Dr. Barry J. Maron on "Current Operative Treatment of Obstructive Hypertrophic Cardiomyopathy," in which he describes the procedural details of the left ventricular myotomy/myectomy operation and added results of 156 patients he operated on after Dr. Morrow's death.[2] In a book chapter in *Current Therapy in Cardiothoracic Surgery*, published in 1989, CLM described in detail the technical aspects of the operation.[3] For some patients with obstructive hypertrophic cardiomyopathy, CLM performed mitral valve replacement and related that experience in an article in 1989.[4] His final first-author paper on the operative treatment of hypertrophic cardiomyopathy concerned the addition of plication of the anterior mitral leaflet to the left ventricular myotomy/myectomy procedure for certain patients, as an alternative to mitral valve replacement.[5] During my 2 years at NIH, CLM had, of course, added coronary artery bypass surgery to septal myectomies and valve replacements, but he did not like to wear loupes, which, of course, would present a challenge to most of us.

In his eulogy to Dr. Morrow given to the Halsted Society, CLM mentioned that Dr. Morrow often said, "Fishing is my real occupation; I only do open heart surgery as a hobby." CLM was also an avid fisherman, joining his mentor on many weekend fishing excursions. He particularly enjoyed fly-fishing his entire life.

Like Dr. Morrow, CLM was also precise with words in his speech and writings. For example, he was sensitive to misuse of the words "surgery" and "operation," and did not hesitate to correct his trainees. Surgery, of course, is a field, like medicine, with 3 parts—preoperative evaluation, the operation, and postoperative care—and should not be used interchangeably with the word "operation," only 1 part. He always ended his operative reports with the statement, "It is hoped that the patient will derive clinical and hemodynamic benefit from the operation."

Industry Executive

By skipping his last 2 years of general surgical training at Illinois, CLM did not meet criteria for board certification in surgery, which therefore excluded him meeting criteria for specialty board certification is thoracic surgery. This meant that his clinical practice would have to be confined to NIH where board certification was unnecessary. As the years passed, the original purpose of having clinical surgery at the National Heart Institute came under review, in light of all the many prestigious medical centers in the USA then doing open heart surgery and cardiovascular surgical research. Eventually, an effort was made by the leadership of NIH to close down the Surgery Branch.

Fortunately, during his 20 years at NIH, CLM had served as a Consultant and later Chairman of the Implantable Cardiovascular Devices Panel of the Federal Drug Administration (FDA). In 1990 at age 52, CLM decided to leave clinical practice and start his own consulting company, "C.L McIntosh & Associates" in Bethesda, Maryland, which offered consultation in clinical trials and FDA interactions. His expert knowledge of the regulatory approval process was unique and highly prized. In the relatively early days of personal computers, his company developed a "Clinical Trial Management System" (the McIntosh system) to help manufacturers meet the FDA demands in reporting their clinical data.

In 2003 at 60 years of age, CLM became a Vice-President of Cook Group of Bloomington, Indiana, with the title of Chief Medical Science and Technology Officer. In this executive position, he supervised innovation at Cook Group and traveled worldwide on behalf of the company to promote and improve its cardiovascular devices. He also

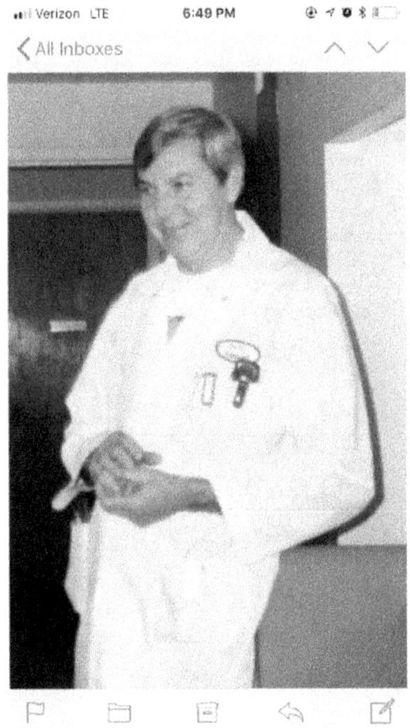

Figure 1. Charles L. McIntosh, MD, PhD, Surgeon at NIH, 1970 to 1990.

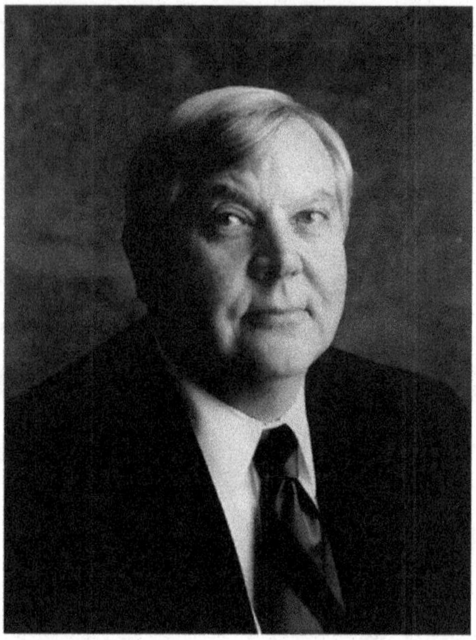

Figure 2. Charles L. McIntosh, MD, PhD, Executive at Cook Group, 2003 to 2016.

continued to attend surgical meetings. With his engaging personality, CLM became friends with the Cook family and with the company President, Mr. Kem Hawkins, a Cook employee of 35 years, who delivered the eulogy at the memorial service for CLM held in Oxford.

The creative side of CLM, which made him particularly effective in industry, was evident early in his surgical career. During his residency he invented a multiple suture holder and reported on it.[6] He also developed blunt-tipped surgical needles for deep tissue closure, to reduce risk to the surgical staff of needle punctures.

In this digital age with the tremendous personal upheaval brought about by mobile devices, CLM's "old ways" of conversation and manners would be considered exceptional. Even his letters, memos, and operative reports were beautifully crafted. Deborah Barbour, his wife, recently sent me a set of photographs from a visit my own family took to their home in Oxford, Maryland, where he displayed his talent as a chef ("Chilean sea bass" was served). CLM was not in any of the photographs. Indeed she can locate but very few images of him. Although modest in manner, however, no one could tell a story better at dinner when given the chance. His "impact factor" is difficult to gage, of course, but those whose lives he touched, in surgery or industry, were always the better for it, for he was an accomplished surgeon who was also a gentleman (Figures 1 and 2).

Charles Stewart Roberts, MD*
Department of Cardiac and Thoracic Surgery, Baylor University Medical Center, Baylor Scott & White Health, Dallas, Texas
* Corresponding author: Tel: 214-820-7100; mobile: 843-725-9847; fax: 214-820-6863. (Charles.Roberts@BSWHealth.org).

1. McIntosh CL, Michaelis LL, Morrow AG, Itscoitz SB, Redwood DR, Epstein SE. Atrioventricular valve replacement with the Hancock porcine xenograft: a five year clinical experience. *Surgery* 1975;78:769–775.
2. McIntosh CL, Maron BJ. Current therapy of obstructive hypertrophic cardiomyopathy. *Circulation* 1988;78:487–495.
3. McIntosh CL. Idiopathic hypertrophic subaortic stenosis.. In: Grillo HC, Austen WG, Wilkins EW, Mathisen DJ, Vlahakes GJ, eds. Current Therapy in Cardiothoracic Surgery, Toronto: B.C. Decker; 1989:391–397.
4. McIntosh CL, Greenberg GJ, Maron BJ, Leon MB, Cannon RO III, Clark RE. Clinical and hemodynamic results after mitral valve replacement in patients with obstructive hypertrophic cardiomyopathy. *Ann Thorac Surg* 1989;47:236–246.
5. McIntosh CL, Maron BJ, Cannon RO III, Klues HG. Initial results of combined anterior mitral leaflet plication and ventricular septal myotomy-myectomy for relief of left ventricular outflow tract obstruction in patients with hypertrophic cardiomyopathy. *Circulation* 1992;86(5 Suppl):I160–I167.
6. McIntosh CL. A multiple suture holder. *Surg Gynecol Obstet* 1968;126:601–602.

Roberts WC. Charles L. McIntosh, MD, PhD (1938 to 2017): NIH surgeon and industry executive. *Am J Cardiol.* 2018;122(7):1278-1280. doi:10.1016/j.amjcard.2018.06.020

23

What Does Woke Heart Surgery Look Like?

[Note: Submitted with the title "Woke Ideology and Heart Surgery." The editors changed the title. This was published under the pseudonym, "William Harvey, MD"]

The American College of Surgeons (ACS), founded in 1912, recently sent its members an email with its Report of Recommendations by its Task Force on Racial Issues. Fresh off the press in November 2020, the report opened with this phrase, "Following the killing of George Floyd"—the holy year zero. Even surgery is now connected to George Floyd. The report recommended an "Office of Diversity" and a "Regental Committee," along with ten other "Critical Enabling Habits." The ACS then created a "Diversity Pillar," one of five pillars of the ACS, to be addressed by a Board of Governors Diversity, Equity, and Inclusion Initiatives Workgroup and a Surgical Workforce Diversity, Equity, and Inclusion Workgroup. The Society of Thoracic Surgeons, a specialty group founded in 1963 that includes heart surgeons, has undertaken similar initiatives.

As a practicing cardiovascular surgeon for 25 years and member of both organizations, I look with deep regret upon the embrace of woke ideology and obsession with skin color. It will lead, I suspect, to diminished membership appeal and prestige, a distracted focus and mission, and less respect for surgical heritage, in time, in both organizations. The elite surgical leaders, working within academia, have ignored the surgical majority in the ACS who do not support this political dogma or identity politics in general.

As a kind of secular religion, woke ideology dictates that a person (in this case, a surgeon or a patient) is considered not as an individual, but rather as a member of a group, a category, based on skin color or sex or both. Woke ideologues reduce all persons in society, it seems, to the simple binary categories of white and non-white skin color, which are defined further as oppressor and victim groups, respectively. A person as an individual becomes irrelevant.

The profession of surgery, in my opinion, needs to disregard this harmful ideology, preserve meritocracy, and maintain race and sex neutrality. To the operating surgeon to the patient in need, individual merit is what matters. Meritocracy is the enemy of woke ideology.

While on a walk on a hot Saturday afternoon, I stopped to chat with a police officer adjusting his new Kevlar vest, waiting for a partner to arrive to search a home. The discussion went to the distinction of treating a person as an individual or as a member of a group, as a category. Indeed, a surgeon treats one individual at a time, does one operation at a time, provides one consultation at a time, sees one clinic patient at a time. We do not operate on a group of one skin color or another, or a victim group one day and an oppressor group the next. These are not even considerations. Woke ideology does not fit the profession of surgery, or, indeed, the field of medicine. All individual lives matter, one at a time. No group is singled out as more or less important.

As every patient would say, my sidewalk consultant also said, "I want the best heart surgeon operating on me." As a heart surgeon at a large institution, I do not hire, fire, train, treat, or refer based on race or gender. While standing over a beating heart draped in an operative field, I could not identify the race or sex of the patient without prior knowledge. The heart of each human being is subject to the same diseases. To a heart surgeon, skin color is irrelevant in the operation and in practice.

No patient asks for a surgeon who is hired because of skin color or sex, or to satisfy a Committee on Diversity, Equity, and Inclusion. Race-based and sex-based policies are detrimental to all parties. No one wins—neither the surgeon nor the patient, neither the majority nor the minority, and certainly not the organization.

No one would wish to be considered a "Diversity Surgeon," which is to say a surgeon preferentially hired or promoted because of non-white skin color or female sex. When this phenomenon happens, and it has, even in historically great programs, referrals for heart surgery crash at that institution. Everyone knows why, and no one dares speak of it. High-quality surgical colleagues migrate elsewhere and let it burn. New surgeons are eventually hired to rebuild and restore reputation. For the "Diversity Surgeon," skin color or sex is the career subject of interest, the topic of talks and articles, a path to the spoils of leadership. Involvement in these diversity matters, indeed for all skin colors and both sexes, is a kind of check box for academic advancement, no matter how disconnected from reality.

The goal of race-based initiatives in surgical societies, it would appear, is to force, or pretend to force, top-down change in surgeons, instead of nourishing bottom-up change in students. Pursuing the former, however, is no remedy for neglect of the latter. If the organizations desire the racial demographic of surgeons to match society, and one supposes that is the goal, then why not address early gaps in family, education, and achievement, which occur long before membership in these surgical organizations is even a possibility? Perhaps the two surgical organizations could start with students in Chicago, the headquarters of both, a city that had 43 gunshot victims last weekend—treated, no doubt, by members of the ACS.

As the saying goes, "one can never be woke enough." It should be added now that "an organization can never be diverse enough"—that is, to satisfy a Committee on Diversity, Equity, and Inclusion. Once established, the committee is here forever. Its chair and members will never, ever close it down. Instead, they will double down, expressing perpetual dissatisfaction. The goal of the committee will remain lofty and vague so that it is never achieved. How many surgeons per skin color group in society, for example, is acceptable to terminate the committee? We will never know.

At a recent coronary bypass operation at my institution, the six team members in the room, half women, were from six different countries—the USA, Peru, Iran, Vietnam, China, and the Czech Republic. Each heart team member brings individual talent to the operating room, together with an individual experience on Planet Earth, as does the patient. Woke ideology, with its skin-color obsession and binary white and non-white categories, is simply irrelevant. In the operating room, diversity of personnel evolves naturally, standards of excellence are applied to all, and individual merit is the only measure.

Harvey W [Roberts CS]. What does woke heart surgery look like? *American Thinker*, June 29, 2021. https://www.americanthinker.com/blog/2021/06/what_does_woke_heart_surgery_look_like.html

---

24

How Important Is 'Equity' When You're Getting Heart Surgery?

[Note: Submitted with the title "Equity or Excellence in Heart Surgery." The editors changed the title.]

A screenshot was sent to me of a social media post by a CEO whose friend was having heart surgery. It read: "I talked to him about three hours before his surgery and his only concern was that he hoped his surgeon wasn't hired to fill a racial or gender quota." This sentiment crystallizes a dilemma currently facing the profession of surgery.

Diversity, Equity, and Inclusion (DEI) initiatives in surgery are ubiquitous. DEI has been embraced by innumerable departments of surgery and societies of surgeons as well as healthcare institutions. Vice chairs of DEI have been appointed, and DEI committees have been created within surgical departments, adding to a costly DEI bureaucracy already established in hospitals and universities. DEI no longer challenges the system; it is the system, and the public is aware.

Perhaps because of cancel culture, discussion of DEI within the ranks of surgeons has been limited. There has been no debate. As an alternative to DEI in academia, Abbot and Marino (two scientists) have proposed a different framework: Merit, Fairness, and Equality (MFE). An open discussion of the two systems, DEI and MFE, is warranted, in my opinion, in the field of surgery.

The basic unit of DEI is the group. Human beings are categorized by skin color or sex, with oppressor or victim status attached to each group, irrespective of individual life experiences. The basic unit of MFE is the individual, and judgment is based on merit. Excellence is considered the highest form of merit.

Perhaps the closest word to "diversity" is "variety." The variety of human beings participating in the field of surgery is enormous; it is a worldwide profession. Equity in DEI means equal outcome. Equality in MFE means equal opportunity. Equity in surgery, as in nature or society, is unachievable. Some surgeons receive more referrals, do more operations, and have fewer complications than others. Compensation among surgeons is also unequal because it is usually based on productivity. In general, surgeons strive to be excellent, not equal.

Inclusion is an admirable goal in surgery if it means inclusion with uncompromised standards. No surgeon would want to be perceived by a patient or colleagues as being "included" with inferior qualifications because of group identification. No party would be served well—patient, surgeon, profession, or institution. Furthermore, if the inclusion of one group is advanced by discriminating against another group, then exclusion is a more accurate term.

Merit, the first word of the MFE framework, is a traditional measure in surgery and other professions. Steve Jobs hired "A Players" at Apple. Jack Welch actively fired "the bottom 10%" at General Electric. Michael E. DeBakey, a founder of cardiovascular surgery, promoted excellence. In an interview in 1996, he stated, "Concentrate on excellence. ... I think you should put your money where the track record shows that it works best—in people who pursue excellence in the field."

A goal of individual excellence in surgery is fundamentally different from a goal of group equity. Though DEI has been rather quickly embraced by leaders in surgery, its general support by members of the profession is questionable.

The academic framework that produces the highest-quality surgeons will eventually prevail. The DEI framework, in my opinion, is so inherently flawed that it will fail. Patients, like the one above, expect their surgeon to be hired not to fill a group quota, but because of individual merit, which is the only reliable measure.

Roberts CS. How important is 'equity' when you're getting heart surgery? *American Thinker,* December 18, 2021. https://vvv.americanthinker.com/blog/2021/12/how_important_is_equity_when_youre_getting_heart_surgery.html

25

Stewart R. Roberts, MD, and the South

Ever since the War between the States, the South [13 States] has been the poorest section of the nation. The richest State in the South ranks lower in per capita income than the poorest State outside the region.... The low-income belt of the South is a belt of sickness, misery, and unnecessary death. Its large population of low-income citizens are more subject to disease than people of any similar area.

—Report on the Economic Condition of the South
Prepared for the President [Roosevelt] by the National Emergency Council, 1938

Between Appomattox (1865) and Pearl Harbor (1941), the South remained a distinct region of the United States of America, unique in its demography, culture, economy, and health (Figure 1). After World War II, the South blended with the rest of the USA, but not before. Within this period of time (76 years) and within this distinct region of the world, Stewart R. Roberts, MD (1878-1941), hereafter SRR, lived and rose to a notable level of medical achievement.

This book comes 28 years after this writer published a slim book on SRR, combining a brief biographical sketch with a selection of quotations gathered from his many published addresses. After an initial sense of satisfaction, the writer began to consider the book inadequate. The chief legacy of SRR, if any, lay in his published articles, none of which were included in the first book. The reprints and photocopies of his articles remained on a shelf, collected carefully in two leather-bound volumes 50 years ago by the second son of SRR, William C. Roberts, MD, the father of this writer.

Most of the published articles, about 100 in all, were addresses to medical groups that were subsequently published. The purpose of the present book is to let his own writings tell the story. The task began when a box of his personal letters came into the writer's hands a year ago, providing greater insight into SRR, and adding a selection of letters to the collection of articles.

The decision to add Osler to the title was not taken lightly. SRR and Osler shall be compared, followed by some thoughts on the life, articles, letters, and legacy of SRR.

The Comparison

Sir William Osler was considered to be the most important physician in the world of his generation. Born in Canada in 1849, Osler earned his medical degree and took his postgraduate hospital training at McGill University in Montreal. His career had four geographic phases—Montreal for the first 10 years, Philadelphia for 5, Baltimore for 12, and Oxford for the final 12. Osler is best known for his single-authored textbook of medicine published in 1878, in which his therapeutic recommendations are limited strictly to those proven by evidence, effectively discarding a vast array of sham remedies. Osler's individual publications are staggering in number; however, with no single major medical discovery is he solely credited.

REPORT TO THE PRESIDENT

ON

THE ECONOMIC CONDITIONS OF THE SOUTH

SECTION 7

HEALTH

For years evidence has been piling up that food, clothing, and housing influence not only the sickness rate and death rate but even the height and weight of school children. In the South, where family incomes are exceptionally low, the sickness and death rates are unusually high. Wage differentials become in fact differentials in health and life; poor health, in turn, affects wages.

The low-income belt of the South is a belt of sickness, misery, and unnecessary death. Its large proportion of low-income citizens are more subject to disease than the people of any similar area. The climate cannot be blamed—the South is as healthful as any section for those who have the necessary care, diet, and freedom from occupational disease.

Several years ago the United States Public Health Service conducted syphilis-control demonstrations in selected rural areas in the South. These studies revealed a much higher ratio of syphilis among Negroes than among whites, but showed further that this higher ratio was not due to physical differences between the races. It was found to be due to the greater poverty and lower living conditions of the Negroes. Similar studies of such diseases have shown that individual health cannot be separated from the health of the community as a whole.

Figure 1. From the 1938 report to President Roosevelt.

As the first chair of medicine at Hopkins, Osler was one of the "Big Four," together with Halsted in surgery, Welch in pathology, and Kelly in obstetrics and gynecology. At Oxford University, Osler was the Regius Professor of Medicine, the highest academic title. As a physician, he was a master clinician whose consultation was widely sought, a prolific author whose publications number some 2000, a teacher of numerous students and trainees who remained devoted to him, a medical historian and bibliophile whose historical writings were not only scholarly but beautifully written, a leader of medical societies who regularly attended meetings at home and abroad, a seasoned correspondent to many in medicine, young and old, and a warm and devoted friend to many, inside and outside of medicine, who loved him dearly in return.

Osler is not a person to whom one advances a comparison lightly. SRR and Osler never met. Osler (1849-1919) was a generation younger than SRR (1878-1941). During the time frame of the medical career of SRR (1902-1941), they lived and worked in different regions of North America (Baltimore and Atlanta) for 10 of those years (1902-1912) and on opposite sides of the Atlantic (Oxford and Atlanta) for 6 years (1912-1919). When SRR went to Europe in 1911 to prepare for his book on pellagra, Osler had not come yet to Oxford, and when he returned to Europe in 1926, Osler had already died. SRR became Professor at Atlanta Medical College in 1912, the year Osler left for England, and was made Professor of Clinical Medicine at the newly established Emory University in 1915. Their paths in life never crossed. The comparison, however, may be justified for these reasons:

1. SRR was apparently called "The Osler of the South" in his lifetime. The letter from Seale Harris, a distinguished leader of Southern medicine, quoted at the beginning of the book and included in the appendix of the book, states that SRR was "frequently called 'the Osler of the South.'"

2. Both were master clinicians. Patients were referred to SRR from many states and, like Osler, he travelled to many states by Pullman railway to visit patients. Doctors consulted him regularly on difficult cases. SRR made rounds daily at 8 AM at Emory University Hospital and then saw patients at the Roberts Clinic downtown beginning at 10 AM.

3. Both were medical writers. SRR was a prolific writer for his time and region; Atlanta was not Montreal. He published >100 medical articles and a book on Pellagra.

4. Both shared an early love of biology. SRR was first appointed Professor of Biology at Emory College and obtained a master of science degree from the University of Chicago while on sabbatical. Osler's early devotion to biology is well known.

5. Both were teachers of students and residents during their entire careers (SRR for 38 years). Like Osler, SRR wrote several articles on medical education, and both received numerous requests to advance the careers of students, trainees, and colleagues through recommendations. Dr. Boland, a surgeon at Emory and President of the Southern Medical Association (1936-7) wrote of SRR in 1925, after SRR had been on a medical faculty for 20 years (10 at Emory): "In all his work, nothing is dearer to him than the instruction of medical students, and hundreds of these throughout the country can attest to his talent for imparting knowledge."

6. Both were medical historians, always members of medical and nonmedical history clubs, regularly giving presentations, some of which were published. On the walls at the Roberts Clinic were pictures of the "Founding Four" of Hopkins, distinguished physicians of Vienna, and Sir James Mackenzie, the Scottish cardiologist, to name a few.

7. Both were bibliophiles who left their libraries to their respective alma maters.

8. Both physicians wrote elegant prose, reflecting a classical and Christian education. The prose of SRR is not inferior to that of Osler.

9. Like Osler, SRR was a member and leader of numerous medical societies, and elected President of three (one local, one regional, and one national). To attend meetings, he traveled widely and regularly by Pullman.

10. The professional correspondence of both physicians was broad; for SRR it included numerous physicians in Georgia, in the South, and in the country. Most correspondents seemed to be friends based on a love of medicine and medical fellowship.

11. The friendships of both men ranged widely: for SRR, a 1st tier of immediate and extended family in Atlanta, Macon, and Oxford, GA; a 2nd tier of lifelong friends, mostly from Emory; a 3rd tier of physicians all over Georgia and the South; and a 4th tier of national colleagues. SRR was known as a "physician's doctor and a preacher's doctor," and he cultivated lifelong relationships, like Osler, with many in medicine and the ministry.

12. Both physicians were well versed in the Bible. The father of Osler was an Anglican minister and the father of SRR was a Methodist minister. Both fathers and both sons had classical and Christian educations, and the writing of SRR and Osler reflects that background.

13. Both shared a love of European heritage, especially English. The Osler family was from Cornwall and the Roberts from Kent. Both loved English poetry, lines from which they each quoted often in essays. While Osler traveled often to Europe and eventually moved to Oxford, England, for his final 12 years, SRR also went to Europe twice for medical purposes, in 1911 and in 1926, perhaps a rare feat among physicians in the poorest region of North America.

SRR made no major discovery and participated in no single monumental clinical event such as a new treatment or operation, but neither did Osler. Both achieved a career status that comes only from decades of scholarly work, combined with a humanitarian quality. Both shared a reverence for those who came before, which is evident in the writings of both, though they lived and worked in altogether different environments in North America.

If there were to be an Osler of the South after World War II, Charles S. Bryan, MD, of Columbia, SC, would be him perhaps. Bryan was a master clinician and scholar whose life and work are comparable to Osler's. The South as a region, however, became less and less distinct after 1945, as the country became more homogenous. The South of SRR's time, Appomattox to Pearl Harbor (1865-1941), was separate, economically and culturally, from the rest of the country.

President Roosevelt commissioned a study of the South on June 22, 1938, writing to "Members of the Conference on Economic Conditions of the South" on July 5, 1938:

> It is my conviction that the South presents right now the Nation's No. 1 economic problem—the Nation's problem, not merely the South's. For we have an economic unbalance in the Nation as a whole, due to this very condition of the South.... It is an unbalance that can and must be righted, for the sake of the South and of the Nation.

The report was published a month later on July 25, 1938. It contained 15 sections on various subjects such as soil, water, population, education, and health. In the first section on economic resources, the last paragraph reads:

> The paradox of the South is that while it is blessed by Nature with immense wealth, its people as a whole are the poorest in the country. Lacking industries of its own, the South has been forced to trade the richness of its soil, its minerals, and forests, and the labor of its people for goods manufactured elsewhere. If the South received such goods in sufficient quantity to meet its needs, it might consider itself adequately paid.

The health section of the report (Figure 1) is a 1938 synopsis of the conditions in which SRR worked as a physician (1900-1941) for 4 decades. These conditions were in some ways different than those in which Osler worked during much of his career, certainly in Montreal and Oxford. Both physicians addressed public health concerns early in their careers, though among population demographics that were vastly different, at least Atlanta compared to Montreal or Oxford. At the annual meeting of the Southern Medical Association and through its publication, *Southern Medical Journal,* certain health issues, such as venereal disease and malaria and pellagra that disproportionately affected the South, were regularly addressed.

The South in those 4 decades (1902-1941) of SRR's medical practice had a binary black-white racial demographic (71% white and 29% black in 1930), and an overwhelmingly rural population (>99% of Southerners in 1930 had been born in rural districts). The state of Georgia, in particular, had a black population percentage in 1900, the year SRR graduated from Southern Medical College, of 47%, and in 1940, a year before his death, it was 35%. In contrast, Pennsylvania in 1890, the approximate time of Osler's practice there, was >99% white, and Maryland in 1900, while Osler was in Baltimore, was 80% white. Montreal and Oxford were >99% white. Thus, the racial demographic in which each physician practiced was quite different, which also distinguished the South from other parts of North America and Europe.

After Osler died in 1919, SRR wrote an essay, *Sir William Osler, Clinician, Teacher,* in which he expressed his admiration for Osler. A *Memorial Volume* of essays on Osler, edited by Maude E. Abbott, MD, was published in 1926. The essay on Osler by SRR appears in this volume (and also in *Southern Medical Journal*), only one of three essays (out of 130) by authors residing south of the Potomac River (*Sir William Osler as Bibliophile* by Leonard L. Mackall of Savannah, Georgia, and *Recollections of Dr. Osler's Method* from Harry T. Marshall, MD, from the University of Virginia).

The Life

Many details of the life of SRR are recounted in the biography published by this writer in 1993. A detailed chronology, however, is given in this book. Briefly, SRR was born in Oxford, GA, in 1878, the eldest of five children, to James William Roberts, a Methodist minister, and his wife, Clifford Rebecca Stewart, a graduate of Wesleyan College in Macon.

James William Roberts and SRR seem to have had a complex relationship. Virtually nothing exists in writing to describe it. The father had graduated first in his class at Emory College in 1877, had been minister at the prominent Trinity Church in Atlanta, and then President of Wesleyan College in Macon. Most of his sermons at Trinity and many events of his life were published in the *Atlanta Constitution* newspaper; indeed, his life would be well chronicled by that newspaper, perhaps to the dismay of his eldest son. In private typed notes "recorded presumably in preparation for a talk," SRR had a heading entitled "Whipping," under which he wrote:

> Justified by "spare the rod and spoil the child." I have to confess with shame that I went about the house for some days with murderous hatred of my father locked within my bosom. Physical punishment not a wise element in the education of proud and sensitive children.

James William Roberts left the ministry after 5 years at Wesleyan College, divorced his second wife (his first wife, Clifford Rebecca Stewart, the mother of SRR, had died of typhoid fever when SRR was 8 years of age), moved to Atlanta and worked with the Asa Candler of *Coca-Cola* to develop Druid Hills. He later remarried his second wife and re-entered the church as a member, both of which events were chronicled by the Atlanta newspapers. His obituary in 1919 appeared on the front page of the *Atlanta Constitution.* His private will gave a smaller share of share estate to SRR, of all his seven children (five with first wife and two with second).

SRR went to Emory College in Oxford in his teens for 2 years but was withdrawn for a period of rest by his father because of "exhaustion." He then enrolled in Southern Medical College for 2 years, graduated, then returned to Emory College for the final 2 years, graduating with first honor, like his father.

SRR was the fourth generation of his family connected to Emory College. His maternal great-grandfather Starr had donated money to found the college in 1837, allowing for future members to attend by scholarship (no record affirms that SRR attended on this scholarship). His maternal grandfather, Joseph Spencer Stewart, graduated from Emory in 1849, the first on both the Stewart (maternal) and Roberts (paternal) lines. In general in these two families, the men went to Emory and the women went to Wesleyan, for both colleges were single gender at the time. In 1915, Emory University was established in Atlanta, and Emory-at-Oxford was subordinated to it. In that year, 1915, SRR was appointed Professor of Clinical Medicine and served Emory in Atlanta for the next 25 years. SRR delivered the Commencement Address to his alma matter in 1925. In that address is a paragraph that later became known as "The Emory Creed." Such was his lifelong love of Emory.

After graduation from Emory College in 1902, SRR was appointed Professor of Biology but took a leave of absence to obtain a master's degree in zoology at the University of Chicago. Upon his return to Emory College in Oxford, he taught biology and was the campus physician. In 1905 he moved to Atlanta and began a lifelong private practice, with part-time academic appointments, which was the customary relationship of practice to academia (full-time professors were exceedingly rare). SRR was associated first with Atlanta Medical College, then Atlanta College of Physicians and Surgeons, and finally, from 1915 to 1941, with Emory University School of Medicine as Professor of Clinical Medicine.

Early in his career, SRR took an interest in public health. On behalf of the Young Men's Christian Association (YMCA), he travelled widely to college campuses to warn students of venereal disease, which was rampant in the South. Later he served as Medical Director of the Atlanta Public Schools. Pellagra, a nutritional deficiency, was ravaging the South, and he went to Italy and Austria in 1911 to study the disease, which led to a published book on pellagra in 1912. When the Great War came, he joined with two of his brothers upon the entry of the USA in 1917 and was appointed Medical Director of Camp Jackson, SC, which was terribly affected by the influenza epidemic. His younger brother, Will, served as a surgeon in the Front in France.

Upon returning to Atlanta after the war, SRR opened The Roberts Clinic and resumed his teaching responsibilities at Emory. It was his custom to attend hospital patients at Wesley Memorial Hospital (now Emory University Hospital) in the morning and see patients at The Roberts Clinic in the afternoon, with a glass of Coca-Cola always on hand between patients.

SRR always participated in local and national medical societies, especially the Southern Medical Association, becoming its President in 1924. He was also involved in the beginning of the American Heart Association, becoming its president in 1932 and a member of the Advisory Editorial Board of its journal, *The American Heart Journal*, from 1926 to 1941.

He married twice, first to Louise MacDonald of Atlanta from 1905 to 1926, and then to Ruby Viola Holbrook, also of Atlanta. With the second wife, he had three sons, one of whom died early. The two other boys became physicians, one at Emory for most of his career in radiology, and one in cardiovascular research at the National Institutes of Health in Bethesda and then Baylor University Medical Center in Dallas.

SRR lived on Ponce de Leon Avenue in the Druid Hills section of Atlanta for most of his adult medical career, but moved to a farm near Stone Mountain, GA, in 1936, at age 56 with his family, close enough to allow for a daily commute to Emory and The Roberts Clinic. SRR succumbed to heart failure at age 61, after two consecutive heart attacks. He was buried among family (Roberts, Stewart, Starr, etc.) at Oxford Memorial Cemetery in Oxford, GA, the original home of Emory College.

SRR was modest in regard to his own abilities. He believed in "making the most of ordinary abilities.... A genius is an ordinary person who works extraordinarily hard." His wife recorded the following remarks:

> No, you are wrong about me. I am only an ordinary person, without special ability in any line. In most things I am only slightly above the average, and in many I am frankly under than over. This is certainly true of my physical equipment. I can't run. I'm only an ordinary walker and only a fair swimmer. I can probably ride a horse better than I can do anything else, but am certainly not a remarkable horseman. Neither am I a good shot. My eyesight is not strong, and I have to be close to my game to get any aim at all. As far as literary gifts are concerned, I am certainly not a brilliant writer. I have written a good deal, but I always have to slave over everything I put on paper.

The Articles

The best single piece of writing in the collection, in this writer's opinion, is "An Ideal of Modern Medicine," which formed a portion of an address called "A Medical Center," delivered on December 16, 1915, as the retiring President of the Fulton County (Atlanta) Medical Society. "An Ideal" was extracted from the address and privately printed in Atlanta. It was republished by his second son in 1969 (Roberts WC. Dr. Stewart R. Roberts' "An Ideal of Modern Medicine." *Annals of Internal Medicine* 1969; 70: 1016-1017). This writer saw it in 1981 framed on the office wall of a pediatric cardiologist at Vanderbilt.

The best full article, in this writer's opinion, is called "The Art and Human Nature," which was an address given at Harvard Medical School in Boston on October 28, 1931 (Roberts SR. The art and human nature. *New England Journal of Medicine* 1932; 206(2): 70-76). The elegant prose draws upon the heart and soul of SRR at 53 years of age, the prime of his career, after three decades in medicine, and reflects a combination of classical and Christian education. His last medical philosophical essay, "The Doctor's Visit," was an address delivered to the graduating medical and nursing classes of the University of Texas at Galveston on May 30, 1936 (Roberts SR. The doctor's visit. *Texas State Journal of Medicine* 1936; 32: 266-271). In correspondence SRR mentioned that he hoped to write a book called "The Doctor's Visit," but it never came to pass. His only book was on pellagra in 1912.

SRR published historical essays on Charcot, William Osler, Benjamin Franklin, William Charles Wells, William C. Gorgas, Vesalius, and Jane Todd Crawford, and unpublished manuscripts were found on George Washington and William Tecumseh Sherman, which were addresses given to the Symposium Club, a literary club in Atlanta. The Osler and Gorgas essays were published in the *Southern Medical Journal* and the William Charles Wells essay was published in the *Boston Medical and Surgical Journal* (which became the *New England Journal of Medicine*). These historical essays combine considerable research with the touch of the artist. The essay on "William C. Gorgas of Alabama," for example, begins:

> In the South the Black Warrior River runs by way of the Tombigbee into the Alabama, the Alabama into Mobile Bay. The Bay is luxuriant with the rich purple of the water hyacinth, the yellow white of the floating lily, and green grace of the willow, and merges unnoticed, "too full for sound or foam," with the warm blue waters of the Gulf. The Gulf reaches to the Caribbean and is the fountain of that mysterious, self-conscious "river of the ocean," which flows round the tip of our new El Dorado upward by the Newfoundland banks beyond the Sargasso Sea to give the English climate what comfort it has and to the English spring its bewitching beauty. Along the north shore of the Gulf is that shadowy line which marks the end of cold and snow which men forego, and the beginning of the longer heat, the rainy season, and the stars of the tropical night.
>
> All along these Southern shores until recently were those two morbid masters, yellow fever and malaria, whose ever recurring human damage was in sad, sharp contrast with Nature's sweet unison of sun and water and flower....

The Presidential Address for the Southern Medical Association in 1925 and for the American Heart Association in 1934 was on medical history—the first on William C. Gorgas and the second on William Withering, a copy of which has, unfortunately, not been located.

SRR wrote several articles on pellagra, the niacin deficiency which affected the South so terribly. His only published book was on pellagra in 1912, a decade before Goldberger fully established the nutritional cause, written after a research trip to Italy and Austria to study the disease where it was also devastating. In the absence of a known cause, SRR focused on its myriad clinical presentations, now expressed often as "the four D's"—diarrhea, dermatitis, dementia, and death. In the first chapter he writes:

> One need not expect to find a typical pellagra. It is a disease of many symptoms and of many variations; its only consistency is its inconsistency; it seems cured and yet recurs; the pellagrin seems to be approaching his end and yet lives for many years; it spreads and is

not contagious; the offspring of the pellagrin receives his mark and yet it is not inheritable; it is not and appears; it is and disappears; it is a morbid entity and yet it contains within itself many lesser entities; it falls with equal right in the sphere of dermatology, neurology, and gastrology, and yet it is a general disease; divers diseases become one, and this one is called pellagra; there is no pellagra—only the pellagrous.

In the Report to the President on "Economic Conditions of the South," even in 1938, 15 years after the cause was known, the disease still affected the South:

> The scourge of pellagra, that affects the South almost exclusively, is a disease chiefly due to inadequate diet; it responds to rather simple preventative measures, including suitable nourishing food; even in southern cities from 60 to 80 percent of the families of low incomes are spending for food less than enough to purchase an adequate diet.

Throughout his medical career, SRR addressed public health matters, including sexually transmitted diseases. Not until 1928 was penicillin discovered by Alexander Fleming, so for nearly three decades of medical practice, SRR did not have antibiotics to prescribe for bacterial infections. Several articles address infectious diseases such as pneumonia and malaria. Other public health articles address disease statistics in Georgia. He was a lifelong advocate for improving the health for the poor, and several articles present his views, which advocate universal health care coverage, a radical view which put him at odds with fellow physicians and public officials, including President Roosevelt.

Teaching was the subject of many articles, for he was a Professor of some category from 1902 to 1941, almost four decades. Like Osler, he believed in the full engagement of the student in the classroom and at the bedside, and not medical learning by lecture in a lecture hall. He encouraged reading and the study of history, and believed a small book is harder for an author to write than a big book.

All but four of the published articles of SRR are single-authored. Only with Dr. Roy Kracke, the distinguished Emory pathologist, did SRR join with other co-authors. These papers on agranulocytosis with Roy Kracke were perhaps the most important scientific articles in the bibliography of SRR; all were published in major journals. Agranulocytosis is a rare acute condition in which the absolute neutrophil (a type of white blood cell) count is < 100 neutrophils per microliter of blood, which makes a person vulnerable to severe infection.

Cardiovascular disease was the subject of 20 articles by SRR, all single-authored. The first in 1916 and the last in 1936 were on hypertension. His first paper on atherosclerosis was called "Angina Pectoris" in 1916, 4 years after James Herrick read his paper on "Clinical Features of Sudden Obstruction of the Coronary Arteries," which is considered a classic on acute myocardial infarction. Several papers of SRR address heart failure, the very condition he suffered from late in life after two myocardial infarctions.

SRR may be considered the first cardiologist in the South (certainly the first *academic* cardiologist in the South) in the opinion of this writer, because he (1) published 20 articles on cardiovascular disease in a 3-decade period, 1916 to 1936; (2) delivered numerous cardiovascular addresses in Atlanta, in Georgia, in the South, and in the country; (3) owned and used the first electrocardiograph machine in Atlanta ("Old Ironhorse," a string galvanometer with 3 leads and floor space as big as a room); (4) served on the first Advisory Editorial Board (12 years, 1925-1937), the only Southerner, of the *American Heart Journal*, the first cardiovascular specialty journal in the USA; (5) served on the early Board of Directors (15 years, 1926-1941), the only Southerner, of the American Heart Association; (6) served as President of the American Heart Association (1933-1934), the first Southerner; (7) was slated to be "grandfathered in" to the new cardiovascular specialty (1941) by the American Board of Medicine, only one of two Southerners; (8) confined his speaking engagements to heart disease after about 1933-1934, his term as President of the American Heart Association ("I have been limiting my talks and papers in the last few years to diseases of the heart and circulation"; Personal letter, October 19, 1936); (9) described himself as "a heart specialist," and an associate at the Roberts Clinic, Dr. Van Buren, stated that he had a "tremendous cardiology practice," was "recognized as a cardiologist," and was a "first to advocate activity for cardiacs; prior to that, they were kept in bed for weeks" (10) held a Heart Clinic on Wednesday mornings at 9 AM at Emory University Hospital. His focus on heart disease was early, academic, sustained, and rare in the South.

The Letters

Two boxes of letters came to this writer, long after the first slim biography was published in 1993. In these boxes were letters from 1935 to 1941; however, no letters were found for 1938 and 1939. It is conceivable that he was recovering from his first heart attack in 1938 and took a year off; however, many letters may simply be missing.

The total number of letters was about 600, but only 121 are included here. They were dictated to his secretary for many years, Miss Mary Mitchell, at the Roberts Clinic. None were handwritten.

Letters give an insight into personality that formal published papers do not. The range of people that SRR corresponded with was wide, from prominent physicians in Boston to local farmers in Georgia. SRR seemed to write to everyone with a particular kindness and warmth. Other physicians were, of course, the main correspondents, and many letters not included here concerned patient care matters.

SRR also had several close epistolary friends, including Dr. James King Hall, a prominent psychiatrist in Richmond who published frequently. Their friendship appeared to be deep and warm. At one time SRR traveled to Richmond at the invitation of Dr. Hall and gave a presentation on "Medical Care at Andersonville Confederate Prison," a subject of great interest to SRR, whose several books on Confederate prisons remained on bookshelves in his widow's home for decades. Dr. Hall gave a two-volume book on the medical history of Virginia to the Fulton County Medical Society in honor of SRR after he passed.

This slice of time of letters of SRR gave this writer an additional insight into his personality. For example, in a letter to Dr. W. R. Houston, a physician who moved from Medical College of Georgia in Augusta to the academic faculty at the University of Texas in Austin, SRR wrote on June 17, 1936, "I certainly agree with you about freedom, only more so. It is why I could never tie myself up with church or educational institution and bend my back to their limitations." In spite of his Christian faith and Emory loyalty, SRR seemed to desire intellectual independence, the freedom to express himself without institutional restrictions.

In several letters, many not published here, one learned certain historical facts. For example, in a reference letter for a nurse dated May 19, 1936, SRR writes that she was "a graduate nurse to the Base Hospital at Jackson, South Carolina in the fall of 1918, for duty in the influenza epidemic that affected Camp Jackson at that time and overflowed the hospital with influenza and pneumonia patients."

The prose in the letters of SRR, presumably typed after direct dictation to his secretary transcribing in shorthand, at the Roberts Clinic, seems to come from a warmth of heart and authenticity of personality in the prime of his life. One reads in them no impatience or hubris, but rather understanding and humility.

The Legacy

SRR may be regarded, not only *during* his life, but perhaps *after* it as well, as "The Osler of the South," it being a distinct region by culture, economy, and demography during the period (Appomattox to Pearl Harbor, 1865-1941) within which SRR lived. He was a Humanist, with a literary style, a clinical mastery, and a warm touch with patients, colleagues, and friends, to match the best of his place and time. To rise to national academic prominence from this region during this period was a notable achievement, perhaps on the same level as becoming a U.S. Senator from a Southern State. In his generation, no one could have been more Southern in heritage than SRR, and yet his similarities to Osler, a Canadian in the British Empire, were manifold. Both were finished products of classical and Christian education who brought honor to the medical profession.

SRR may also be considered "the first cardiologist" in the South, in the opinion of this writer, based on his numerous cardiovascular writings and addresses, and his involvement in the initial years of the American Heart Association and its journal, *American Heart Journal.* The specialty of cardiology arose during his lifetime and SRR embraced it as his own in the 30s, his last decade. Emory continued to have a rich history in cardiology, primarily through the educator, J. Willis Hurst, MD, who edited a textbook, *The Heart,* from 1966 through many editions.

The family legacy of SRR will be, of course, that he was the first of many Roberts and Stewarts to pursue the profession of medicine. He was the original. Apart from medicine, he reflected his heritage of six generations in the South and its educational emphasis. His English prose, such as these last lines from "An Ideal of Modern Medicine," may also serve to remind future physicians and surgeons in the family of the wisdom and beauty of humility:

> May I remember that I am heir to the same diseases as my patients, must meet the same death, must pass with them beyond the River, and may I go with a smile.

Life Chronology

1878 Born in Oxford, GA [home of Emory College], 36 miles from Atlanta center
Oldest of five children (mother died of typhoid along with sixth child)
Father: James William Roberts (A.B., Emory College, 1877, 1st Honor), Pastor at Trinity Church, Atlanta, across from State Capital and later President, Wesleyan College, Macon, GA, 1887-1902
Mother: Clifford Rebecca Stewart (A.B., Wesleyan College, 1875)

1887 Moved to Oxford along with four siblings when his mother dies of typhoid fever
"Miss Emmie" Stewart of Oxford, his mother's sister, takes over motherhood

1887-93 Palmer Institute, Oxford, GA and West End Academy, Atlanta, GA

1892-4 Preparatory Department, Emory College, under his father-in-law,
Joseph Spencer Stewart [A.B., Emory College, 1849], the Superintendent

1894 Emory College (led class both freshman and sophomore years)

1896 Withdrawn for 1 year by his father for "exhaustion" and "overwork"
Worked in the railroad office in Atlanta

1897 Enrolled in Southern Medical College, Atlanta

[Southern Medical College merged with Atlanta Medical College that year to become Atlanta College of Physicians and Surgeons]

1900 MD degree, Atlanta College of Physicians and Surgeons

1900-2 Emory College for junior and senior years (led class both years)
Served as Student Health Physician to Emory College
Kappa Alpha Order (Epsilon Chapter founded at Emory College in 1869) [By 1897, Kappa Alpha Order was the largest fraternity in the South with 39 chapters. James William Roberts, Jr., younger brother of SRR, Emory class of 1908, joined as well.]
Few Literary and Debating Society (after Ignatius Few, the first President of Emory). President as a student (1901-2); gave "Alumni Address" as a faculty member (1904). [Debates were held with Phi Gamma, the alternative "sister society"]
Omicron Delta Kappa (known as The Circle), national leadership honor society
Minister's Sons Club (Motto: "We have but one life to live, why not live it.")
Prize for the best Senior English Class essay on the poetry of Paul Hamilton Hayne, Charleston poet of the Confederate cause
Debating Champion his junior and senior years

1902 A.B. (Bachelor of Arts) degree, 1st Honor (like his father), Emory College

1902-6 Professor and Chair of Biology, Emory College, Oxford ($1500/y)
Joined The Oxonians, literary club of Emory's faculty

1902-3 Academic leave of absence granted for "2 terms" (1 year) to further studies in biology

1903 Pierce Hall of Science, Emory College, completed ($35,000) for Departments of Biology (Roberts), Chemistry (Duncan), and Physics (Bonnell). "Over 6000 dollars has been spent … n making this building one of the best equipped electrical laboratories in the South."
Lecture on "Bacteria" (Newton County Teachers Institute, May 1905)
Awarded scholarship to Brooklyn Academy of Arts and Science (Long Island biological station), 50-a-year nationwide, but one through the University of Chicago, which he received [June 18, 1903, *Atlanta Constitution*]

1904 S.B. and S.M. degrees (Bachelor and Master of Science), The University of Chicago
Dissertation submitted "August 2004" to Department of Zoology entitled: "A Comparison of the Cervical and Brachial Plexuses in Certain Reptiles"
Post-Graduate Course in Physiology, Harvard Medical School (summer term) "prepared to fill the chair of physiology and zoology"

1905 (May) Lecture on "Bacteria," Newton County Teachers Institute
In charge of "Alumni Department" of the *Emory Phoenix* (periodical)

1905-8 Frequently invited speaker on health and "the venereal peril," sponsored by the YMCA ["an experience of about 3 years in speaking and conversing with thousands of college students throughout the Southern States on this subject," 1908]

1906 (January) Presiding Chairman, Emory College debates (Few versus Phi Gamma societies] "Resolved, That it is wrong to Flirt." Roberts found in favor of the negative (an innocent pastime).

Faculty of University Summer School (for teachers), University of Georgia, Athens, GA

1906 Moved from Oxford to Atlanta, GA

1905-9 Professor of Physiology and Instructor of Neurology, Atlanta School of Medicine
School established in 1905, as a second new medical school in the city
SRR began part of his time in Atlanta in 1905 and moved permanently in 1906, resigning his faculty position at Emory College
Became certified by the American Board of Internal Medicine
Joined the American Medical Association

1906-29 Marriage to Martha Louise Welch, no children; "Aunt Louise" to family.
Daughter of M.M. Welch, prominent in civic and religious circles
Granddaughter of Henry McDonald, Pastor of 2nd Baptist Church, Atlanta
Ms. McDonald, as a widow, lived with them, until they separated in 1927

1908 Appointed Juror in Coca-Cola Trial (12 Scientists from USA appointed to determine if Coca-Cola contained opiates; finding no opiates, Coca Cola won the lawsuit)

1909-11 Director of Medical Examiners for Atlanta Public Schools
Resigned professorship and held position for 2 years
Address, "School Child: Food and Hygiene," to Federation of Women's Clubs and Fulton County Medical Society in Joint Meeting, December 1910
Address, "The Cause of Extreme Mortality Among the Negroes" (tuberculosis foremost) to "the assembled Negroes at 4 PM" (students from Atlanta Baptist College, Morris Brown College, and Gammon Theological Seminary) at Tuberculosis Exhibit, Atlanta, April 23, 1909

1910 Joined Druid Hills Methodist Church (with 10 other original members)
[Edward G. Mackay was first pastor and a lifelong friend]
Superintendent, Church Sunday School, Druid Hills Methodist Church, 1910-2

1910-3 Associate Professor of Principles and Practice of Medicine, Atlanta College of Physicians and Surgeons (his alma mater)

1911-5 Visiting Physician, Wesleyan Memorial Hospital (40 beds and 1 operating room)
[Visiting Neurologist 1911-2], later Emory University Hospital

1911 (April) Took the stand in another Coca-Cola trial
"He declared he could find no harmful effects from the use of the beverage."

1911 Research sabbatical to Europe (Italy and Austria) and to Boston (Harvard)
Visited the Ospitale Maggiore in Milan, Italy, and the Pellagrosario at Roverto, Austria (town in the Tyrol at the foot of the Alps)
The triple cause of pellagra in Europe: "peasant life, poverty, and polenta"

1912 Book published, *Pellagra* (C.V. Mosby) during the peak of pellagra malady in the South [before the pursuit and discovery of its nutritional etiology by Goldberger, 1914-27]

1913 Speaker, Laymen's Missionary Convention, Memphis, TN

Laymen's Missionary Movement since 1906 (a nationwide Protestant Church movement) "on the social evil in our great cities"
Founding member, Druid Hills Golf Club, near Emory campus

1913-5 Professor of Clinical Medicine, Atlanta Medical College

1914 Post-Graduate Course at Harvard Medical School

1914-5 Assistant Visiting Physician, Grady Hospital
Secretary, Section on Medicine, Southern Medical Association Annual Meeting held in Dallas, November 8-11, 1915

1915-16 **President, Fulton County Medical Association** (Atlanta)
Presidential Address on "A Medical Center"

1915-41 Professor of Clinical Medicine, Emory University School of Medicine
[first title, Professor of Medicine and Clinical Medicine, 1915-21, then simplified]
For 25 years, SRR taught Emory medical students
The original senior clinical professors at Emory, in addition to SRR: William S. Kendrick, MD, C. W. Strickler, MD, and later, J. Edgar Paullin, MD
The first "full-time" professor and chair (1942-1946) was Eugene Stead, MD

1916-20 Member, House of Delegates, American Medical Association

1916 Appointed to Board of Trustees, Emory University

1916 "An Ideal of Modern Medicine" privately printed (part of "A Medical Center")

1916 Post-Graduate Course at Harvard Medical School

1916-7 Elected 1st Vice-President, Southern Medical Association (Birmingham, AL) at Annual Meeting held in Atlanta, November 13-16, 1916

1917 Chief of Medical Service, and Major, Medical Reserve Corps, U.S. Army
Base Hospital #43 (Emory) during organizational phase (World War I)

1918 Commanding Officer and Lieutenant Colonel, Medical Reserve Corps, U.S. Army
Base Hospital, Camp Jackson (now Fort), Columbia, SC (January-December)
Granted leave of absence from Professorship at Emory
1st case of Spanish flu on October 19, 1918.
Peak number 1800 troops died

1919-41 The Roberts Clinic, Atlanta (near Fox Theater)
20 Ponce de Leon Avenue (1919-26) then 768 Juniper Street (1927-41)
First partners were L. B. Robins, J. A. McGarity, and W. G. Geffcken
Later two partners were Vernon E. Powell and Lila M. Bonner (1927)
[continued as **Roberts Memorial Clinic** after his death in 1941]
First ECG in Atlanta

c1919-41 Member, Symposium Club (oldest literary club for men in Atlanta)
[only 12 members, monthly presentations, one a year per member]

1921 Gave tribute to Seale Harris, MD, at the Annual Meeting,
Southern Medical Association, Hot Springs, AR, November 14-17.

He is that man of this generation who has done more to uphold Southern medicine than any man among us, or any man who has ever lived in Southern medicine to this day. —SRR on Seale Harris, MD, retiring Editor of Southern Medical Journal

1922 Attending staff, *new* Wesley Memorial Hospital, Emory campus
[renamed Emory University Hospital in 1932]

1922-5 Founding Editor, *The Emory Medical Review* (quarterly), only five issues published

1923-8 Founding member, Emory University Medical Historical Club held monthly (8 PM, 4th Monday) at Wesley Memorial Hospital
(SRR gave several papers and served as president in 1924)

1924 Guest of the Texas Medical Association to advise on establishing a group, Internal Medicine of Texas, changed to The Texas Club of Internists (1938), Luncheon meeting held on April 23 at the St. Anthony Hotel in San Antonio. SRR was a member of the Southern Interurban Clinical Club, which formed the basis of his expertise in forming a specialty group.

1924-5 President, Southern Medical Association
Elected on November 27, 1924, at Annual Meeting in New Orleans
"The Larger View of Heart Disease," received much media attention
Presided over Annual Meeting in Dallas, November 9-12, 1925
Presidential Address, "William C. Gorgas of Alabama," Monday, November 9, at First Baptist Church, Main Auditorium, Dallas followed by Clinical Program in Medicine, Baylor Hospital. SRR was discussant for two addresses (one Monday and one Wednesday): "Clinical Demonstration of Diseases of the Heart" by George Carlisle of Dallas; "Myocardial Insufficiency; The Importance of its Early Recognition" by Allan Eustis of New Orleans, Wednesday November 11
Reception followed by a Ball in the Baker Hotel, Tuesday, November 10
Alumni receptions Wednesday, November 11 (Emory at Adolphus Hotel)
Curtice Rosser, Shelton Horsley, Evarts Graham, Charles Mayo gave addresses
Thereafter SRR served on Board of Trustees, as retiring President

Southern Interurban Clinical Club met at Mayo Clinic, Rochester, MN

SRR invited to San Antonio, TX, for Texas Medical Association, as guest to guide the establishment of the Texas Club of Internists (the first specialty group in Texas)

1925 Elected 1st President of Atlanta Chapter, Emory Alumni Association (300 members). SRR was an Alumni Trustee for 3 earlier years.
At Charter Day Banquet celebrating the Alumni Association
Largest attendance by his Emory class of 1902

Elected to Board of Directors, Gorgas Memorial Institute of Tropical and Preventive Medicine, Chicago, IL (proposed $5 million center for the study of tropical diseases)

Consulting Physician to Henry Grady Hospital, Atlanta

1925-37 Member of Advisory Editorial Board, *The American Heart Journal* [October 1925, Volume 1, Number 1, to December 1937, Volume 14, Number 6, 12 years]

1926-41 Board of Directors, American Heart Association (15 years)

1927 (March/April) Visited London, England, and Edinburgh, Scotland Purchased numerous books (eight at *B. F. Stevens & Brown*, four Trafalgar Square)

1927 Baccalaureate Address, Emory University, titled "Emory After 25 Years"
Containing three paragraphs which became "Emory's Creed" ("Emory's Creed" was republished in *Emory Alumnus* in 1932 and 1941)
This year was the 25th anniversary of his graduation from Emory College.
Address at opening of Tampa Municipal Hospital, Tampa, FL, November 6:

> The people of Tampa have gotten more value for their hospital investment than any other city I have ever visited. Square foot for square foot, I have never seen a more magnificent institution.... May your splendid building and its personnel be preserved from the influences of ward politics, thus falling into the evil ways that have ruined so many municipal hospitals in this country.

1928 Vice-President (one of two), American College of Physicians, Annual Convention in New Orleans

1929-41 Marriage to Ruby Viola Holbrook (1903-1994), age 26 (he was 51)
Wedding on December 14, 1929, at St. Andrews Church, New York City
She graduated from Commercial High School, Atlanta, in 1920.
She was his secretary and understood the medical profession.
Daughter of Parks Bell Holbrook (16 children) and Aurora Hardman of Georgia
Lived at 2126 North Ponce de Leon Avenue (Druid Hills near Emory)
then briefly at 1105 Lullwater Road, before moving to farm in 1935
Separate quarters established for Miss Emmie Stewart, his "second" mother
Three children were born:
Stewart R. Roberts, Jr., (October 2, 1931)
William Clifford Roberts (September 11, 1932)
Ross Holbrook Roberts (1935-1966)

1931 Address, "Nervous and Mental Influences in Angina Pectoris,"
Annual Scientific Session, American Heart Association, Pennsylvania Hospital, Philadelphia, PA. June 9, 1931

1931 Address, "The Art and Human Nature," delivered at Harvard Medical School,
October 28, 1931, published in *The New England Journal of Medicine*
First son born on his dad's birthday (October 2)
Stewart Ralph Roberts, Jr. (became radiologist)

1931-6 Chairman, Board of Directors, Atlanta Academy of Medicine and Dentistry

1932 Presided over "Seale Harris Testimonial Breakfast" at the Tutwiler Hotel, Annual Meeting, Southern Medical Association, Birmingham, AL, November 17 (7 speakers, 150 physicians present)

1933-4 President, American Heart Association
Annual Meeting held at the Hotel Cleveland, Cleveland, OH, June 12, 1934
Presidential Address on "William Withering"
[similar talk given earlier, on February 27, 1928, "Withering and Digitalis," to Emory Medical History Club]

1934 Address, "Medical Care at Andersonville Confederate Prison,"

First Annual Banquet, History of Medicine Section, Richmond Academy of Medicine, Richmond, VA (invited by Dr. J. K. Hall, a prominent psychiatrist and his personal friend)

Delivered Founders' Day Lecture at Medical College of South Carolina, Charleston, SC, on November 8 (110th anniversary)

Appointed to **Medical Advisory Council** to the Committee on Economic Security; among eight physicians appointed by President Roosevelt in November 1934: Harvey Cushing, Stewart R. Roberts, George Crile, Thomas Parran, Jr., James Alexander Miller, Walter L. Bierring, Robert B. Greenough, and George M. Piersol

1935 Move from Atlanta to Stone Mountain, GA [7 miles from hospital, 12 from office]
Farm of 118 acres called "Goodacres" on unpaved Redan Road (October)
Built a three-story farmhouse with a large front porch and a large back "farm room" to handle the dairy, chicken, and farm products, some sold to Emory
Employed tenant farmer and his family, including children

> I hope to improve my health, and to let the children grow up with good bodies and happy hearts. Practice pushes me continually. I seem to have little time for such cultural aspirations as I may have, and I realize I am doing less studying than I should.... I have made up my mind to read one cultural and informing book all the time. (Age 57, Letter to W. R. Houston, MD, September 28, 1935)

Guest speaker, Florida Medical Association banquet, Ocala, FL, May 13-15

Memorial Day address in Danville, KY, honoring Jane Todd Crawford, the patient of Ephraim McDowell, who submitted to and survived the world's first ovariotomy in 1809

Reunion Chair, Emory University School of Medicine, Class of 1900

Chairman, Committee on Medical Education, Fulton County Medical Society

1938 First heart attack, treated at Emory University Hospital then confined to home for a year (still paid by his partners at the Roberts Clinic)
Brother, James William Roberts, Jr., MD, Emory surgeon, dies of lung cancer
Both brothers were being treated at Emory University Hospital at the same time
("Dr. Will" referred patients to his brother, "Dr. Stewart," and vice versa)

1939 Commencement, "The Doctor's Visit," University of Texas Medical School, Galveston [consideration given to a book called "The Doctor's Visit]

1940 Address, "Dr. Calhoun as Author and Teacher"
In honor of Ferdinand Phinizy Calhoun, MD, of Atlanta, President of American Ophthalmological Society, Fulton County Medical Society, Piedmont Driving Club, Atlanta, GA, July 12, 1940 (200 Georgia physicians attended)

1941 Appointed by Paul Dudley White, MD, to the Executive Committee of the Board of Directors, American Heart Association. (10 of the 27 Directors), the only Southerner

1941 Died April 14 (age 62) of heart failure at his home, Stone Mountain, GA
Funeral at Glenn Memorial Methodist Church, Emory Campus
Service officiated by Dr. Nat G. Long (Glenn Memorial Methodist Church) and Dr. Edward G. Mackay (Druid Hills Methodist Church)
Buried in Roberts Section in Oxford Memorial Cemetery, Oxford, GA
Age of sons: Stewart, Jr., 9; William, 8; and Ross, 5

After 1941

1942 Stone Mountain Farmhouse burns down; Mother and two sons move to Atlanta [922 Woodcrest Avenue, Brookwood Hills, for 50 years]

1941-1994 **Ruby Holbrook Roberts**, single working mother, 1941-1974 (33 years)

1941-1947 Executive Secretary, Fulton County Medical Society, now Atlanta Academy of Medicine, National Register

1947-1974 Owner, *Medical Placement and Mailing Service* [office in Roberts Memorial Clinic]. The second business of its kind in the country, the first located in Chicago. Fully supported both sons financially through college and medical school

1994 Died at age 91; also buried at Oxford Memorial Cemetery, Oxford, GA

Children of SRR and Ruby Holbrook Roberts:

Stewart R. Roberts, Jr., MD (1931-2022): Associate Professor of Radiology, 1977-2000, and Assistant Professor of Medicine (Pulmonary), 1973-1991, Emory University School of Medicine, Atlanta, GA. Author of "The Chest X-Ray" and "Approach to the Radiographic Examination of the Abdomen," in: Walker HK, Jr., Hall WD, Hurst, JW (eds): *A Problem-Oriented Approach to History, Physical, and Laboratory Examination.* Second Edition, Boston, Butterworths, 1980. [3 children]

William Clifford Roberts, MD (1934-2023): Executive Director, Baylor Heart & Vascular Institute, Baylor University Medical Center, Dallas, TX, 1993-2023. Recipient of the Distinguished Alumni Award (1996) from Southern Methodist University and the Distinguished Medical Achievement Award from Emory Medical Alumni Association (1984). Recipient of 1978 Gifted Teacher Award, 2004 Master Award, and 2016 Lifetime Achievement Award of the American College of Cardiology. [4 children]

Ross Holbrook Roberts (1935-1966): Parietal lobe injury with forceps delivery. Institutionalized at age 5 (Stewart Home near Frankfort, KY, then in Augusta, GA) Buried at Oxford Memorial Cemetery, Oxford, GA.

Professional Achievements

1. Master clinician (internal medicine practice for 36 years in Atlanta) [widely consulted on heart disease, pellagra, neurology, etc.]
2. Established Roberts Clinic (1919-41; became Roberts Memorial Clinic in 1941)
3. Professor of Clinical Medicine at Emory University (25 years, 1915-41) [earlier positions: Professor and Chair of Biology, Emory College, 1902-6; Professor of Physiology, Atlanta School of Medicine, 1906-1908; Associate Professor of Medicine, Atlanta College of Physicians and Surgeons, 1911-3; and Professor of Clinical Medicine, Atlanta Medical College, 1913-5]
   Taught students at college (4 years) and medical school (35 years)
4. Author of 100 published articles (all but 4 single-authored) [7 in JAMA, 3 in New England Journal of Medicine, 15 in Southern Medical Journal]
5. Author of a book on pellagra (1912, before Goldberger research, 1914-27)

6. First cardiologist in the South (first ECG in Atlanta, 20 cardiovascular articles)
7. President (9th), American Heart Association, 1933-4 (first Southerner)
8. Member, Board of Directors, American Heart Association, 1925-1941 (first Southerner)
9. Advisory Editorial Board (22 original members), *American Heart Journal*, 1925-37 (official journal of the American Heart Association until 1952)
10. Member, Committee on the Cost of Medical Care (only Southerner), sponsored by NY foundations, 1925
11. Member, Medical Advisory Council (only Southerner of 11 physicians), formed to advise Committee on Economic Security, under President Roosevelt, 1934-5
12. Member, Board of Directors, Gorgas Memorial Institute for Tropical Diseases and Preventive Medicine, Chicago, IL (1925-41)
13. Commanding Officer, Base Hospital, Camp Jackson, 1918 (influenza epidemic)
14. Author of "An Ideal of Modern Medicine" (from "A Medical Center," 1915)
15. Author of "Emory's Creed" (from Emory Baccalaureate Address, 1926)
16. President (18th), Southern Medical Association (1924)
17. Vice-President and Member, Board of Regents, American College of Physicians
18. One of two Delegates from Georgia, American Medical Association (1916-20)
19. President, Fulton County (Atlanta) Medical Society (1913)
20. Chairman of the Board, Atlanta Academy of Medicine
21. Founding Editor, *Emory Medical Review* (1923-5)
22. Medical Historian (numerous addresses and publications, e.g. "William Charles Wells of Charleston and London," Boston Medical and Surgical Journal)
23. Bibliophile with a large medical library (500 books donated to Emory)
24. President, Emory University Medical History Club
25. Harvard Medical School address, "The Art and Human Nature," 1932 (New England Journal of Medicine)
26. Wide correspondence regionally and nationally (Paul Dudley White, George Crile, Louis Hammon, etc.)
27. European trips for medical education and research (1911 and 1927)
28. Appointed jurist ("12 of the most distinguished chemists of America"), Coca-Cola Trial, 1910
29. Public health and hygiene advocate (beginning as YMCA speaker, 1902, and then Inspector of Atlanta Public Schools, 1909-11)
30. Classically educated with powerful speaking and writing style
31. Trustee, Emory College and Emory University (at various times)
32. First President, Atlanta Chapter, Emory Alumni Association (1925)
33. Emory University student distinctions
    Graduated 1st Honor from Emory College, Oxford, 1902
    Phi Beta Kappa, Founder at Emory College
    Few Literary Society (debating society named after Ignatius Few),
    President, Alpha Omega Alpha (then Atlanta College of Physicians and Surgeons)

Society Memberships

Medical Alpha Omega Alpha, Emory Chapter, Class of 1900
Fulton County Medical Association [President, 1915, and Chairman, Committee on Education, 1935]

Atlanta Academy of Medicine [Chairman, Board of Directors, 1931-1937]
Emory Medical History Club [President and Founding Member, 1923]
Atlanta Heart Club [President]
Atlanta Neurological Club
Medical Association of Georgia [Vice-President]
Southern Medical Association [Vice-President (1917-8), President (1924-5)]
American Clinical and Climatological Association [member]
Southern Interurban Clinical Society [Fellow and Secretary]
Gorgas Memorial Institute of Tropical and Preventive Medicine [Board of Directors, 1925-1941]
American Society of Tropical Medicine & Hygiene
American Heart Association [President (1932-3) and Board of Directors (1925-41, including Executive Committee, 1941)]
Advisory Editorial Board, *American Heart Journal* (1925-37)
American College of Physicians [Fellow, Vice-President, and member, Board of Regents]
American Medical Association [one of two delegates from Georgia, 1916-20]
American Board of Medicine [certified without exam, 1937 (first year of existence)] [Cardiovascular Certification (without exam), 1941 (its first year), pending at time of death]

Nonmedical

Kappa Alpha Order [fraternity, initiated in 1894-6, Emory College]
Omicron Delta Kappa [Emory College, national leadership honor society]
Few Literary and Debating Society [Emory College], President, 1901-2
Minister's Sons Club [Emory College]
Phi Beta Kappa [Founded the Emory Chapter], Class of 1902
The Oxonians, literary club of Emory College faculty, 1902-6
Fraternal Order of Masons
Atlanta Chapter, Emory Alumni Association, First President
Emory Alumni Board of Trustees [first Emory College, later University]
Druid Hills Methodist Church [Founding Member (1/10), 1910-1933, Edward G. Mackay, Pastor]
Glenn Memorial Methodist Church [Member, 1933-41, Nat G. Long, Pastor]
Independent Methodist Club
Druid Hills Golf Club [Founding Member, 1913]
Symposium Club [one of 12 in one of oldest Atlanta literary club]
Atlanta Historical Society

Addresses in Cardiovascular Disease (1914-1937) (an incomplete list based primarily on published articles)

1. Syphilis of the Heart. Section on Medicine, Southern Medical Association, 8th Annual Meeting, Richmond, VA, November 9-12, 1914
2. Arteriosclerosis and High Pressure. Annual Meeting of the 9th District of Medical Association of Georgia, Hoschton, GA, May 15, 1916
3. Angina Pectoris. Meeting of Medical Association of Georgia, Columbus, GA, 1916
4. A Study of Arterial Sounds. Session on Practice of Medicine at 68th Annual Session of the American Medical Association, New York, NY, June 1917
5. Hyperpressure. Meeting of Medical Association of Georgia, Augusta, GA, 1917

6. The Failing Heart. Meeting of 9th District Medical Society of Georgia, Gainesville, GA, September 21, 1921
7. A Study in Hypotension. Section on Practice of Medicine at the 73rd Annual Session of the American Medical Association, St. Louis, MO, May 1922
8. The Influence of Malaria on the Circulation. 18th Annual Meeting of the American Society of Tropical Medicine, Washington, DC, May 2-3, 1922
9. Arterio-Sclerosis in its Relation to Blood Pressure. Fall Clinic (for North Texas Doctors), Parkland Hospital, Dallas County Medical Society, Dallas, TX, September 1922
10. Digitalis in its Relation to the Classification of Heart Disease. 74th Annual Convention, Medical Association of Georgia, Savannah, GA, May 3, 1923
11. The Larger View of Heart Disease. Section on Medicine, Southern Medical Association, 18th Annual Meeting, New Orleans, LA, November 24-7, 1924
12. The Clinical Relation of Hypotension and Hypertension to Mortality. Medical Section of the American Life Convention, Chattanooga, TN
13. Heart Disease ("…is now a general in the army of death, while pneumonia is a mere captain"), American Congress on Internal Medicine, Washington, DC, March 10, 1925
14. Discussant: "Clinical Demonstration of Diseases of the Heart" by George Carlisle of Dallas at the Annual Meeting, Southern Medical Association, Dallas, November 9, 1925
15. Discussant: "Myocardial Insufficiency: The Importance of its Early Recognition" by Allan Eustis of New Orleans at the Annual Meeting, Southern Medical Association, Dallas, November 11, 1925
16. The Heart Muscle. The Jerome Cochran Lecture before the Alabama State Medical Association, Mobile, AL, April 28, 1926
17. Functional Pressure Versus Structural Sclerosis. 80th Annual Meeting of Ohio State Medical Association, Toledo, OH, May 11-12, 1926
18. Relation of Obesity to Heart Disease. American College of Physicians (or AMA or other), Washington, DC, May 20, 1927
19. The Rheumatic Heart. Virginia State Medical Society, Petersburg, VA, October 18-20
20. Withering and Digitalis. Emory Medical History Club, Wesley Memorial Hospital, February 27, 1928
21. Heart Failure. Semi-annual meeting, 10th District Medical Society, Louisville, GA, March 23, 1928
22. Treatment of Organic Heart Disease. Academy of Medicine, Atlanta, GA, June 7, 1928 [Emory Alumni Week]
23. Nonvalvular Diseases of the Heart. 3rd District Medical Society, Greenwood, GA
24. The Diagnostic Relations Between the Gall Bladder and the Heart. Oration on Medicine, 79th Annual Meeting of Illinois State Medical Society, Peoria, IL, May 21-3, 1929
25. Hypertension. Semi-Annual Meeting, 9th District, Medical Association of Georgia, Commerce, GA, March 19, 1930
26. The Circulation in Pregnancy. General Clinical Session, 24th Annual Meeting, Southern Medical Association, Louisville, KY, November 11-14, 1930
27. The Thyroid Heart. Inter-State Post Graduate Assembly, 1931
28. Neuroses as a Cause of Hypertension. 82nd Annual Convention, Georgia Medical Association, 1931

29. Nervous and Mental Influences in Angina Pectoris. Annual Meeting of the American Heart Association, Philadelphia, PA, June 1931
30. Cardiovascular Disease. Joint Program of Emory University and University of Georgia, Athens, GA, June 19, 1931
31. The Heart. 5th District Medical Society, Emory University Hospital, Atlanta, GA, October 21, 1931
32. Coronary Occlusion—Its Relations and Treatment. Guilford County Medical Society, King Cotton Hotel, Greensboro, NC, February 28, 1933
33. The Relation of Heart to Surgery. 5th Annual Banquet, Southeast Surgical Congress, Nashville, TN, March 6, 1934 [Emory surgeon Frank Boland was President in 1932]
34. The Heart. Fulton County Medical Society Program. Report of the American Medical Association Meeting in Cleveland, Atlanta, GA, July 5, 1934
35. William Withering. Presidential Address, Annual Meeting, American Heart Association, Cleveland, OH, 1933-4
36. Tachycardia. 85th Annual Convention, Georgia Medical Association, Augusta, GA, May 9, 1934
37. Treatment of Congestive Heart Failure. 5th District Medical Society Program, Academy of Medicine, Atlanta, GA, March 29, 1935
38. Cardiovascular Renal Disease. Annual Meeting, Southern Medical Association, Baltimore, MD, November 17-20, 1936
39. Recent Research on Hypertension. Fulton County Medical Society Program, Atlanta, GA, 1937

Roberts CS. Stewart R. Roberts, MD, and the South. In: *Selected Articles and Letters of Stewart R. Roberts, MD (1878-1941)*. Newcastle upon Tyne, UK: Cambridge Scholars Publishing; 2022: 1-18.

26

The Physician Legacy of Stewart R. Roberts, MD (1878–1941), "The Osler of the South"

Charles S. Roberts, MD*

A legacy in medicine in one Southern family began with a single physician, Stewart R. Roberts, MD, who was born in Oxford, Georgia, in 1878, and became the first cardiologist in the South.[1] In a letter to Richard Foster, the President of the University of Alabama, dated March 22, 1940, Dr. Seale Harris (1870–1957), a contemporary Birmingham physician who had been President of the Southern Medical Association and editor of the *Southern Medical Journal* for 12 years, began with this paragraph:

> *I am enclosing a letter which I received from my friend, Dr. Stewart Roberts, Professor of Medicine in Emory University, Atlanta. I may add that Dr. Roberts is one of the ablest men in American medicine and is frequently called the "Osler of the South."*

A comparison of Stewart R. Roberts[1], MD, to the great Sir William Osler (1849–1919) is not the purpose or argument of this article. Virtually no one compares to Osler, who was considered the greatest physician of his generation in the English-speaking world. His single-authored medical textbook of 1892 was a tremendous achievement.[2] The career path of Osler, from Montreal to Philadelphia to Baltimore, and finally to Oxford, England, never crossed that of Roberts, who was born a generation later and spent his entire medical career in the South, peculiar in its agrarian tradition and racial demography and, by far, the most economically depressed region in the United States for decades after the Civil War.

Born and bred on the same continent, both physicians, nevertheless, shared certain characteristics: (1) both were the sons of Christian ministers of English ancestry and both had a Classical and Christian education; (2) both studied biology intensely before pursuing medicine; (3) both specialized in internal medicine and enjoyed a large private practice with in-state and out-of-state referrals; (4) both published extensively (though of course, Osler's number of articles was extraordinary), wrote elegant prose, and were frequently invited medical speakers; (5) both wrote on humanitarian subjects and each was considered a "Renaissance Man"; (6) both taught medicine to students, residents, and colleagues for decades and supported the careers of many; (7) both enjoyed medical fellowship at society meetings, corresponded widely with physicians beyond their locale, and traveled widely for medical purposes (Roberts visited Europe twice for extended periods); (8) both were bibliophiles who read extensively outside of medicine, and both donated their large personal medical libraries to their respective institutions; (9) both spoke and wrote often on the history of medicine; and finally (10) both were intensely loyal to their respective institutions, although always keeping a certain intellectual independence.

Born in 1878 in Oxford, Georgia, Roberts graduated from Emory College in Oxford with first honor in 1902, after graduating from Atlanta College of Physicians and Surgeons in 1900. He earned a master's degree in zoology at the University of Chicago in 1904, then served briefly as Professor of Biology at Emory at Oxford, before moving to Atlanta in 1906 to begin a practice of internal medicine. When Emory University was established in the Atlanta area in 1915, Roberts was appointed Professor of Clinical Medicine, a position he held until his death from heart failure in 1941.

Roberts published more than 100 articles, and all but 4 were single authored. In 1912, at the age of 34, he published a book on pellagra, a vitamin deficiency disease of unknown etiology at the time, which was ravaging the South.[3] Roberts later focused most of his clinical attention on heart disease and is considered the first cardiologist in the South (although he used the term "heart specialist" because the term "cardiologist" had not appeared). Roberts published 20 articles specifically on cardiovascular disease, the first and last on systemic hypertension, and others on angina pectoris and heart failure. He had the first electrocardiographic machine in Georgia, which occupied an entire room in The Roberts Clinic on Juniper Street in Atlanta.

In many ways, Roberts participated in the birth of the specialty of cardiology. He was the first and only Southerner to serve on the early Board of Directors of the American Heart Association (1925 to 1941), and from 1933 to 1934, he served as its President. His Address at the annual meeting held in Cleveland was on "Withering and Digitalis," although no written copy has been found. After that year, until his death in 1941, he confined his speaking engagements to heart disease. Documentation of some 39 talks on cardiovascular disease were found among his papers.

Roberts was also the first and only Southerner on the original Editorial Advisory Board of the *American Heart Journal* (he served 12 years, 1925 to 1937), which, at the time, was the official journal of the American Heart Association and the only American cardiovascular journal. He corresponded with numerous leaders of the American Heart Association for 15 years. One of his last letters, a month before his death in 1941, was to Paul Dudley White of Boston, the newly elected President of the American Heart Association who had just appointed him to its Executive Committee. When the specialty of cardiology set out to establish a board certification process, Roberts was one of 2 Southerners invited to be certified without examination,

---

Department of Cardiac Surgery, Baylor University Medical Center, Dallas, Texas. Manuscript received June 5, 2021; revised manuscript received and accepted September 8, 2021.

See page 196 for disclosure information.

*Corresponding author: Tel: 469-800-7760; fax: 469-800-7770.

E-mail address: Charles.Roberts@bswhealth.org

0002-9149/© 2021 Published by Elsevier Inc.
https://doi.org/10.1016/j.amjcard.2021.09.007

although he died before the certification process was finally established.

The influence of Roberts during his nearly 4 decades as a professor (the last 26 years at Emory University School of Medicine) was widely felt among medical students and residents and colleagues. They were perhaps his chief immediate legacy. He taught students and residents in the classroom and on the wards throughout his career and wrote letters of recommendation for numerous applicants to medical school, for medical students seeking residency positions, and for colleagues deserving of awards or advancement or in search of a new position.

The influence of Roberts, however, was also felt within his own family, nuclear and extended, contemporaneously and in his descendants, direct and indirect. Although no physician in his family in Georgia came before him, multiple physicians, all related by blood, came after him (the first, his younger brother, Will, graduating 12 years after him). He was the original. Several family physicians were influenced by him personally, before his death in 1941, and others, such as the present author, by gaining a familiarity with his life and writings. The writing and speaking ability of Roberts reflected his Classical and Christian education in Georgia. Perhaps the best example of his writing is "An Ideal of Modern Medicine," reprinted here[2], written when he was 37 years of age, as part of his departing address as President of Fulton County (Atlanta) Medical Society in 1915.[4]

All 12 of these physicians were connected to the state of Georgia by either birth or education or both. The closest friend of Roberts was his younger brother Will, a surgeon in Atlanta with an office across the street from the Roberts Clinic. Roberts was eager to help his own family members, including, for example, Lamar Roberts, a nephew interested in medicine. His letter of recommendation for Lamar, reprinted here[3], was written while Roberts was in severe heart failure 2 months before he died. Lamar was accepted to Duke Medical School and had a distinguished career in neurosurgery, including a 10-year period at the Montreal Neurological Institute with Wilder Penfield, who, similar to Osler, was another famous Canadian.

The private family anecdotes of Roberts are many, but one in particular pertaining to a Stewart physician (his maternal side) found its way into publication. It was written by Franz H. Stewart, MD, his first cousin, who became a prominent internist in South Florida and served as editor of the *Journal of the Florida Medical Association*, in which this piece was published in February 1969:

I'm Glad You Come

Stewart Roberts was a great physician and leader. Many of us still look up to him with affection and are proud he was our preceptor. Once he visited a small house on a by-road not far from Atlanta. Two or three children were playing in the yard. The husband met him at the door and after a conference and a careful examination, plans were made together to care for the medical problem with the best means available.

As the doctor left, the husband took his hand and said, "I'm glad you come."

I understand this better since a loved one was ill last spring. A fine physician, with all paramedical help needed, accepted the problem, sought additional aid and together they made plans to care for the medical problem with the best means available. Even before the favorable results appeared, I understood well—"I'm glad you come."

List of Physicians in the Family

Stewart R. Roberts, MD (1878–1941): THE FIRST
Atlanta College of Physicians and Surgeons (now Emory), MD, 1900 (Alpha Omega Alpha)
Emory College (Oxford), AB, 1902 (Phi Beta Kappa, Omicron Delta Kappa, Kappa Alpha Order)
University of Chicago, MS (Zoology), 1904
Author, Pellagra *(St. Louis, C.V. Mosby, 1912)*
Commanding Officer, Camp Jackson Base Hospital, South Carolina, World War I
Professor of Clinical Medicine, Emory University School of Medicine, 1915 to 1941
President, Fulton County Medical Society (Atlanta), 1915
President, Southern Medical Association, 1925
President, American Heart Association, 1933 to 1934

James William (Will) Roberts, Jr., MD (1886–1938): younger brother
Emory College (Oxford), PhB (Bachelor of Philosophy), 1909 (Kappa Alpha Order)
Emory University, MD, 1913
Trained at Grady Hospital (Atlanta), Mayo Clinic (Rochester), and Barnes Hospital (St. Louis)
Captain, Emory Unit, Base Hospital 43, The Western Front, World War I, 1917 to 1918
Associate Professor of Surgery, Emory University

Stewart R. Roberts, Jr., MD (1931–present): son
Emory University, AB, 1953 (Alpha Tau Omega)
Emory University, MD, 1959 (Alpha Omega Alpha)
Military Service, Fort Jackson, South Carolina, Camp Gordon, Georgia, and Fort Hood, Texas (1953 to 1955)
Trained in medicine and cardiology at Duke 1959 to 1963, then practiced medicine for 5 years
Trained in radiology at Emory, 1968 to 1971, then on radiology staff, 1973 to 2000
Associate Professor of Radiology, Emory University, 1977 to 2000

William Clifford Roberts, MD (1932–present): son
Southern Methodist University, AB, 1954 (Phi Delta Theta) (Distinguished Alumni Award, 1996)
Emory University, MD, 1958 (Emory Alumni Distinguished Medical Achievement Award, 1984)
(Alpha Omega Alpha, Georgetown University, 1986)

Cardiovascular Researcher at National Institutes of Health (Bethesda) and then Baylor (Dallas)
Editor, The American Journal of Cardiology *(1982–present)*
Editor, Baylor University Medical Center Proceedings *(1994–present)*
Gifted Teacher Award, American College of Cardiology, 1978
Master, American College of Cardiology, 2004
Lifetime Achievement Award, American College of Cardiology, 2016

Charles Stewart Roberts, MD (1960–present): grandson
Vanderbilt University, BA, 1981 (Kappa Alpha Order)
Emory University, MD, 1986
Surgical training at University of North Carolina and Royal Brompton Hospital, London
Author, Stoking the Fire, A Surgical Memoir of London *(Armonk, New York, Futura, 1998, 192 pages)*
Chair of Cardiac Surgery, Baylor University Medical Center, Dallas (2018 to present)
Clinical Professor of Surgery, Texas A&M College of Medicine (2018 to present)

Carey Camille Roberts, MD (1991–present): great-granddaughter (married surname Lindheim)
University of Georgia, BS, 2013 (Phi Kappa Phi [Honor Society], Kappa Delta)
Georgetown University, MD, 2017 (Alpha Omega Alpha)
Resident in Anesthesiology, New York-Presbyterian Hospital, New York City, 2017 to 2021
Fellow in Thoracic Anesthesiology, Memorial Sloan-Kettering Cancer Center, 2021 to 2022

H. Lamar Roberts, MD (1919–1978): nephew
Emory University (attended) (Phi Delta Theta)
University of Texas, BA, 1941 (Phi Delta Theta)
Duke University, MD, 1944 (and his surgical residency)
McGill University, MSc, 1949, and PhD, 1952 (on speech defects and neurological localization)
(Sigma Xi, the Scientific Research Honor Society)
Lieutenant, Medical Corps, United States Naval Reserve, 1945 to 1946 and 1953 to 1954
Co-author with Wilder Penfield, Speech and Brain Mechanisms *(Princeton University Press, 1959)*
First Chief of Neurosurgery, College of Medicine, University of Florida, Gainesville, 1958 to 1971

Katherine Ann Roberts, MD (1961–present): grandniece (married surname Fitton)
University of Florida, BA, 1982 (Kappa Alpha Theta)
Georgia State University (pre-med courses after 8 years in banking)
Medical College of Georgia (Augusta), MD, 1997
Trained at Virginia Commonwealth University (Medical College of Virginia, Richmond)
Fellow, American Association of Clinical Endocrinology
First endocrinologist in Williamsburg, Virginia ("Williamsburg Endocrinology")

Thomas Lewellyn Ross, Jr., MD (1908–1983): nephew
Mercer University, BS, 1926
Emory University, MD, 1930
Spent 2 years (1933 to 1935) in practice with his uncle, Dr. Roberts, at the Roberts Clinic
Colonel, US Medical Corp, 1942 to 1946, serving in Army Hospitals in China (Kunming and Shanghai)
Founded Macon Heart Clinic of Medical Center of Central Georgia
President, Georgia Heart Association and a Director, American Heart Association
Heart of the Year Award, Georgia Heart Association, 1975

Joseph Spencer Stewart, Jr., MD (1895–1974): first cousin
University of Georgia, AB, 1915
Medical College of Georgia (Augusta), MD, 1918 (6 students)
U.S. Army *Surgeon, European Theater, World War I*
Division Surgeon (Colonel), Air Transport Command, European Theater, World War II
Chief of Staff and Director of Surgery, Jackson Memorial Hospital, Miami
(Gastric Resections and Vagotomies... American Surgeon *1951;17:202–208,* and *Congenital Extrinsic*

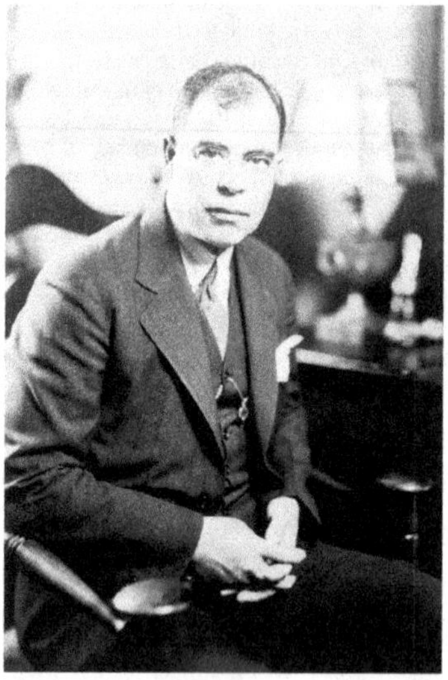

Figure 1. Stewart R. Roberts, MD (1878 – 1941), Professor of Clinical Medicine, Emory University School of Medicine, 1915 to 1941.

An Ideal of Modern Medicine

WHENEVER and wherever my work, by day or night, in peace or war, on land or sea, in laboratory or office, home or hospital, class room or open field, may I be patient, poised and thorough; loyal to science and to men, unselfish in labor and pure in life. May I hold that science is better than gold and men than greed, that service is proportionate to preparation, and reward to labor. May I use drugs only when indicated, diagnose before I treat or operate, clean before I deliver, use my laboratory, preserve a sense of proportion, respect but not worship my own opinion, seek consultation often, be slow to judgment and cautious in word and deed, and mingle in mind and touch with medical men. In the laboratory may I keep my records, in clinical cases my histories, and between them and me preserve the accuracy of truth. May I be strong with the weak, righteous with the wicked, wise with the foolish, honest with myself and kind to all men. May I avoid professional comparisons and sensitiveness, speak well of those of the household of medical faith, shun jealousy and eschew envy, follow progress, beware lest the demands of life chill my enthusiasm for study and knowledge, play sometimes and wander when I may. May I take injustice gracefully, disappointment easily, fight disease cheerfully, death hopefully, believe victory and defeat equally a part of the larger plan, and rise from both fresh for repeated conflicts. May I remember that I am heir to the same diseases as my patients, must meet the same death, pass with them beyond the River, and may I go with a smile.

ATLANTA
JANUARY 1916

STEWART R. ROBERTS

Figure 2. A medical oath written by Stewart R. Roberts, MD, when he was 37 years of age.

*Duodenal Obstruction in the New Born...*Southern Surgeon *1948;14:15–33)*

President, Dade County Medical Society, Miami

President, Florida Medical Association (founded in 1874)

President, Florida Chapter, American College of Surgeons (founded in 1913)

President, Southeastern Surgical Congress, 1951 to 1952 (founded in 1930)

Franz Hahr Stewart, MD (1906–2000): first cousin

University of Georgia, BS, 1928

Emory University, MD, 1932 (Alpha Omega Alpha, University of Miami, 1960)

Completed training at Presbyterian Hospital (Columbia University), New York (1932 to 1935)

First Lieutenant of Cavalry, U.S. Army 1931, then Lieutenant, Naval Reserve 1935

U.S. Navy Physician (Commander in Medical Corps), Pacific Theater, World War II (1941 to 1946)

Chief of Medical Service at 5 Miami hospitals, Jackson Memorial, Baptist, Mercy, Variety, Doctors

Professor and Chair Pro Tempore ("for the time being") during the search for the first Chair;

Department of Medicine, University of Miami School of Medicine, Miami, Florida

Author of 75 to 100 published articles

Laureate (highest honor), Florida Chapter, American College of Physicians

Editor, Bulletin of the Dade County Medical Association, *1949 to 1953 (and President, 1947)*

Editor, Journal of the Florida Medical Association, *1968 to 1970*

(*Malaria: Practical Aspects in Management. Southern Medical Journal* 1947;40:359–382 and *Dengue. Analysis of the Clinical Syndrome at a South Pacific Base.* United States Naval Medical Bulletin 1944;42:1233–1240).

Franz Hahr Stewart, Jr., MD (1936–present): nephew

Emory University, BA, 1958

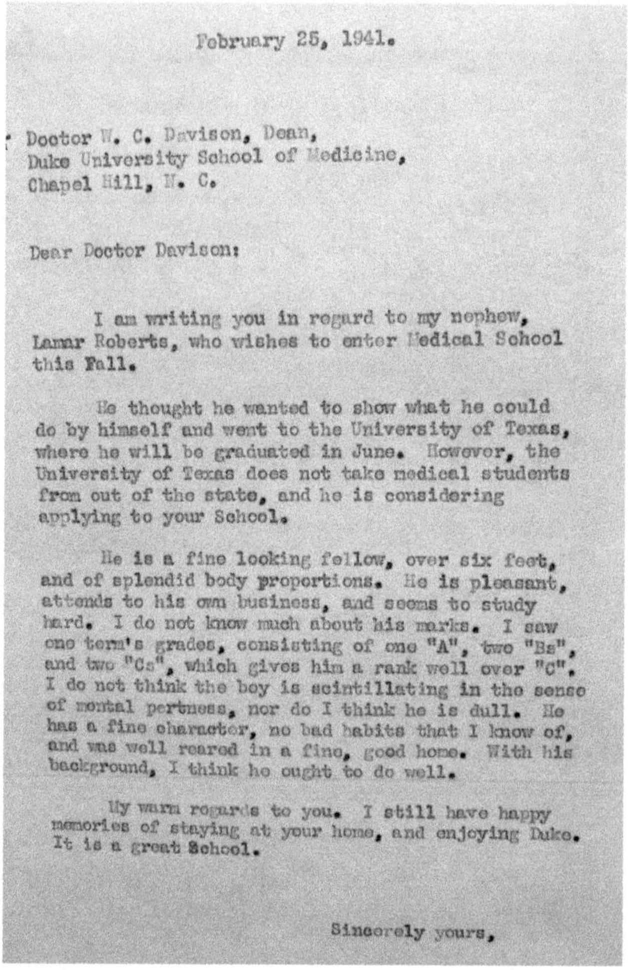

February 25, 1941.

Doctor W. C. Davison, Dean,
Duke University School of Medicine,
Chapel Hill, N. C.

Dear Doctor Davison:

I am writing you in regard to my nephew, Lamar Roberts, who wishes to enter Medical School this Fall.

He thought he wanted to show what he could do by himself and went to the University of Texas, where he will be graduated in June. However, the University of Texas does not take medical students from out of the state, and he is considering applying to your School.

He is a fine looking fellow, over six feet, and of splendid body proportions. He is pleasant, attends to his own business, and seems to study hard. I do not know much about his marks. I saw one term's grades, consisting of one "A", two "Bs", and two "Cs", which gives him a rank well over "C". I do not think the boy is scintillating in the sense of mental pertness, nor do I think he is dull. He has a fine character, no bad habits that I know of, and was well reared in a fine, good home. With his background, I think he ought to do well.

My warm regards to you. I still have happy memories of staying at your home, and enjoying Duke. It is a great School.

Sincerely yours,

Figure 3. Letter from Dr. Stewart R. Roberts to his friend, the Dean of Duke Medical School in support of his nephew Lamar Roberts, who was later accepted, and became a distinguished neurosurgeon. Letters of recommendation in this period in American history, it seems necessary to state, had less hyperbole, and a grade of C in college was, in fact, average.

Columbia University, MD, 1962

Medical residency and cardiology fellowship at Jackson Memorial Hospital, Miami, United States. Army flight surgeon in Viet Nam (>75 combat helicopter missions) (awarded Bronze Star Air Medal and 2 Oak Leaf Clusters, Army Commendation Medal, Vietnamese Cross of Gallantry)

Internal Medicine Practice in Miami (together with his father for 18 years)

President of Medical Staff, Mercy Hospital (1991) and Doctors' Hospital (1982 to 1984)

Board of Directors, Mercy Hospital and Doctors' Hospital, Miami

Earl Spencer Stewart, MD (1938–2013): nephew
Emory University, BS, 1960
University of Miami, MD, 1964

Trained at Jackson Memorial Hospital, Miami (2 years), then Presbyterian Hospital, New York (4 years)

US Naval Surgeon for 2 years (1971 to 1972), including 6 months in Viet Nam and 8 months as Chief of Surgery at 8th Naval District at Corpus Cristi, Texas

Fellow, American College of Surgeons and American College of Physicians
Vascular Surgeon, Ocala Regional Medical Center, Ocala, Florida (from 1987) Fig 1-fig3

Disclosures

The authors have no conflicts of interest to declare

1. Roberts CS. *Life and Writings of Stewart R. Roberts, MD: Georgia's First Heart Specialist*. Spartanburg: The Reprint Company Publishers; 1993.
2. Osler W. *The Principles and Practice of Medicine. Designed for the Use of Practitioners and Students of Medicine*. New York: D. Appleton; 1892.
3. Roberts SR. *Pellagra: History, Distribution, Diagnosis, Prognosis, Treatment, Etiology*. St. Louis: C.V. Mosby; 1912.
4. Roberts WC. Dr. Stewart R. Roberts' "An Ideal of Modern Medicine.". *Ann Intern Med* 1969;70:1016–1017.

Roberts CS. The physician legacy of Stewart R. Roberts, MD (1878-1941), "the Osler of the South". *Am J Cardiol.* 2022;162:191-196. doi:10.1016/j.amjcard.2021.09.007

27

PROC (BAYL UNIV MED CENT)
2022;35(3):397

https://doi.org/10.1080/08998280.2022.2030176

Taylor & Francis
Taylor & Francis Group

Education in the operating room

Bryana N. Baginski, MD[a], and Charles S. Roberts, MD[b]

[a]Department of Surgery, Baylor University Medical Center, Dallas, Texas; [b]Department of Cardiac Surgery, Baylor University Medical Center, Dallas, Texas

Coronary artery bypass grafting (CABG) is an operation on the first two branches of the aorta that requires a dedicated, expert team. Several specific roles in the operating room are allied to achieve success, including the circulating nurse, scrub nurse, anesthesia technicians, anesthesiologists, perfusionists, physician assistants (PA), and the operating surgeon and assistants. Expertise in these roles requires education, usually on an individual basis during an operation, over the course of weeks, months, or years, depending on the role, until the trainee is fit to be independent.

Baylor University Medical Center is home for daily medical education in numerous settings, of course, including the operating room. One October morning in a CABG operation, five separate mentor/mentee sessions were simultaneously occurring. As listed in *Table 1*, teaching was occurring between the primary surgeon and the surgical resident, the anesthesiologist and the anesthesia resident, the experienced PA and the new PA, the perfusionist and his student, and the nurse circulator and nurse intern. Only the scrub nurse at this operation was not actively teaching. Thus, five of the six principals in a CABG operation were actively engaged in teaching. The six roles, overall, are depicted in *Figure 1*. Maintaining excellence in surgery necessitates that the next generation is prepared.

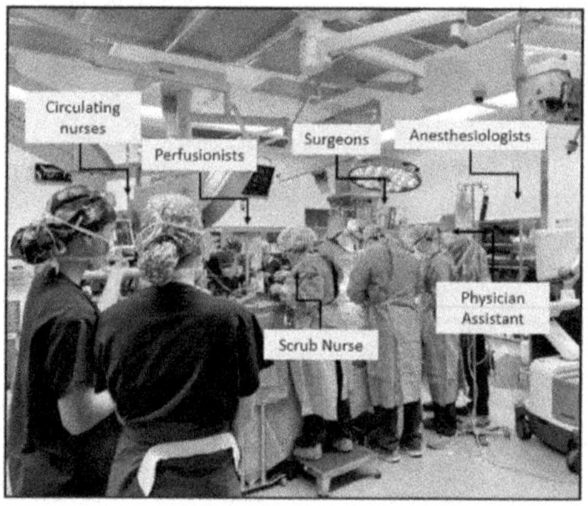

Figure 1. Education is necessary in six roles in the operating room in coronary artery bypass grafting.

Table 1. The mentor-mentee relationships in one cardiac operation

Role	Mentor (years of experience)	Mentee (educational level)
Surgeon	Charles S. Roberts, MD (25)	Bryana N. Baginski, MD (PGY-1 surgery resident)[a]
Anesthesiologist	Simon Choi, MD (5)	Cheng Yang, MD (PGY-4 anesthesia resident)[b]
Physician assistant	Gabriel Schlebach (12)	Christine Triporo (<1 y in cardiac)
Perfusionist	Murphy L. Rayle (7)	Francesca G. Henrichs (master in perfusion science)[c]
Circulating nurse	M. Caroline Klingenberg (4)	Samantha Haddad (nurse intern)

[a]Baylor University Medical Center.
[b]Brooke Army Medical Center.
[c]University of Nebraska.

Corresponding author: Charles S. Roberts, Department of Surgery, Baylor University Medical Center, Dallas, Texas (e-mail: charles.roberts@bswhealth.org)
Received November 29, 2021; Accepted January 13, 2022.

Baginski BN, Roberts CS. Education in the operating room. *Proc (Bayl Univ Med Cent).* 2022;35(3):397. doi:10.1080/08998280.2022.2030176

28

PROC (BAYL UNIV MED CENT)
2022;35(4):572–574

https://doi.org/10.1080/08998280.2022.2057156

Taylor & Francis
Taylor & Francis Group

A perspective on first assisting in cardiovascular operations

Charles Stewart Roberts, MD[a], and Lauren Zammerilla Westcott, MD[b]

[a]Department of Cardiac Surgery, Baylor University Medical Center, Dallas, Texas; [b]Department of Surgery, Baylor University Medical Center, Dallas, Texas

ABSTRACT
The quality of surgical assistance is an important factor affecting surgical performance and outcomes. This article gives a perspective on key principles of first assisting, specifically during cardiovascular operations. The principles start with operative techniques, then expand into concepts relating to the surgical field and operating room. By adhering to the described principles, the first assistant may enhance a surgical operation, benefiting the surgeon, the operating room team, and, most important, the patient.

KEYWORDS Cardiovascular surgery; first assisting; surgical principles

Excellent first assisting adds efficiency, elegance, and quality to a surgical operation. Poor surgical assistance has been identified as a key intraoperative stressor for the primary surgeon, potentially affecting his or her surgical performance and contributing to complications.[1] During an operation, a part of the primary surgeon's mind tracks the first assistant: What action is he or she performing? How well is the action being done? Is the action advancing or impeding the operation? The primary responsibility of a first assistant, in our view, is "do no harm." The second responsibility is to facilitate the flow of the operation by helping the primary surgeon. The "perfect surgical assistant" has been described as "calm, confident, competent, and courageous."[2] In addition to these attributes, the following principles, in our opinion, may be useful to consider, specifically when assisting in cardiovascular operations *(Figure 1)*.

OPERATING PRINCIPLES

Be gentle with tissues

This is a primary surgical principle, from which most others originate. Dr. William Halsted (1852–1922) of The Johns Hopkins Hospital was an early advocate of minimizing tissue trauma. Due to the improvements of anesthesia during his era, the rapid and violent handling of tissue was no longer necessary, and it became possible to dissect carefully, ligate blood vessels individually, and close incisions neatly in layers. Modern surgery is gentle surgery. Instruments and devices applied roughly cause unnecessary tissue trauma. The first assistant should keep this in mind when using various tools. The suction, for example, should be used lightly, like a bird, especially when suctioning around delicate venous grafts or vascular anastomoses. Suctions used as blunt retractors can be too rough and noisy at times, when forceps will do. Self-retaining retractors should be opened slowly and narrowly at first, with gradual expansion to allow full exposure.

Displace instead of grasp, when possible

When either exposing or sewing, gentle displacement of the tissue with closed forceps will often suffice instead of grasping and crushing with forceps. For example, the three-layer soft tissue closure anterior to the sternum can usually be accomplished without grasping subcutaneous tissue. Simple displacement causes less tissue trauma. If grasping is necessary, it should be done delicately and gently. Although considered to be an "atraumatic" instrument, the DeBakey forceps can cause damage to tissue, especially blood vessels.

Preserve the intima

Blood vessels have three layers: the intima, media, and adventitia. Virchow's triad states that thrombosis may be a consequence of one or more of three conditions: hypercoagulability, stasis, and intimal injury. Intimal damage in a

Corresponding author: Charles S. Roberts, MD, Department of Cardiac Surgery, Baylor University Medical Center, 621 North Hall St., Suite 120, Dallas, TX 75226 (e-mail: charles.roberts@bswhealth.org)
The authors report no funding or conflicts of interest.
Received October 30, 2021; Revised March 14, 2022; Accepted March 21, 2022.

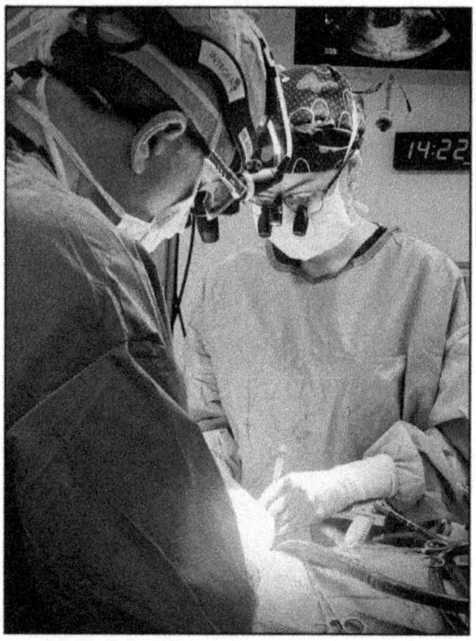

Figure 1. The junior author (LZW) assisting the senior author (CSR) in a coronary artery bypass grafting operation.

cardiovascular operation can be minimized if one handles blood vessels with delicacy by grasping the adventitia only.

Sew with the curve of the needle

Introduce the needle into tissue at 180° and advance it with the curve of the needle. When using a standard needle holder, this requires an ability to "palm"; that is, open and close the needle holder without fingers in the slots. "Palming" is necessary to pronate the wrist sufficiently to achieve the desired 180°. When fingers are fixed in the needle-holder, direction is limited, and needles are often inserted at inappropriate angles. When removing the needle from tissue, "push, push, pull" is often useful, or simply "push, pull." This means gently pushing the needle from the posterior body with the needle driver. The needle should be allowed to rest where it lands and not be held up under tension during retrieval. It can then be grasped anteriorly with the needle driver and pulled out of the tissue, always along the curve of the needle. Tension in either needle or tissue when sewing is to be avoided.

Cut the suture at the desired level in a timely fashion

The assistant should know the level above the knot the surgeon desires the suture strands to be cut (the preference of the senior author is 1 cm for braided suture and 2 cm for monofilament suture) and should be prepared to cut with the tips of the scissors only. The senior surgeon prefers to hold the suture until cut and pass off the strands himself, so that the assistant's hand does not suddenly block his field of vision. It should be unnecessary for the surgeon to say "cut" after completing the knots if the assistant is already poised to do so.

OPERATIVE FIELD PRINCIPLES

Keep eyes focused on the operative field

Despite one's best intentions or efforts, the hands inevitably move when the eyes look away. If the surgeon is performing an anastomosis and the first assistant is holding the vein with forceps, a momentary look away by the first assistant, to find the suction, for example, will move the vein. Either keep both eyes and hands focused on the field or remove them. Although one is expected to make eye contact during conversations in social settings, it is contraindicated and dangerous while operating. When communication is necessary, it should be done without averting the eyes from the field. The message can then be relayed through the appropriate channels (surgical scrub technician to circulating nurse, anesthesia providers, etc.).

Utilize basic hand signals for basic instruments

Simple, silent hand signals to the nurse or surgical scrub technician keep things quiet and peaceful. Use three signals routinely: scissors are the straight index and middle fingers coming together and apart; forceps are the index fingertip and thumb tip brought together repeatedly; and needle holder (with suture) is a closed hand moving with a slight twist repeatedly, as if placing a stitch. These three hand signals are universal and lessen the verbal sensory input at the table.

Optimize the surgeon's perspective first

The primary surgeon's and first assistant's visual perspectives are different, as each one views the field from a different angle. The assistant may have to adjust his or her body to obtain the appropriate visual field to assist the primary surgeon. Given this, it is helpful for the assistant to be familiar with the various steps of the operation and the goals of each step. For example, when performing aortic cannulation for cardiopulmonary bypass, the surgeon will need to place a stitch on the aorta. To assist with exposure and facilitation of this step of the operation (via suctioning or tissue retraction), the assistant will need to lean forward (and toward the head) from the left side of the table and peer under the shelf of the divided sternum. This will allow the assistant to see what the surgeon sees.

Mind the planes of separation when working

When adjusting one's body as in the above situation, it is important to maintain spatial awareness. Knocking heads is to be avoided. Spatial awareness should also be maintained when performing simultaneous tasks. For example, when closing a midline wound together from each end, avoid placing hands and instruments in the way of the surgeon closing from the opposite direction.

Minimize disruptive movements

Try to minimize any sudden movement, including shaking of the table, that may be disruptive to the operation. Periodically jarring the table to lean in, for example, can also be distracting. The best endoscopic harvesters of vein in the leg, to use one example, are economical in movement. Endoscopic probe manipulation, trauma to the vein and the leg, and harvest time are minimal.

OPERATING ROOM PRINCIPLES

Scrub in before the surgeon

The assistant should be scrubbed in and ready prior to the surgeon. This will allow the assistant adequate time to prepare and become comfortable (adjust lights, request a step stool, etc.) prior to the commencement of the operation. This can minimize disruptions during the case and allow the circulating nurse and surgical scrub technician to focus on the surgeon and the operation itself. In addition, scrubbing in before the surgeon conveys a message of enthusiasm, initiative, and respect to the surgeon.

Tend toward quiet

Subdue personality to the task at hand. Let the surgeon lead when it comes to initiating conversation and follow his or her cues. If the surgeon is totally focused, a friendly question such as "How was your weekend?" may be untimely. During critical parts or transition phases of an operation, be silent. For example, in a cardiac operation, when cannulating and de-airing, when going on or coming off cardiopulmonary bypass, or during application of an aortic cross-clamp, extraneous communication can be distracting and dangerous. Personal noises such as singing, humming, yawning, and sighing can also distract.

Ask permission to do anything unusual

Any change in routine justifies a discussion with the primary surgeon, who may or may not wish to add a new variable to the operation. For example, although both the surgeon and first assistant may love to teach, the surgeon should decide whether a first assistant can delegate a task to another. In addition, if the first assistant is aware that he or she will have to leave during part of the operation (as may happen in a surgical training program given conference requirements), the primary surgeon should be notified prior to starting the operation so that arrangements can be made.

Share clinical opinions judiciously

Good surgeons appreciate input, especially, for example, when pondering a challenge or posing a question, but only to a point. Routine maneuvers require no comment or advice. It should be emphasized, however, that if the assistant notices something abnormal or an error about to be committed, he or she should point this out, in line with the duty to "do no harm."

Be an agent of harmony

A positive personality provides an intangible benefit to the surgeon and team. The operating room is no place to introduce sensitive, provocative, or negative subjects. Discussing previous complications or other patients is to be avoided. Stressful moments may occur in major surgical operations but will pass with peaceful silence and complete focus. "Keep it clinical" is a good conversational motto to follow if personal conflicts arise.

CONCLUDING PRINCIPLE

There is always something to do

During a fellowship year abroad, the senior author once stood motionless at the surgeon position and was reminded of this final principle by a senior anesthesiologist. The junior author recalls her surgical mentor saying that "idle hands are the devil's workshop" early in her training when she stood with no instruments in her hands. They both are indeed right. There is always something to be done. From wheels-in to wheels-out of the operating room, the assistant should be proactive, anticipating how he or she can facilitate the progress of the operation. The primary surgeon will be deeply grateful for constant attentiveness. By adhering to this concept along with the above principles, the first assistant can greatly enhance a surgical operation, benefiting the surgeon, the operating room team, and, most important, the patient.

ORCID

Lauren Zammerilla Westcott http://orcid.org/0000-0002-4776-2745

1. Anton NE, Montero PN, Howley LD, Brown C, Stefanidis D. What stress coping strategies are surgeons relying upon during surgery? *Am J Surg*. 2015;210:846–851. doi:10.1016/j.amjsurg.2015.04.002.
2. Hall S, Quick J, Hall AW. The perfect surgical assistant: calm, confident, competent and courageous. *J Perioper Pract*. 2016;26:201–204. doi:10.1177/175045891602600903.

Roberts CS, Westcott LZ. A perspective on first assisting in cardiovascular operations. *Proc (Bayl Univ Med Cent)*. 2022;35(4):572-574. doi:10.1080/08998280.2022.2057156

29

WCR 90: Aspects of the Life and Work of William C. Roberts, MD

Charles Stewart Roberts, MD

The following images were assembled to describe the life of William Clifford Roberts, MD (hereafter WCR) who is presently 90 years of age. He was born in 1932 in Atlanta, Georgia. His early youth was spent on a farm in Stone Mountain, Georgia. After his father died, when he was 8 years of age, the family moved back to Atlanta where he graduated from Henry Grady High School in 1950. He went to Southern Methodist University in Dallas for 4 years, then Emory University School of Medicine in Atlanta where he graduated in 1958.

The next 6 years he spent training in various specialties, first a year in medicine at Boston City Hospital, then 3 years in anatomic pathology at the National Institutes of Health (NIH) in Bethesda, then another year in medicine at The Johns Hopkins Hospital, followed by a year at NIH as a Clinical Associate, 6 months in cardiology and 6 months in cardiac surgery.

From July 1964 to the present, January 2023, nearly 60 years, WCR has focused his time and energy on the study of cardiovascular disease. In the first 30 years (1964-1993), he served as Chief of Pathology in the National Heart, Lung, and Blood Institute of NIH in Bethesda, and in the second 30 years (1993-2023), as Executive Director of the Baylor Heart and Vascular Institute at Baylor University Medical Center in Dallas.

During these 60 years, spent equally at 2 institutions, WCR remained focused on the study of anatomical specimens of the heart and blood vessels, obtained either from the autopsy suite or the operating room. Study of these anatomical specimens yielded >1300 medical publications

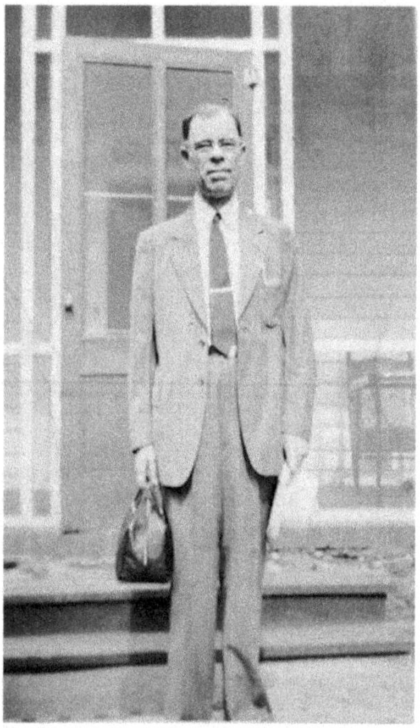

Figure 1. Stewart R. Roberts, MD [1878-1941], the father of WCR, was Professor of Clinical Medicine at Emory University School of Medicine for 25 years (1915-1941). He was frequently called "The Osler of the South,"[3] for he published about 100 medical articles, most of which were addresses given to medical societies, and was author of a book on pellagra.[4] In this photograph, he is in front of his home in Stone Mountain, Georgia. Born in Atlanta on September 11, 1932, WCR lived at Stone Mountain from age 3 to 10. His father died of heart failure in 1941, when WCR was 8 years of age.

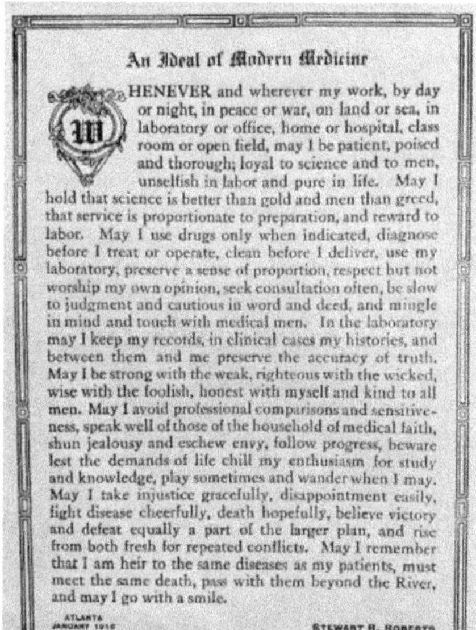

An Ideal of Modern Medicine

WHENEVER and wherever my work, by day or night, in peace or war, on land or sea, in laboratory or office, home or hospital, class room or open field, may I be patient, poised and thorough; loyal to science and to men, unselfish in labor and pure in life. May I hold that science is better than gold and men than greed, that service is proportionate to preparation, and reward to labor. May I use drugs only when indicated, diagnose before I treat or operate, clean before I deliver, use my laboratory, preserve a sense of proportion, respect but not worship my own opinion, seek consultation often, be slow to judgment and cautious in word and deed, and mingle in mind and touch with medical men. In the laboratory may I keep my records, in clinical cases my histories, and between them and me preserve the accuracy of truth. May I be strong with the weak, righteous with the wicked, wise with the foolish, honest with myself and kind to all men. May I avoid professional comparisons and sensitiveness, speak well of those of the household of medical faith, shun jealousy and eschew envy, follow progress, beware lest the demands of life chill my enthusiasm for study and knowledge, play sometimes and wander when I may. May I take injustice gracefully, disappointment easily, fight disease cheerfully, death hopefully, believe victory and defeat equally a part of the larger plan, and rise from both fresh for repeated conflicts. May I remember that I am heir to the same diseases as my patients, must meet the same death, pass with them beyond the River, and may I go with a smile.

ATLANTA
JANUARY 1916

STEWART R. ROBERTS

Figure 2. Stewart R. Roberts, MD, the father of WCR, was educated at Emory College in Oxford, Georgia, in a Classical and Christian tradition, which was reflected in his speech and writing. WCR republished this essay by his father in a brief article in 1969.[5]

Department of Cardiac Surgery, Baylor University Medical Center, Dallas, Texas. Manuscript received February 22, 2023; revised manuscript received and accepted February 25, 2023.

Abbreviations: AJC, *American Journal of Cardiology*; BUMC, Baylor University Medical Center; NIH, National Institutes of Health; WCR, William Clifford Roberts.

E-mail address: charles.roberts@bswhealth.org

https://doi.org/10.1016/j.amjcard.2023.02.018

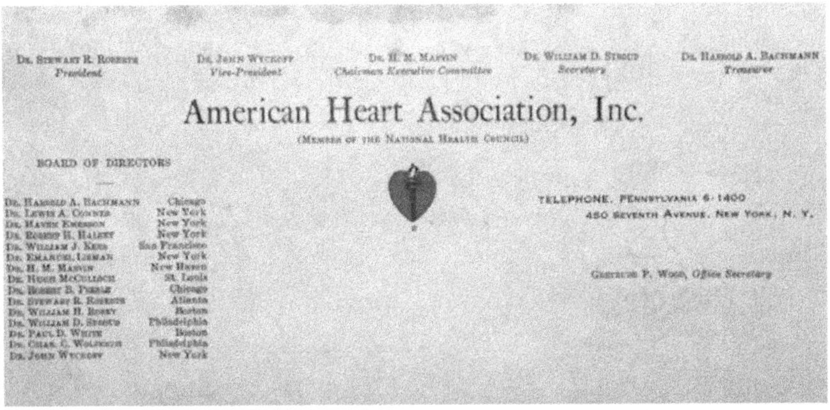

Figure 3. Stewart R. Roberts, MD, the father of WCR, was the first cardiologist in the South. He published 20 articles on cardiovascular disease from 1916 to 1936 and delivered numerous cardiovascular addresses in Atlanta and in the South and in the USA.[6]

(PubMed), together with numerous books and book chapters. Most publications involved collaboration with students, trainees, and staff members (including 2 sons and 1 granddaughter who spent summers in his laboratory).

As his expertise in cardiovascular disease developed, WCR traveled widely for speaking engagements, including 46 countries. Some 50 of his talks were downloaded on YouTube. Photography both in his laboratory and when traveling became a passion.

In addition to his primary pursuit, WCR also served as editor in chief of 2 journals, *The American Journal of Cardiology* (1982-2022) and the *Baylor University Medical Center Proceedings* (1994-2022). His own mastery of manuscript preparation and publication gave him an expertise and understanding in interacting with authors submitting their own work to these journals.

From 1972 to 2019 (46 years), WCR hosted a medical meeting in the first week of December in Williamsburg, Virginia. He invited superb speakers on cardiovascular disease. Several speaker and numerous attendees came year after year.

WCR was married for 36 years to the late Carey Cansler Roberts [1935-2016] of Charlotte, North Carolina. She had attended Agnes Scott College in Atlanta and was the author of 4 published novels. They had 4 children and now 11 grandchildren and 4 great-grandchildren. WCR hosted large family gatherings in December and June for 20 years. He started The Roberts Foundation in 2019 to support Heath and Heritage endeavors.

W. Bruce Fye, MD, cardiologist and medical historian, conducted an interview of WCR which was published in 2007 in the *Baylor University Medical Center Proceedings.*[1] In the same year (15 years ago), this writer also published an interview of WCR in the *American Journal of Cardiology.*[2]

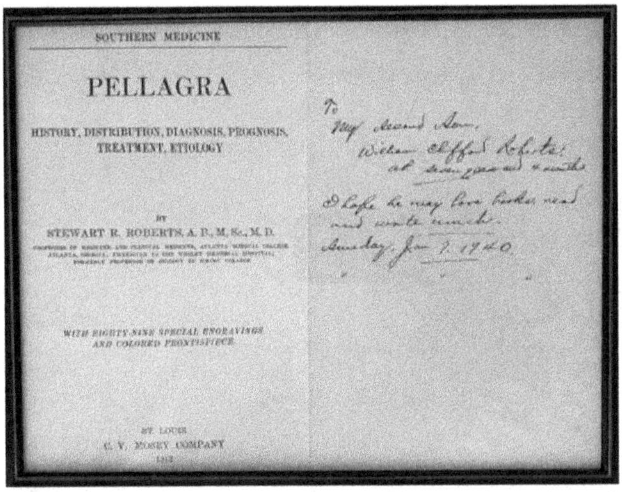

Figure 4. Stewart R. Roberts, MD, father of WCR, published a book and 7 articles on pellagra. His inscription to his second son, written a year before his death from heart failure, was prescient.

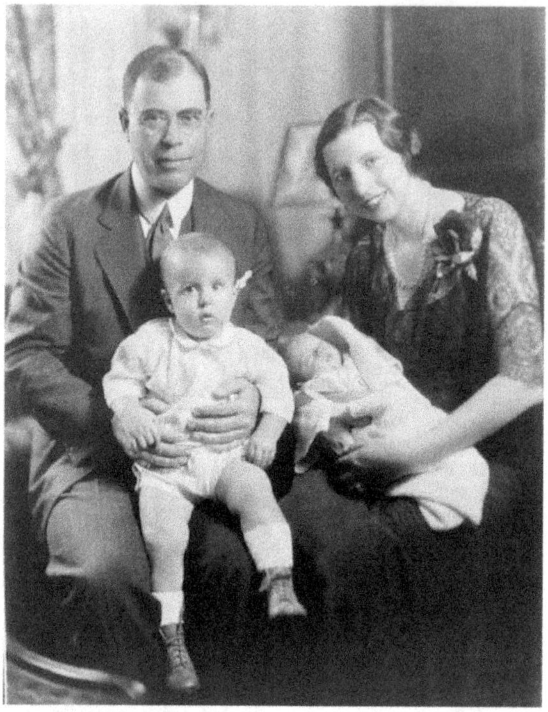

Figure 5. Dr. Stewart R. Roberts and his wife, Ruby Holbrook Roberts, with their first two sons. WCR was raised from age 8 on by his mother, who established a business called "Medical Placement and Mailing Service." She covered the entire cost of college and medical school for both boys in this photograph.

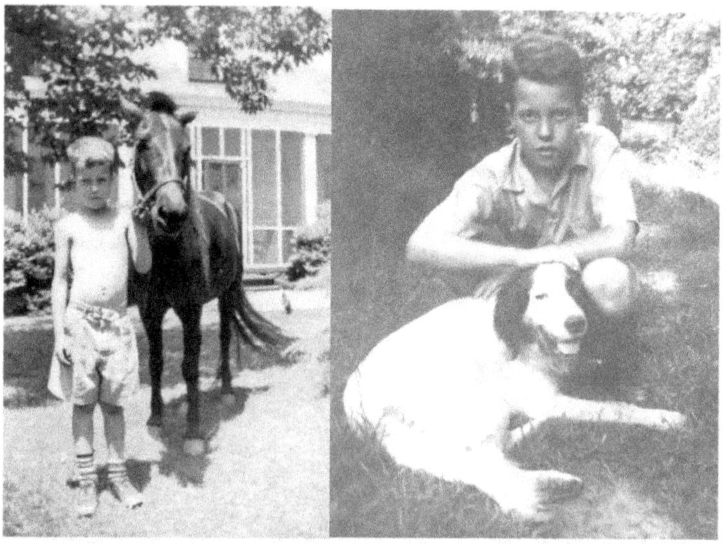

Figures 6. WCR with his pony, left, at the farm in Stone Mountain, Georgia, and older, right, with his dog at his home in the Brookwood Hills section of Atlanta.

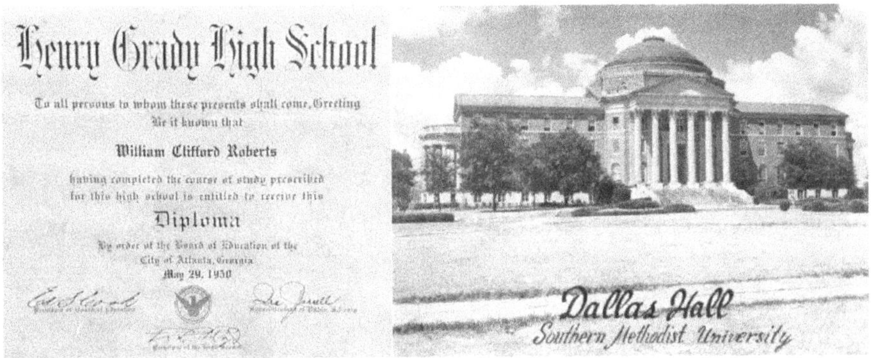

Figures 7. WCR graduated from Henry Grady High School in Atlanta, Georgia, in 1950, then went for 4 years to Southern Methodist University in Dallas, Texas, where he joined Phi Delta Theta fraternity and majored in English.

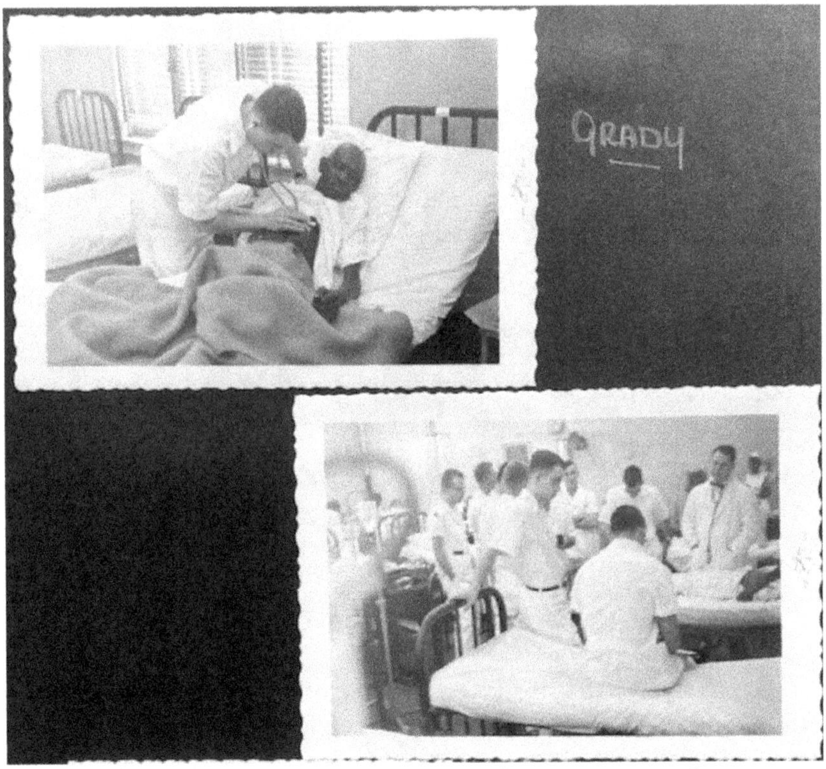

Figure 8. WCR went to Emory University School of Medicine from 1954-1958. He was 4th generation at Emory and 2nd generation in medicine. His older brother Stewart R. Roberts, Jr., MD, also went to Emory University School of Medicine, though a year behind WCR because of military service, and he became a radiologist at Emory University Hospital. Grady Memorial Hospital opened when WCR was a senior. Linton Bishop, MD, was the rounding physician.

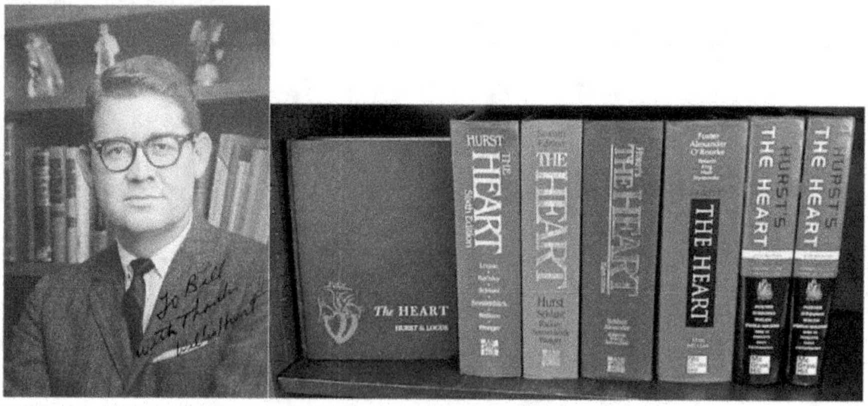

Figures 9. J. Willis Hurst, MD [1920-2011] became chair of medicine at Emory University School of Medicine in 1957, and the next year, he helped WCR secure an internship in straight medicine at Boston City Hospital. WCR had strongly considered surgery, but the influence of Hurst and his late father, Stewart R. Roberts, MD, was great. WCR and Dr. Hurst remained lifelong friends and WCR contributed chapters to several editions of *The Heart*, first published in 1966 and edited by J. Willis Hurst, MD, and R. Bruce Logue, MD (1st edition only).

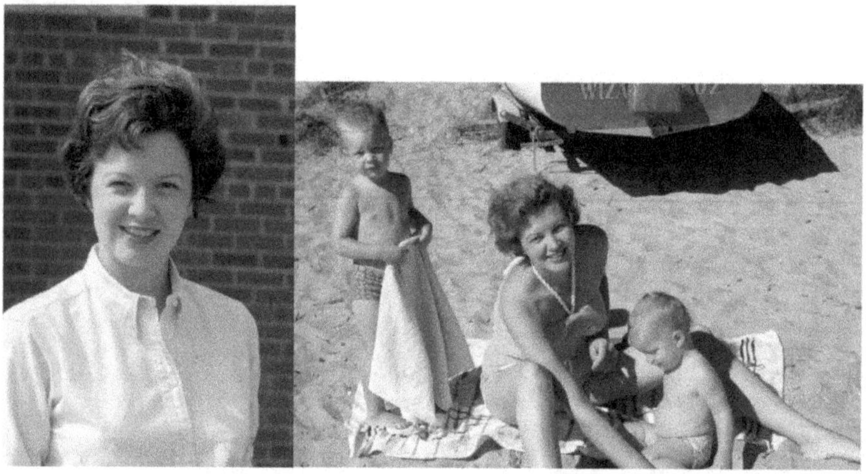

Figures 10. Carey Cansler [1936-2016] and WCR were married in Atlanta in 1955, after his first year of medical school. She was attending Agnes Scott College. They had 4 children. Carey stayed home to raise the children until 1975, then went into marketing at a bank, then a hospital. Throughout she was a freelance writer and published 4 novels. She and WCR shared a love of books and learning.

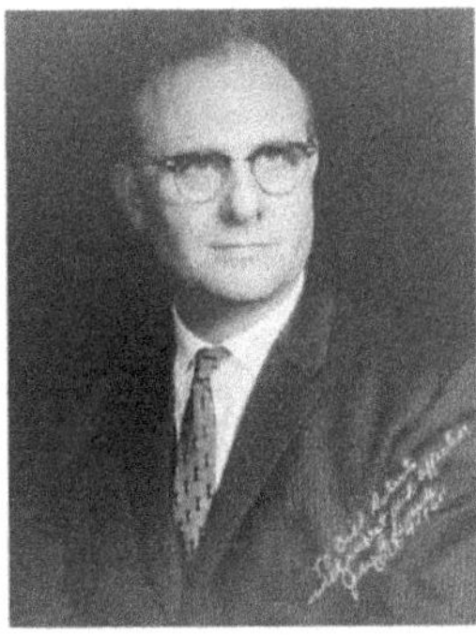

Figures 11. Jesse E. Edwards, MD [1911-2008], above left, was perhaps the main academic mentor of WCR in cardiovascular pathology. After an internship in Boston, WCR went to the NIH for a 3-year residency in Anatomic Pathology, where he began an intense study of the cardiovascular publications of Edwards, who contributed numerous chapters to Gould's edited book on *Pathology of the Heart and Blood Vessels (1st edition, 1953)* which WCR pored over. After his 3-year residency, but before arriving at Hopkins, WCR visited Edwards in St. Paul. Edwards opened the heart according to the flow of blood, while WCR opened the heart according to the disease, sometimes cutting transversely or longitudinally or obliquely, to capture the telling photograph. Both physicians attracted a gathering of trainees and students around the table when examining a heart.

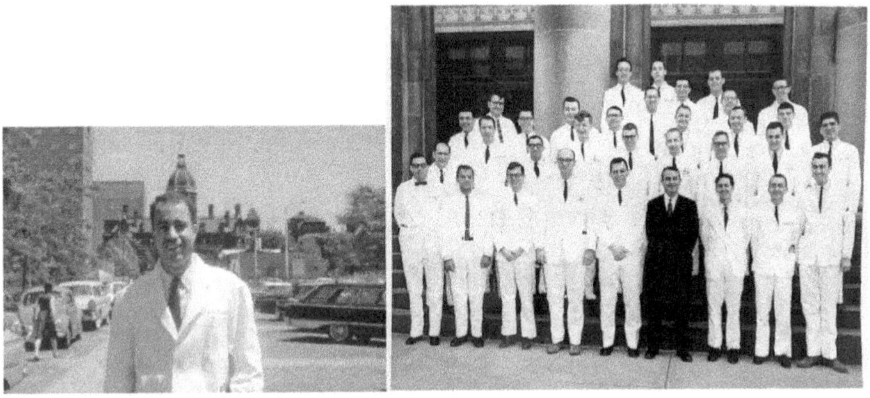

Figure 12. WCR, left, at Hopkins and right, 2nd row, 2nd from left. WCR spent one year on the Osler Service at The Johns Hopkins Hospital. The Chair of Medicine was A. McGhee Harvey (dark suit) and to his right was Gottleib Christian Freisinger, the chief resident, who later became chief of cardiology at Vanderbilt.

THE JOHNS HOPKINS HOSPITAL
MEDCIAL STAFF ROUNDS
SEPTEMBER 22, 1962
HURD HALL
10:00 A.M.

CASE PRESENTATIONS

E. D.	#77 76 65	Arthritis	Dr. Werner
B. G.	#104 44 11	Acute Renal Failure	Dr. Roberts
D. P.	#104 42 14	Fever of Undetermined Origin	Dr. Hathaway
P. K.	#73 57 79	Pernicious Anemia	Dr. Roberts

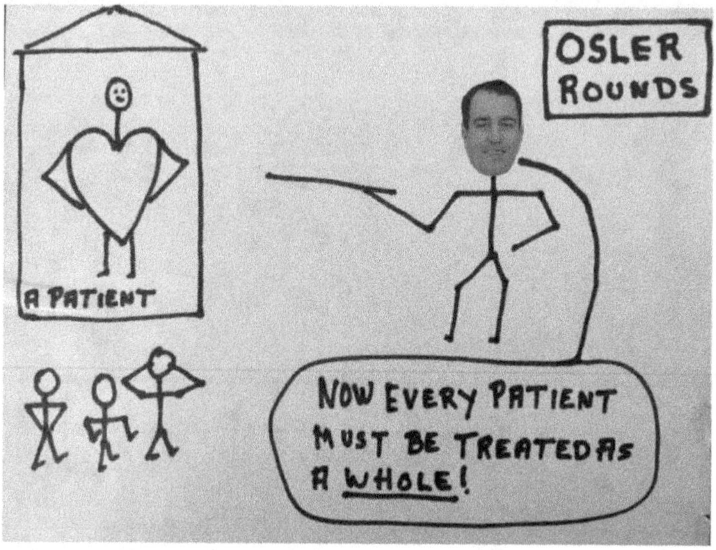
A PATIENT
OSLER ROUNDS
NOW EVERY PATIENT MUST BE TREATED AS A WHOLE!

Figure 13. Above, case presentations by WCR during his year on the Osler Service at Hopkins, and below, a cartoon made by a colleague that year emphasizing the focus by WCR on the heart even then.

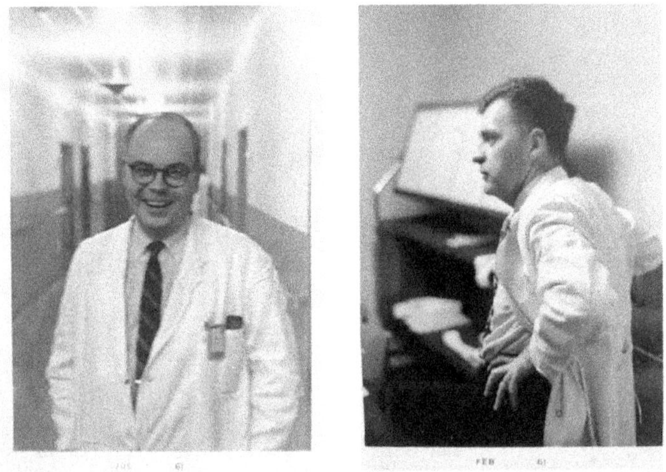

Figure 14. Left, Andrew Glenn Morrow, MD [1922-1982], had trained under Alfred Blalock at Hopkins and was the first chief of cardiac surgery at NIH, appointed in 1953. He offered WCR a position in the Surgery Branch of the Heart Institute to begin in July 1963, to establish a Pathology Unit, which later became a Pathology Branch, on par with the Surgery Branch and Cardiology Branch. Right, Eugene Braunwald, MD, [1929, Vienna, Austria] served as Chief of Cardiology at NIH, then at University of California at San Diego, and finally at the Brigham and Women's Hospital in Boston. WCR's first publication was with Morrow and Braunwald in 1961.[7]

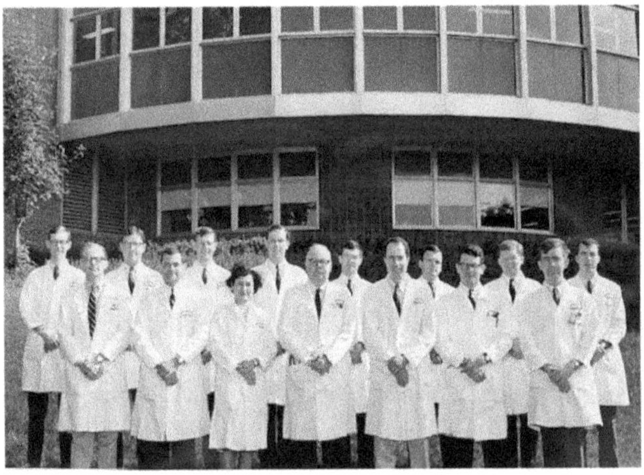

Figure 15. This photograph is of the Surgery Branch of the Heart Institute. WCR is front row, 3rd from right, standing to the left of Dr. Morrow, the Chief. To the right of Dr. Morrow is Nina Braunwald, MD, a cardiac surgeon and wife of Eugene Braunwald. The Surgery Branch had a 2 year program of Clinical Associates, usually taking 2 years out from the 5 year surgery tracks. These positions were prestigious and many department chairs came from this NIH program. Morrow helped train > 125 clinical associates from 1953 to 1982.

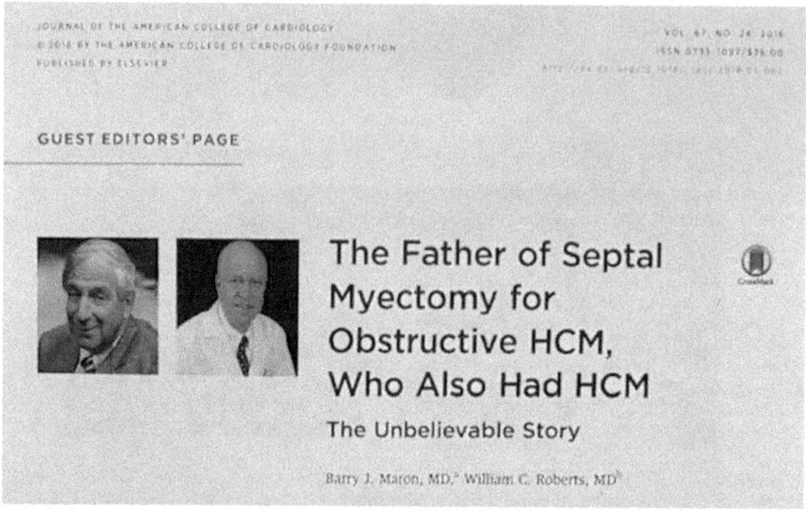
JOURNAL OF THE AMERICAN COLLEGE OF CARDIOLOGY
© 2016 BY THE AMERICAN COLLEGE OF CARDIOLOGY FOUNDATION
PUBLISHED BY ELSEVIER

VOL. 67, NO. 24, 2016
ISSN 0735-1097/$36.00

GUEST EDITORS' PAGE

The Father of Septal Myectomy for Obstructive HCM, Who Also Had HCM

The Unbelievable Story

Barry J. Maron, MD,[a] William C. Roberts, MD[b]

Figure 16. WCR collaborated on numerous papers with Barry J. Maron, MD, the world's expert on hypertrophic cardiomyopathy after Braunwald.[5] Dr. Morrow first conceived of the operation, septal myectomy, or "left ventricular septal myotomy and myectomy," as it was referred to at NIH, and later known as "The Morrow Operation." As the article above states, Morrow had hypertrophic cardiomyopathy and WCR subsequently examined his heart at necropsy.

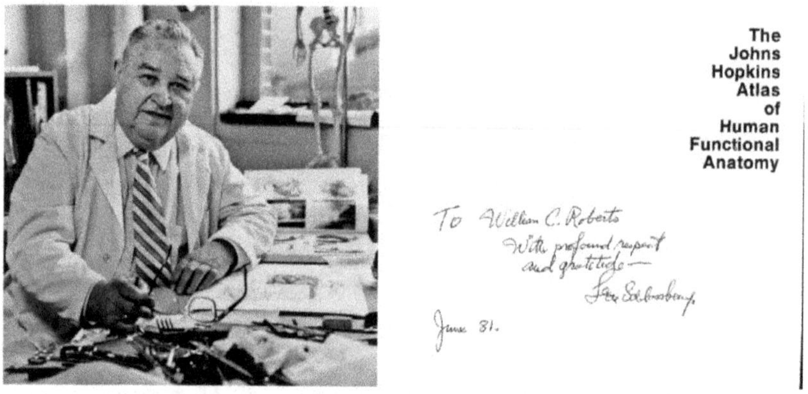

Figure 17. Leon Schlossberg of Hopkins was the premier medical illustrator of his generation. WCR met with him at NIH monthly for many years. Together they prepared exquisite illustrations, nearly all of which were published in cardiovascular articles.

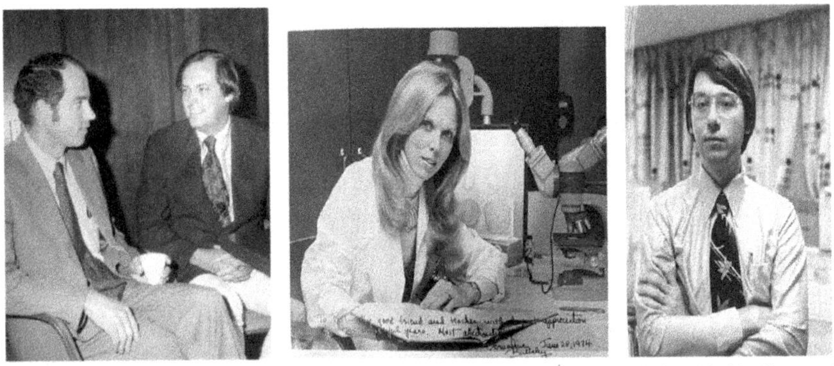

Figure 18. WCR with D. Luke Glancy, MD [1935-2022], who was his first fellow for 2 years at NIH. The were friends and the 2 families were close for many years. Dr. Glancy became Chief of Cardiology at Louisiana State University in New Orleans in 1974 and was Medical Director of Cardiology at Hotel Dieu (now University Hospital) for 18 years. He was editor-in-chief of the *Journal of the Louisiana State Medical Society* for 20 years and published > 400 articles. He trained many of the cardiologists in Louisiana. Both reared in Atlanta, WCR and Luke Glancy were perhaps best friends professionally for 6 decades. WCR had 40 fellows during the 30 years at NIH. Left, Bernadine Healy, MD [1944-2011], a fellow from 1972-4, became a cardiologist and was Director of the NIH from 1991-1993. Right, Thomas L. Spray, MD, a fellow from 1975-1977, was a surgery resident under David Sabiston at Duke at the time and became a world-renown pediatric cardiac surgeon at the Chidren's Hospital of Philadelphia.

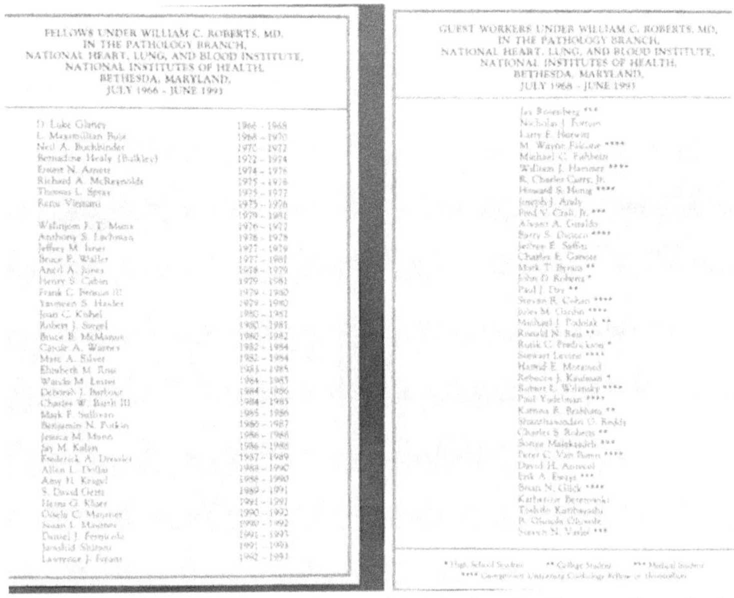

FELLOWS UNDER WILLIAM C. ROBERTS, MD,
IN THE PATHOLOGY BRANCH,
NATIONAL HEART, LUNG, AND BLOOD INSTITUTE,
NATIONAL INSTITUTES OF HEALTH,
BETHESDA, MARYLAND,
JULY 1966 - JUNE 1993

D. Luke Glancy	1966 - 1968
L. Maximilian Buja	1968 - 1970
Neil A. Buchbinder	1970 - 1972
Bernadine Healy (Bulkley)	1972 - 1974
Ernest N. Arnett	1974 - 1976
Richard A. McReynolds	1975 - 1976
Thomas L. Spray	1975 - 1977
Renu Virmani	1975 - 1976
	1979 - 1981
Walinjom F. T. Muna	1976 - 1977
Anthony S. Lachman	1976 - 1978
Jeffrey M. Isner	1977 - 1979
Bruce F. Waller	1977 - 1981
Ancil A. Jones	1978 - 1979
Henry S. Cabin	1979 - 1981
Frank C. Brosius III	1979 - 1980
Yasmeen S. Hasler	1979 - 1980
Joan C. Kishel	1980 - 1982
Robert J. Siegel	1980 - 1981
Bruce B. McManus	1980 - 1982
Carole A. Warnes	1982 - 1984
Marc A. Silver	1982 - 1984
Elizabeth M. Ross	1983 - 1985
Wanda M. Lester	1984 - 1985
Deborah J. Barbour	1984 - 1986
Charles W. Barth III	1984 - 1985
Mark F. Sullivan	1985 - 1986
Benjamin N. Potkin	1986 - 1987
Jessica M. Mann	1986 - 1988
Jay M. Kalan	1986 - 1988
Frederick A. Dressler	1987 - 1989
Allen L. Dollar	1988 - 1990
Amy H. Kragel	1988 - 1990
S. David Gertz	1989 - 1991
Heinz G. Klues	1990 - 1991
Gisela C. Mautner	1990 - 1992
Susan L. Mautner	1990 - 1992
Daniel J. Fernicola	1991 - 1993
Jamshid Shirani	1991 - 1993
Lawrence J. Ferans	1992 - 1993

GUEST WORKERS UNDER WILLIAM C. ROBERTS, MD,
IN THE PATHOLOGY BRANCH,
NATIONAL HEART, LUNG, AND BLOOD INSTITUTE,
NATIONAL INSTITUTES OF HEALTH,
BETHESDA, MARYLAND,
JULY 1968 - JUNE 1993

Jay Rosenberg ***
Nicholas J. Fortuin
Larry E. Horwitz
M. Wayne Falicov ****
Michael C. Fishbein
William J. Hammer ****
R. Charles Curry, Jr.
Howard S. Hong ****
Joseph J. Andy
Fred V. Crall, Jr. ***
Alvaro A. Giraldo
Barry S. Dicicco ****
Jeffrey E. Saffitz
Charles E. Ganote
Mark T. Byrnes **
John D. Roberts *
Paul J. Dry **
Steven R. Cohen ****
Jules M. Gardin ****
Michael J. Podolak **
Ronald N. Bass **
Ruth C. Fredrickson *
Stewart Levine ****
Hamid E. Mozaned
Rebecca J. Kaufman *
Robert L. Wilensky ****
Paul Yudelman ****
Karmen R. Brabham **
Shanthasundari O. Reddy
Charles S. Roberts **
Sonya Malekzadeh ***
Peter C. Van Buren ****
David H. Aronow
Erik A. Evayt ***
Brian N. Glick ****
Katharine Berezowski
Toshiko Kurihayashi
R. Chandra Chowdhury
Steven N. Vaidel ***

* High School Student ** College Student *** Medical Student
**** Georgetown University Cardiology Fellow or [illegible]

Figure 19. During this NIH period, WCR had numerous fellows, beginning with D. Luke Glancy. The fellows came from various backgrounds, including pathology residents, cardiology fellows, and surgery residents. In addition, numerous students spend summers and various periods with him. Renu Virmani spent 2 separate fellowships with WCR and was extremely productive. Jeffrey M. Isner, MD, was also prolific during his 2 years and remained a dear friend of WCR until his premature death. Two children of WCR, Charles and John, each spent a summer in his laboratory and one grandchild, Camille Roberts, spent 5 summers with him later at BUMC. After the NIH years, many fellows and summer students continued to work with WCR at BUMC.

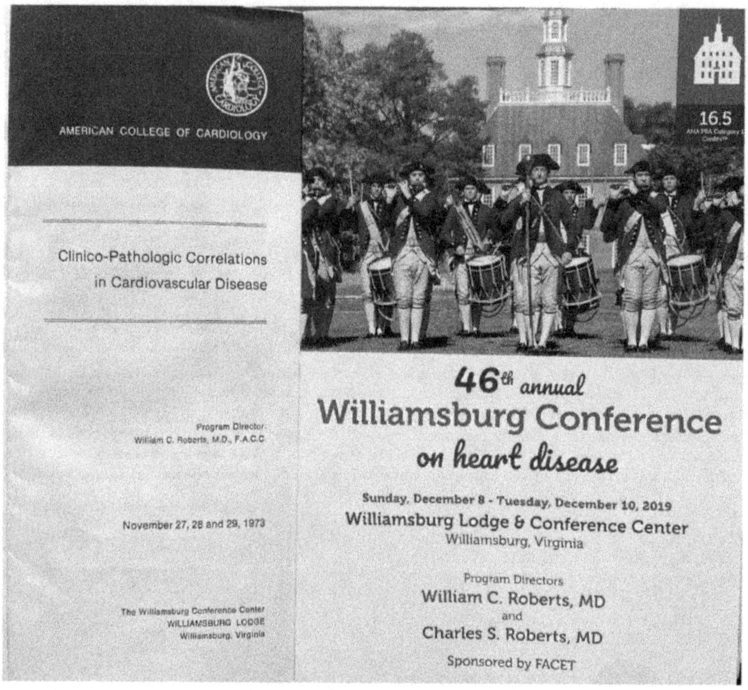

Figure 20. For 46 years WCR hosted an annual medical meeting on cardiovascular disease in Williamsburg, Virginia. Many of the speakers, such as Robert Bonow and Barry Maron, came year after year. The structure was rather unusual in that the speakers were asked to use 90 minutes, usually 75 for the talk and 15 for questions. The Roberts family came to know Williamsburg very well.

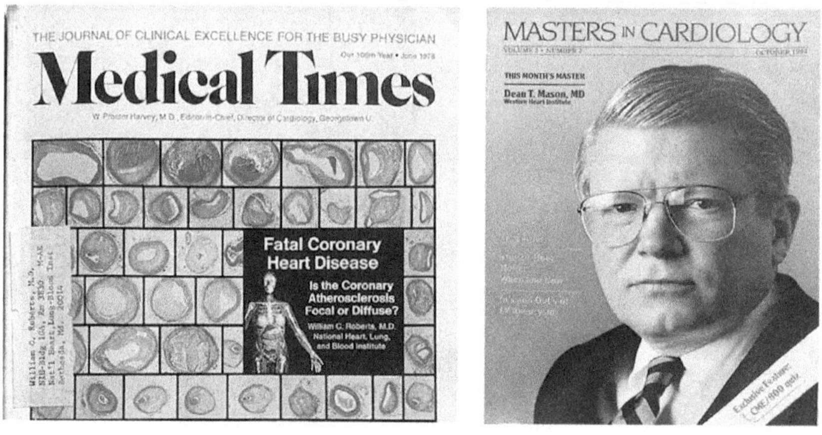

Figure 21. W. Proctor Harvey, MD, was Director of Cardiology at Georgetown University and was an early strong supporter of WCR who was given an academic appointment at Georgetown. Harvey held a cardiology conference every Thursday evening which WCR attended habitually. He was a superb teacher, especially in auscultation and he was Editor-in-Chief of the *Medical Times* (left). Dean T. Mason, MD, (right) was a good friend of WCR for many years, beginning at NIH. At one time, Mason and WCR had outlined a book on "Principles of Cardiology," but it never came to pass. Mason became editor in chief of *The American Heart Journal*. They supported each other's careers quite loyally.

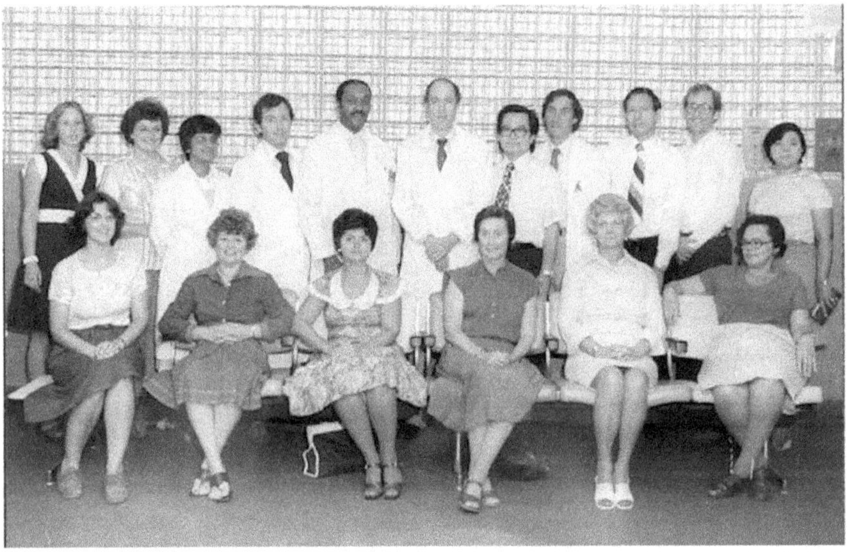

Figure 22. WCR as Chief of the Pathology Branch of the National Heart, Lung, and Blood Institute of NIH in Bethesda, Maryland. During his 30 years as Chief, WCR had numerous fellows, usually 4 at a time.

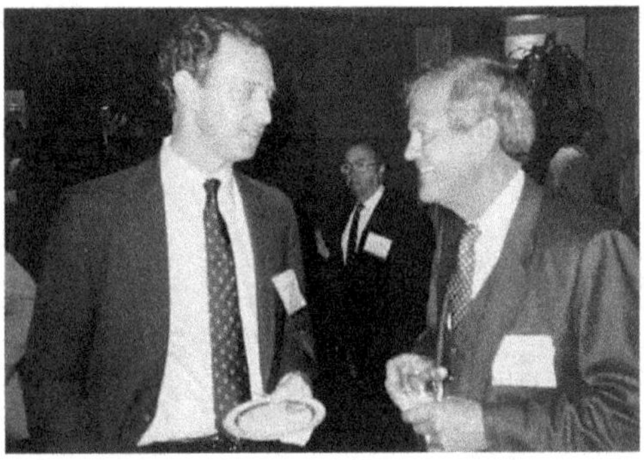

Figure 23. Robert O. Bonow, MD, left, current editor in chief of *JAMA Cardiology* and Kenneth M. Kent, MD, right, who was the first interventional cardiologist in Washington, DC, and a pioneer in coronary angioplasty. They were all colleagues at NIH and remained so in subsequent years.

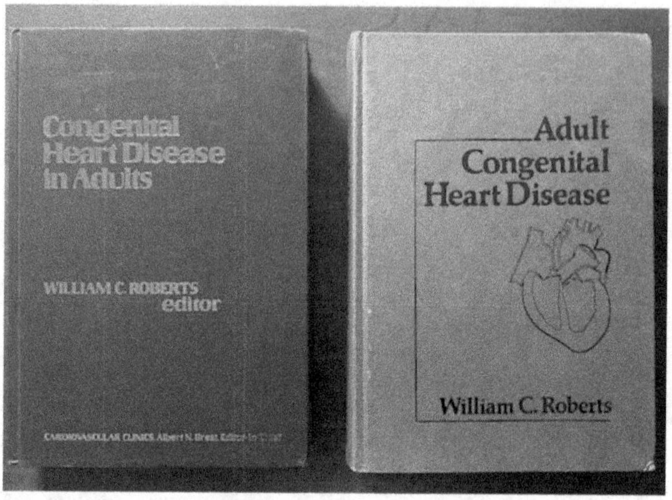

Figure 24. Much of the early career of WCR involved congenital heart disease. He was one of 6 members of the Committee on Coding and Classification for Congenital Heart Disease of the National Heart and Lung Institute, chaired by James W. DuShane, MD, of the Mayo Clinic, which produced a "Classification of Heart Disease in Childhood" in 1970. His two books on congenital heart disease in adults appeared in 1979 and 1987, respectively.

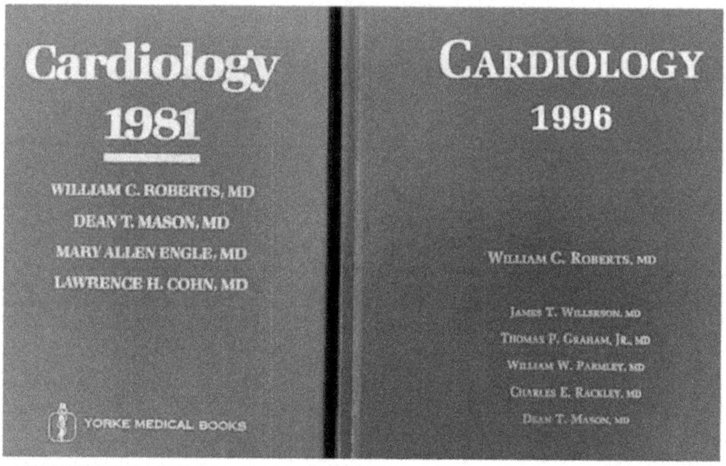

Figure 25. For 16 years (1981-1996), WCR edited an annual review of cardiology, and for 3 more years he was associate editor for James T. Willerson, MD [1939-2020]. Dean T. Mason, MD was associate editor of all 16 volumes.

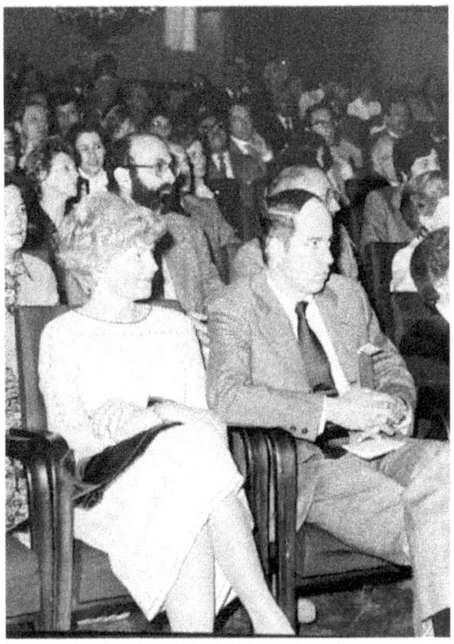

Figure 26. WCR and Carey traveled to many foreign countries together, including this trip to Florence, Italy. As his children grew up, WCR would invite them to join him. Before college, this writer joined him on several trips, domestic and international, including to New York City, to London and Amsterdam, and to France and Switzerland.

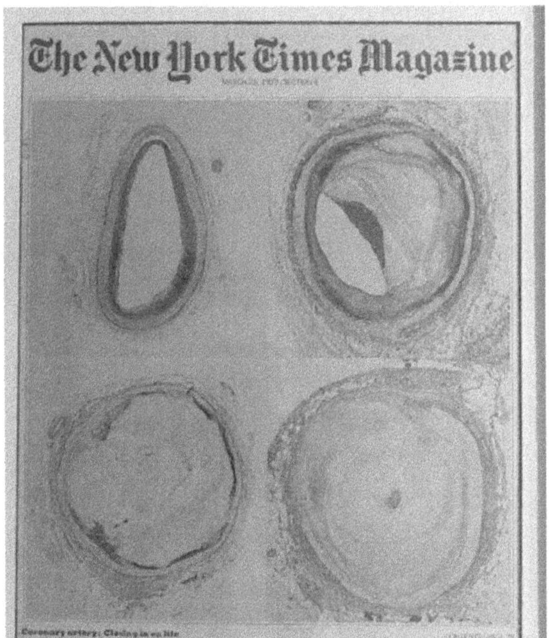

Figure 27. WCR pursued all areas of cardiovascular disease, but perhaps the dominant disease of research was coronary atherosclerosis. Photographs from his laboratory appeared in this *New York Times Magazine* cover published in 1973. When examining a heart from a necropsy patient with coronary atherosclerosis, he would remove the coronary arterial tree and divide it into 5 mm sections which would be examined by microscopy. In this way, he came to the view that coronary atherosclerosis was a diffuse, not focal disease. He advocated prevention by lowering serum cholesterol levels. He became a pescatarian at age 52 and was an early advocate of statin therapy.

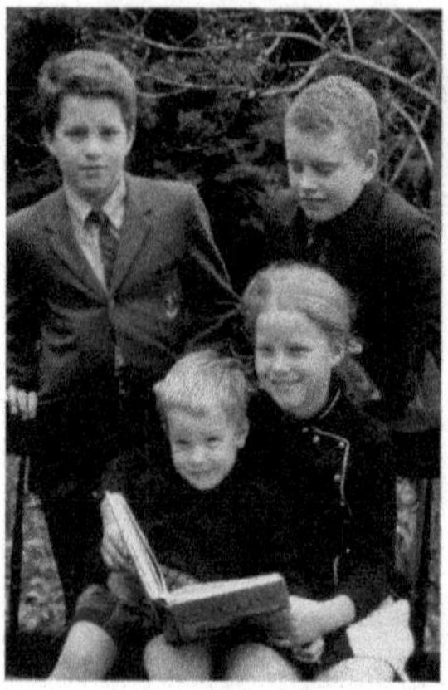

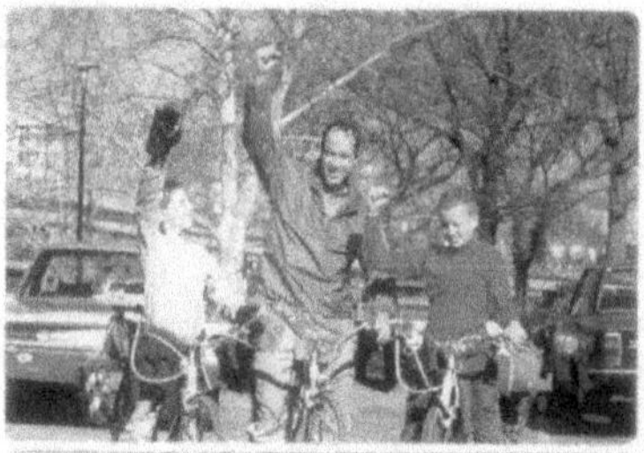

Figure 28. *Left*, WCR and his wife of 36 years, Carey Cansler Roberts, had 4 children (Chuck and Cliff in the back and John and Cay in the front). The home was always full of books. Both parents shared a love of learning. The family of 6 would visit numerous places in the Washington, DC, area— the battlefields, plantations, monuments, museums, and galleries. It was a weekly education for the children before college and an activity that both parents fully supported. Carey knew Virginia and English history well and published on those subjects. WCR also took an interest in natural history . *Right*, WCR and 2 sons after a memorable 5 day bicycle trip on the towpath of the Chesapeake and Ohio Canal.

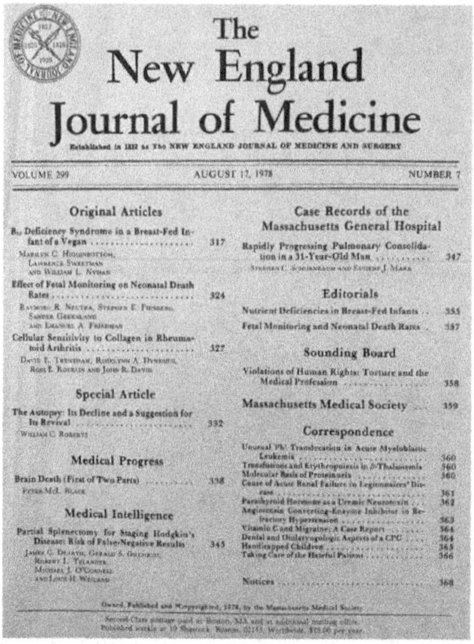

The New England Journal of Medicine

Established in 1812 as The NEW ENGLAND JOURNAL OF MEDICINE AND SURGERY

VOLUME 299 AUGUST 17, 1978 NUMBER 7

Original Articles

B_{12} Deficiency Syndrome in a Breast-Fed Infant of a Vegan ... 317
Marilyn C. Higginbottom, Lawrence Sweetman and William L. Nyhan

Effect of Fetal Monitoring on Neonatal Death Rates ... 324
Raymond R. Neutra, Stephen E. Fienberg, Sander Greenland and Emanuel A. Friedman

Cellular Sensitivity to Collagen in Rheumatoid Arthritis ... 327
David E. Trentham, Roselynn A. Dynesius, Ross E. Rocklin and John R. David

Special Article

The Autopsy: Its Decline and a Suggestion for Its Revival ... 332
William C. Roberts

Medical Progress

Brain Death (First of Two Parts) ... 338
Peter McL. Black

Medical Intelligence

Partial Splenectomy for Staging Hodgkin's Disease: Risk of False-Negative Results ... 345
James G. Dearth, Gerald S. Gilchrist, Robert L. Telander, Michael J. O'Connell and Louis H. Weiland

Case Records of the Massachusetts General Hospital

Rapidly Progressing Pulmonary Consolidation in a 31-Year-Old Man ... 347
Stephen C. Schoenbaum and Eugene J. Mark

Editorials

Nutrient Deficiencies in Breast-Fed Infants ... 355
Fetal Monitoring and Neonatal Death Rates ... 357

Sounding Board

Violations of Human Rights: Torture and the Medical Profession ... 358

Massachusetts Medical Society ... 359

Correspondence

Unusual Ph¹ Translocation in Acute Myeloblastic Leukemia ... 360
Transfusions and Erythropoiesis in β-Thalassemia ... 360
Molecular Basis of Proteinuria ... 360
Cause of Acute Renal Failure in Legionnaires' Disease ... 361
Parathyroid Hormone as a Uremic Neurotoxin ... 362
Angiotensin Converting-Enzyme Inhibitor in Refractory Hypertension ... 363
Vitamin C and Migraine: A Case Report ... 364
Dental and Otolaryngologic Aspects of a CPC ... 364
Handicapped Children ... 365
Taking Care of the Hateful Patient ... 366

Notices ... 368

Owned, Published and Copyrighted, 1978, by the Massachusetts Medical Society

Second-Class postage paid at Boston, MA and at additional mailing office. Published weekly at 10 Shattuck, Boston, 02115. Worldwide, [illegible] per year.

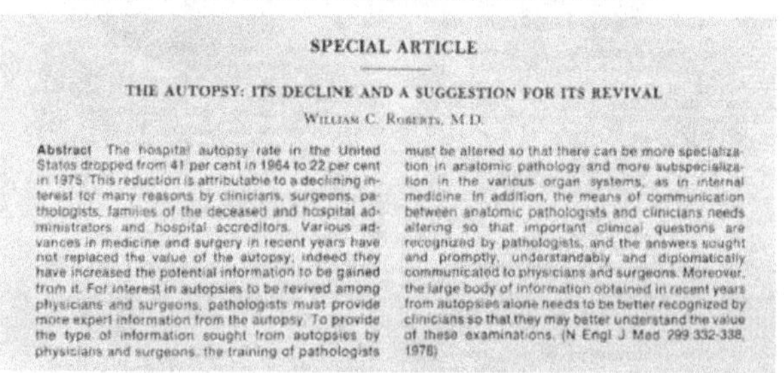

SPECIAL ARTICLE

THE AUTOPSY: ITS DECLINE AND A SUGGESTION FOR ITS REVIVAL

William C. Roberts, M.D.

Abstract The hospital autopsy rate in the United States dropped from 41 per cent in 1964 to 22 per cent in 1975. This reduction is attributable to a declining interest for many reasons by clinicians, surgeons, pathologists, families of the deceased and hospital administrators and hospital accreditors. Various advances in medicine and surgery in recent years have not replaced the value of the autopsy; indeed they have increased the potential information to be gained from it. For interest in autopsies to be revived among physicians and surgeons, pathologists must provide more expert information from the autopsy. To provide the type of information sought from autopsies by physicians and surgeons, the training of pathologists must be altered so that there can be more specialization in anatomic pathology and more subspecialization in the various organ systems, as in internal medicine. In addition, the means of communication between anatomic pathologists and clinicians needs altering so that important clinical questions are recognized by pathologists, and the answers sought and promptly, understandably and diplomatically communicated to physicians and surgeons. Moreover, the large body of information obtained in recent years from autopsies alone needs to be better recognized by clinicians so that they may better understand the value of these examinations. (N Engl J Med 299:332-338, 1978)

Figure 29. This article on "The Autopsy..." was published in 1978. The work of WCR, apart from surgical specimens, depended on the autopsy. For 3 decades, he collected hearts from multiple hospitals in the Washington, DC, area.

FROM THE EDITOR

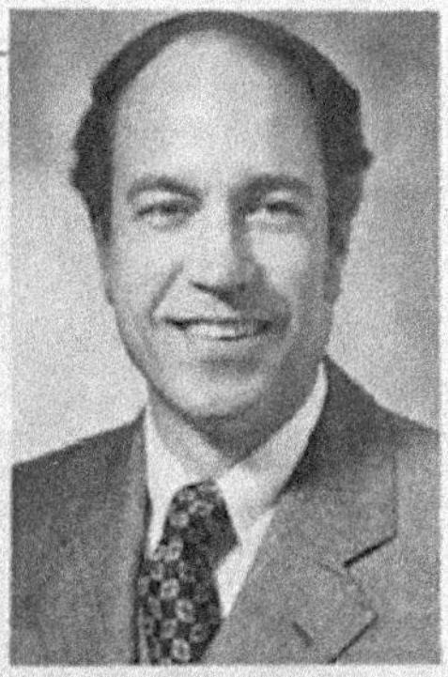

A Few Words From the *Journal*'s Second Editor

I am pleased and at the same time humbled to be the *Journal*'s new editor.* I am well aware of the enormous responsibility of an editor of a major journal today, and will do my best not to abuse or misuse that power. Editors, of course, play major roles in governing the fate of ideas and of their creators. I intend to seek advice and counsel from many quarters.

The *Journal* seeks your finest manuscripts. I pledge to those so submitting that their manuscript will be processed and reviewed expeditiously, that the authors will be treated respectfully, courteously and fairly, and that the interval from submission to acceptance or rejection will be held to a minimum. I have 2 suggestions for authors submitting papers: (1) that they include a *letter* to me stating precisely and concisely the significance and uniqueness of the work in their view, and (2) that they provide several *names* of nonlocal experts who they believe could give objective and informed reviews of their work. These suggested reviewers will be carefully considered along with other experts in the field. Additionally, I would listen if authors occasionally provided the name of an investigator they consider unlikely to give an objective or fair review of their work.

The focus of the *Journal* will remain strongly clinical. I welcome suggestions from readers at any time.

William C. Roberts

William C. Roberts, MD
Editor-in-Chief

Figure 30. WCR followed Simon Dack as the second Editor in Chief of The *American Journal of Cardiology*. He set up an editorial office in Bethesda, near the campus of NIH. As the AJC was not associated with a cardiology society, there were no automatic subscriptions for society members. Subscriptions depended entirely on quality which he strove to achieve. Competition was intense.

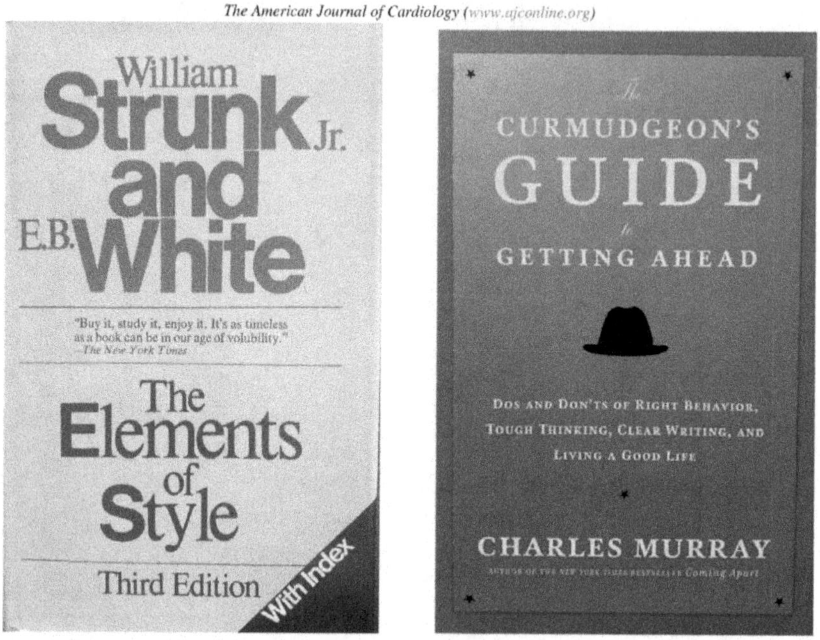

Figure 31. WCR was particular and precise about the English language. Routinely at night he read poems to his children at bedtime. The style book he routinely consulted was Strunk and White. In his library he had multiple shelves of books on the English language, writing, and editing. Charles Murray's short book he bought in bulk and gave to many people. The Bible was also part of his education early in life. His major at SMU was English. His library, medical and nonmedical, was enormous. His mother had donated most of his father's medical library to Emory. WCR collected many books on medical history, particularly by and about Sir William Osler.

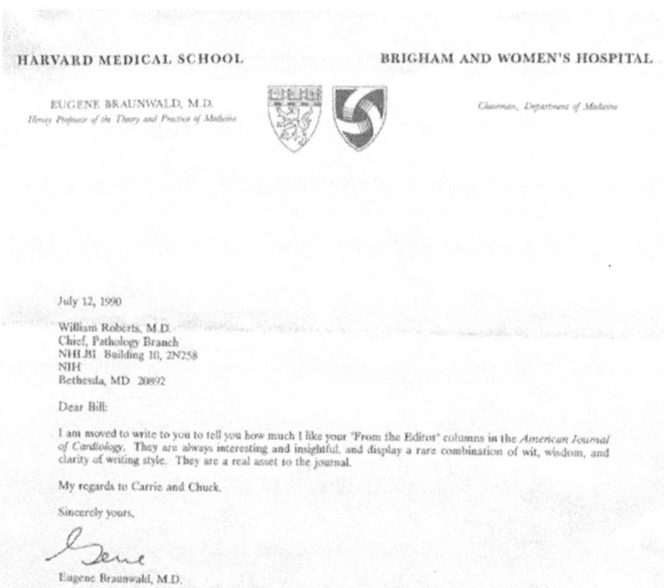

HARVARD MEDICAL SCHOOL BRIGHAM AND WOMEN'S HOSPITAL

EUGENE BRAUNWALD, M.D.
Hersey Professor of the Theory and Practice of Medicine

Chairman, Department of Medicine

July 12, 1990

William Roberts, M.D.
Chief, Pathology Branch
NHLBI Building 10, 2N258
NIH
Bethesda, MD 20892

Dear Bill:

I am moved to write to you to tell you how much I like your 'From the Editor' columns in the *American Journal of Cardiology*. They are always interesting and insightful, and display a rare combination of wit, wisdom, and clarity of writing style. They are a real asset to the journal.

My regards to Carrie and Chuck.

Sincerely yours,

Gene

Eugene Braunwald, M.D.

Figure 32. WCR wrote numerous "From the Editor" columns for the AJC and received this letter from Eugene Braunwald.

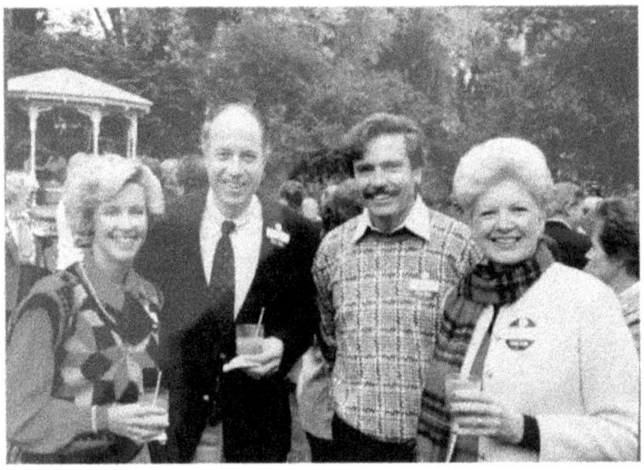

Figure 33. WCR traveled widely within the USA for speaking engagements, often to Hershey, Pennsylvania. In this photograph from left to right, is Margaret Anne Thorton Gruntzig (1956-1985), WCR, Andreas Roland Gruntzig (1939-1985), and Carey Roberts. At that meeting, Dr. Michael E. DeBakey mentioned to WCR that he wished Dr. Gruentzig did not fly his airplane for the danger involved. Gruentzig and his wife died in an airplane crash flying from the Georgia coast to Atlanta in a storm. WCR was close to numerous contemporaries at Emory in Atlanta, beginning with J. Willis Hurst.

```
7/91

                         VISITING HOSPITAL SCHEDULE

WCR            Howard University
HU                  1st Monday..each month @ 1 pm
                         Pathology - (202)806-6307 Angela Bates
                         (202) 806-6306
                         Chairman (Vivian Finn) (202) 636-6306
                         Edna - (202) 865-6309 or (202) 865-1353
Susan          Washington Hospital Center
WHC                 1st Wednesday..each month @ 10:30 am
                         Dr. Joseph Lindsay - (202) 877-7597
                                   (Joyce)
WCR            George Washington University (Grand Rounds)
GWU                 1st Wednesday..each month @ 5 pm
                         Dr. Allen Ross, Cardiology 202-994-3777
                         or x5098 (Contact Jean Hicks)
                         Dr. Richard Katz - 202-994-4183 schedule
---------------------------------------------------------------------

Dan            Georgetown University Medical Center
GT                  every Thursday @ 4pm
                         Pathology Dept. 202-784-3614
                         Paging Operator 202-687-7243
Gisela         Suburban Hospital
SH                  2nd Tuesday..each month @ 8 am
                         Pathology - 530-2566 (Pam or Marsha)
Jamshid        DC Medical Examiner's Office
DCMEO               last Monday..each month @ 1:15 pm
                         Dr. Kim - 202-724-4330 or Margie
                         Dr. Okoye (Mrs. Yvonne Barnes-727-9462)
Jamshid        DC General Hospital
DCGH                last Monday..each month @ 2:30 pm
                         Dr. Kaviani (Robin Mitchell)-675-7176
---------------------------------------------------------------------

Susanne        DC Veterans Administration Hospital
DCVAH               4th Tuesday @ 2 pm
                         Lab service - 202-745-8281
                         Pathology - Drs. Patterson & Saini
                         202-745-8284 or x7497 (Rm. #GB 141)
Susanne        DC Children's Hospital
DCCH                4th Tuesday @ 4 pm
                         Dr. Thomas Hougen, Chairman, Cardiology, 745-2090
                         (BJ), Dr. Frank Midgely, Chief, Cardiac Surgery 745-
                         2137, Dr. Roma Chandra, Chief, Pathology 745-2051
Dan            National Naval Medical Center
NNMC                4th Wednesday..each month @ 4 pm
                         Pathology resident 295-2829 or 295-2520
                         Cardiology - Dr. Baker 295-1075
                         Medical Records - 295-1134
                         Morgue - Norman Oldenburgh 295-2509
                         Dr. Orgorzaleck - 295-0088
WCR            Franklin Square Hospital
FSH                 3 times yearly
                         Dr. Ernest Arnett (301) 391-3900 or x7136
```

Figure 34. This was a schedule of WCR's visits to 11 hospitals in the Washington, DC, area. One of his fellows would usually accompany him and carry back to NIH the yellow buckets with the hearts. A conference would be given at the hospital on each visit for the local staff. In this way, WCR accumulated thousands of hearts to study for his research.

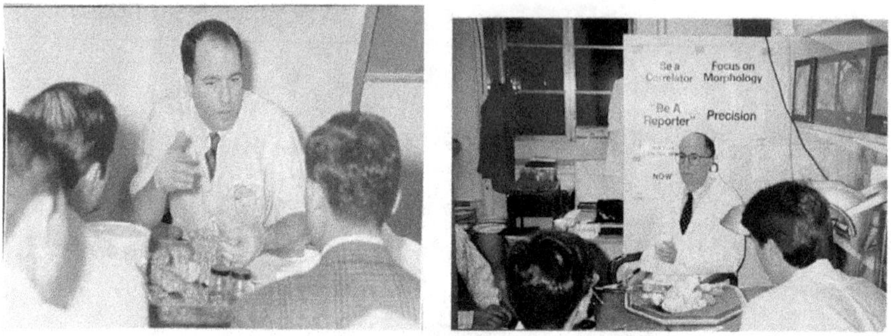

Figure 35. Left, WCR giving a conference at the Bethesda Naval Hospital which was across the street from NIH. Right, WCR at his weekly conference in his laboratory at NIH. These conferences could be rather stressful for the fellows as WCR posed questions frequently and expected clear answers.

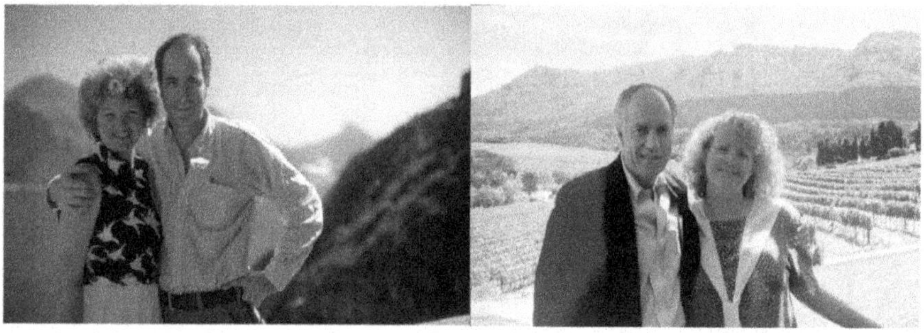

Figure 36. WCR went to South Africa twice. Left, with his wife, Carey in 1974, and right, with his daughter Frances in 1993. They had dinner with Professor John Barlow (of Barlow's Syndrome) and his wife at their home in Johannesburg.

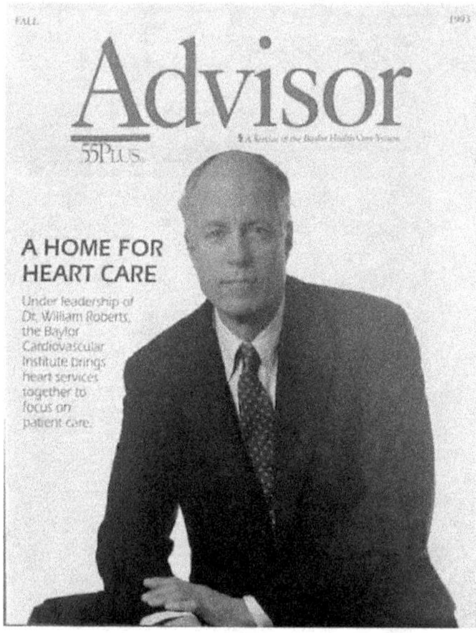
Advisor
55Plus
A HOME FOR HEART CARE
Under leadership of Dr. William Roberts, the Baylor Cardiovascular Institute brings heart services together to focus on patient care.

Figure 37. This began the second period of his career at age 61 in 1993, another 30 years. He managed to withdraw from administrative activities over time and devote his energy to cardiovascular research.

TELEDYNE MINERALS

March 14, 1994

Dr. William C. Roberts
Executive Director
Baylor Cardiovascular Institute
3500 Gaston Avenue
Dallas, Texas 75246

Dear Bill:

Jane and I enjoyed the dinner and your talk the other night at the Old Warsaw. You are certainly right - your data on cholesterol lowering drugs, diet, and exercise need to be communicated to doctors as well as their patients. You have been a big help to me.

Please note that I have a new office address.

Regards,

Jack

Jack H. Hamilton

Figure 38. The building in which WCR has his office is the Jack and Jane Hamilton Heart and Vascular Hospital, now called Baylor Heart and Vascular Hospital.

FROM THE EDITOR

Obtaining and Maintaining an Ideal Body Weight

Immediately following the 71st Scientific Session of the American Heart Association in November 1998, I flew to Tokyo. The 209 passengers were 90% Japanese returning home after the meeting. While observing the boarding process, I did not see a single Japanese passenger who was overweight!

In contrast, think what they saw in the USA, the heaviest nation in the world and yet a nation whose population is fixated on weight. A large percentage of our population is constantly dieting. Leanness is an obsession, but the minority of our population ≥20 years of age are lean. Indeed, 60% of adults in the USA are overweight and 30% are obese (>20% over ideal body weight). No nation in the history of the planet has witnessed overweightness to the extent as that in the USA. Only the Bible sells better in America than do diet books. The most common New Year's resolution in the USA is to lose weight. (Most are broken within 2 weeks.) Many men and women in the USA seem to have their plan for obtaining and maintaining an ideal body weight. Here's mine:

1. I weigh myself every morning upon arising. My number is 170 pounds (I am 72 inches tall), which means that if I am over that number I am particularly careful that day. I have good scales, like those found in physicians' offices, and, therefore, I believe the number. Weighing daily helps to prevent the sudden 5-pound gain. Having a weight number and not changing that number as the weight increases is crucial.

2. I usually eat a light breakfast, consisting, for example, of bran cereal with skim milk or a banana, both with a glass of grapefruit juice. Often on weekends I skip breakfast.

3. For lunch I usually have 3 vegetables.

4. I usually eat whatever I like at supper. If I have flesh, it is fish.

5. I rarely eat anything between meals. When we have these long "starvation periods" between meals, that's when we eat our anterior panniculus.

6. I make desserts on special occasions, such that I eat no more than about 1 dessert a week.

7. I drink water with most meals and avoid the high-caloric cokes. Stone-age men and women drank essentially only water. I drink coffee black and tea as it is served. The caloric cost (7 calories/g of alcohol) is taken into consideration.

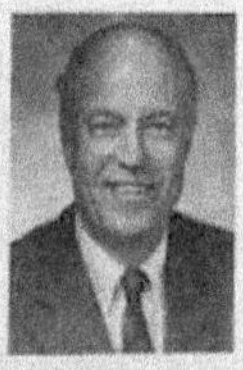

8. I plan for festive occasions (or long, usually foreign, plane rides) so that I can eat heartily if I wish. If I'm going to a party or a Thanksgiving feast I eat very little preceding or immediately following the event. I try to count calories by the week, not by the day or by the meal. It's important to be able to "cheat" occasionally. Calories need to be budgeted by the week, just like money. In this way the particularly good meal can be fully enjoyed.

9. I virtually never eat at bedtime.

Vigorous exercise of course allows for a higher caloric intake, but exercise, unless it is frequent and not followed by a Big Mac, is a difficult way to lose pounds. One has to walk or run 35 miles to lose 1 pound! I try to avoid elevators and to walk rapidly around the hospital. Sometimes, I purposely park my automobile a distance from my destination so that I am required to walk.

Thus, weighing myself daily, limiting consumption of flesh and desserts, avoiding snacks, limiting intake of high-caloric liquids, walking rapidly and using stairs seems to work for me.

I welcome your methods and recommendations.

William C. Roberts

William Clifford Roberts, MD
Baylor University Medical Center
Dallas, Texas 75246

Figure 39. Throughout his career, WCR advocated ideal body weight. The obesity epidemic hit the USA in the last decade of the 20th century. He observed hearts become increasingly covered in adiposity. Those fatty hearts would float in water, whereas those with minimal adiposity would sink.

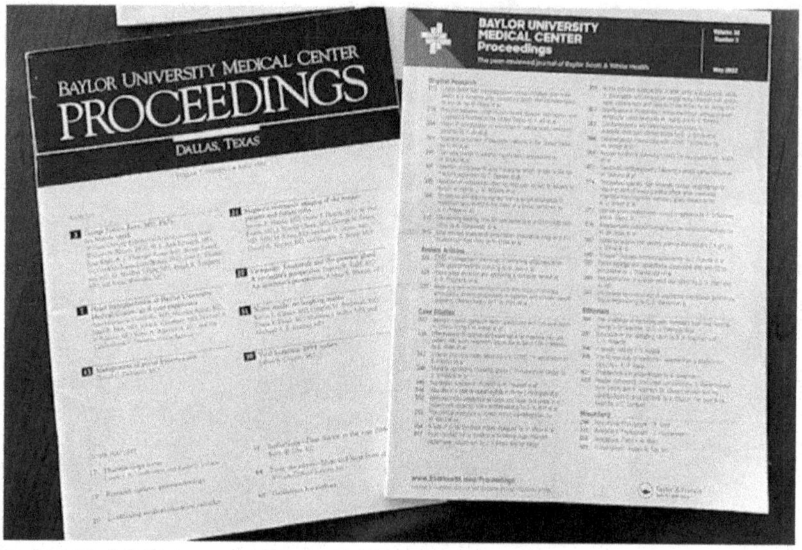

Figure 40. Shortly after arriving in Dallas, he was offered the editorship of the *Baylor University Medical Center Proceedings*, following George Race. During the 28 years of his editorship, the Proceedings was added to PubMed and became published by an international company, Taylor & Francis. Owing to his relationships with many colleagues nationally and internationally, WCR was able to attract manuscripts in areas such as medical history from authors presenting papers at the American Osler Society. Although manuscripts were sent out for review, WCR was, in many respects, a one-man committee when it came to editorial matters. For many years, he personally solicited manuscripts on the Dallas campus of BUMC. By the end of his tenure, over half of the manuscripts submitted to *BUMC Proceedings* came from other institutions. For many years, WCR wrote a column called, "Facts and Ideas from Anywhere," which he dictated from his wide reading.

Roberts Family Gatherings
Supported by William C. Roberts, MD
1998-2020 [23 years]

YEAR	SUMMER	WINTER
1998	Gracie Inn, New York, NY	Greenbrier, White Sulfur Springs, WV
1999	Montreal, Canada	Greenbrier, White Sulfur Springs, WV
2000	Swissotel, Boston, MA	Greenbrier, White Sulfur Springs, WV
2001	Swissotel, Chicago, IL	Greenbrier, White Sulfur Springs, WV
2002	Button Wood Square, Philadelphia, PA	Greenbrier, White Sulfur Springs, WV
2003	University Club,San Francisco, CA	Greenbrier, White Sulfur Springs, WV
2004	Cosmopolitan Club, New York, NY	Greenbrier,White Sulfur Springs, WV
2005	Homestead, Hot Springs, VA	Greenbrier, White Sulfur Springs, WV
2006	Homestead, Hot Springs, VA	Greenbrier, White Sulfur Springs, WV
2007	Homestead, Hot Springs, VA	Greenbrier, White Sulfur Springs, WV
2008	Homestead, Hot Springs, VA	French Lick Resort, French Lick, IN
2009	High Hampton, Cashiers, NC	Greenbrier, White Sulfur Spring, WV
2010	High Hampton, Cashiers, NC	Cosmos Club, Washington, DC
2011	High Hampton, Cashiers, NC	Cosmos Club, Washington, DC
2012	High Hampton, Cashiers, NC	----------------------------------
2013	High Hampton, Cashiers, NC	Renaissance Hotel, Charleston, SC
2014	High Hampton, Cashiers, NC	Hyatt Regency, Savannah, GA
2015	High Hampton, Cashiers, NC	Melrose Hotel, Dallas, TX
2016	Grove Park Inn, Asheville, NC	Mansion of Forsyth Park, Savannah, GA
2017	High Hampton, Cashiers, NC	The Lexington Hotel, New York, NY
2018	High Hampton, Cashiers, NC	Four Seasons Hotel, Austin, TX
2019	Omni Barton Resort, Austin, TX	Grand Hyatt, New York, NY
2020	Warwick Melrose, Dallas, TX	(COVID pandemic)

Figure 41. For 2 decades, WCR hosted large family gatherings twice a year. When his grandchildren were young, the summer trip was usually to a city where the daily activity was educational. The two primary destinations were The Greenbrier during New Years and High Hampton in June.

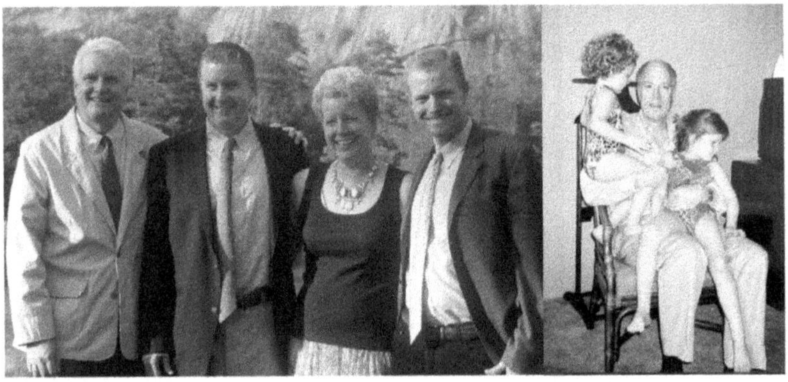

Figure 42. Left, The 4 children of WCR (Cliff, Chuck, Cay, and John) Right, WCR with two granddaughters, Amelia on the right and Camille on the left. He was regarded by all as the "Patriarch."

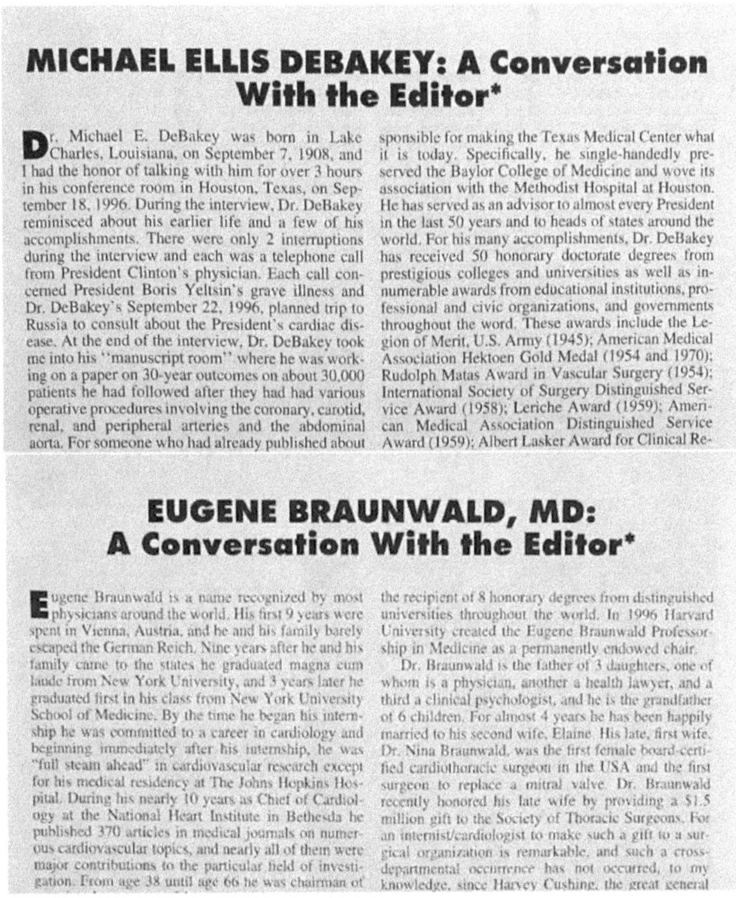

MICHAEL ELLIS DEBAKEY: A Conversation With the Editor*

Dr. Michael E. DeBakey was born in Lake Charles, Louisiana, on September 7, 1908, and I had the honor of talking with him for over 3 hours in his conference room in Houston, Texas, on September 18, 1996. During the interview, Dr. DeBakey reminisced about his earlier life and a few of his accomplishments. There were only 2 interruptions during the interview and each was a telephone call from President Clinton's physician. Each call concerned President Boris Yeltsin's grave illness and Dr. DeBakey's September 22, 1996, planned trip to Russia to consult about the President's cardiac disease. At the end of the interview, Dr. DeBakey took me into his "manuscript room" where he was working on a paper on 30-year outcomes on about 30,000 patients he had followed after they had had various operative procedures involving the coronary, carotid, renal, and peripheral arteries and the abdominal aorta. For someone who had already published about sponsible for making the Texas Medical Center what it is today. Specifically, he single-handedly preserved the Baylor College of Medicine and wove its association with the Methodist Hospital at Houston. He has served as an advisor to almost every President in the last 50 years and to heads of states around the world. For his many accomplishments, Dr. DeBakey has received 50 honorary doctorate degrees from prestigious colleges and universities as well as innumerable awards from educational institutions, professional and civic organizations, and governments throughout the word. These awards include the Legion of Merit, U.S. Army (1945); American Medical Association Hektoen Gold Medal (1954 and 1970); Rudolph Matas Award in Vascular Surgery (1954); International Society of Surgery Distinguished Service Award (1958); Leriche Award (1959); American Medical Association Distinguished Service Award (1959); Albert Lasker Award for Clinical Re-

EUGENE BRAUNWALD, MD: A Conversation With the Editor*

Eugene Braunwald is a name recognized by most physicians around the world. His first 9 years were spent in Vienna, Austria, and he and his family barely escaped the German Reich. Nine years after he and his family came to the states he graduated magna cum laude from New York University, and 3 years later he graduated first in his class from New York University School of Medicine. By the time he began his internship he was committed to a career in cardiology and beginning immediately after his internship, he was "full steam ahead" in cardiovascular research except for his medical residency at The Johns Hopkins Hospital. During his nearly 10 years as Chief of Cardiology at the National Heart Institute in Bethesda he published 370 articles in medical journals on numerous cardiovascular topics, and nearly all of them were major contributions to the particular field of investigation. From age 38 until age 66 he was chairman of the recipient of 8 honorary degrees from distinguished universities throughout the world. In 1996 Harvard University created the Eugene Braunwald Professorship in Medicine as a permanently endowed chair.

Dr. Braunwald is the father of 3 daughters, one of whom is a physician, another a health lawyer, and a third a clinical psychologist, and he is the grandfather of 6 children. For almost 4 years he has been happily married to his second wife, Elaine. His late, first wife, Dr. Nina Braunwald, was the first female board-certified cardiothoracic surgeon in the USA and the first surgeon to replace a mitral valve. Dr. Braunwald recently honored his late wife by providing a $1.5 million gift to the Society of Thoracic Surgeons. For an internist/cardiologist to make such a gift to a surgical organization is remarkable, and such a cross-departmental occurrence has not occurred, to my knowledge, since Harvey Cushing, the great general

Figure 43. After arriving in Dallas in 1993, WCR had little data to work with in the early years at BUMC, so he spent time interviewing pioneers in cardiovascular disease, including Drs. DeBakey and Braunwald. WCR was offered the position of Chair of Pathology at Baylor in Houston by DeBakey. WCR eventually turned down the offer to stay at NIH, but they remained friends for decades.

Commonalities among interviewees

- Parents devoted to children
- Love abundant from parents
- Education stressed by parents
- Enormous curiosity to learn
- Superb students
- Passion for medicine
- Worked exceedingly hard
- Slept little (<6 hours)
- Incredibly focused on goals
- Good writers
- Good teachers and mentors
- Competitive
- Strong character
- Good capacity for friendship
- Little or no alcohol

Figure 44. After interviewing numerous prominent physicians (146 published interviews over a 30-year period), WCR summarized many of the qualities shared by these distinguished and successful physicians.[9]

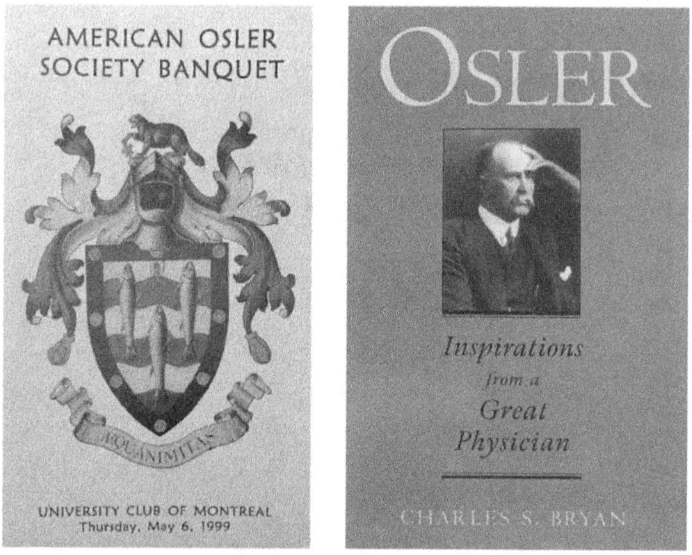

Figure 45. In 1999, WCR joined the American Osler Society. BUMC had the largest contingent, including Marvin J. Stone, MD, and Michael Emmett, MD. WCR also became friends with Charles S. Bryan, MD, a distinguished physician in Columbia, South Carolina, who was author of numerous books and articles on Osler.

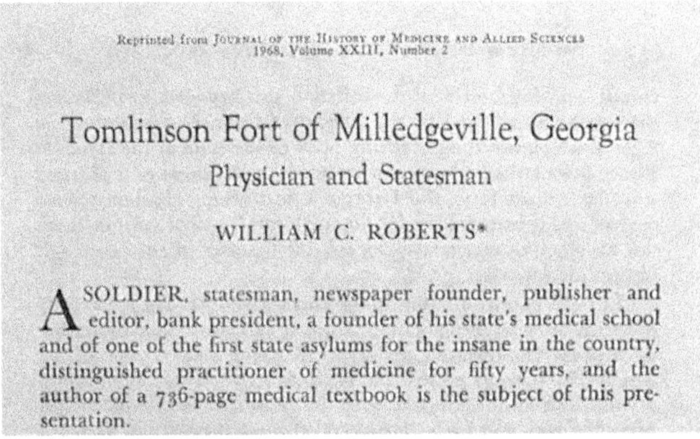

Reprinted from JOURNAL OF THE HISTORY OF MEDICINE AND ALLIED SCIENCES
1968, Volume XXIII, Number 2

Tomlinson Fort of Milledgeville, Georgia

Physician and Statesman

WILLIAM C. ROBERTS*

A SOLDIER, statesman, newspaper founder, publisher and editor, bank president, a founder of his state's medical school and of one of the first state asylums for the insane in the country, distinguished practitioner of medicine for fifty years, and the author of a 736-page medical textbook is the subject of this presentation.

Figure 46. WCR had a lifelong interest in medical history which was often reflected in his writings. The above article was his first and only "formal" or academic medical history paper, published in 1968.[10] Many editorials discuss medical history, however, and WCR had a special interest in Sir William Osler, particularly his observations on the bicuspid aortic valve and infective endocarditis.

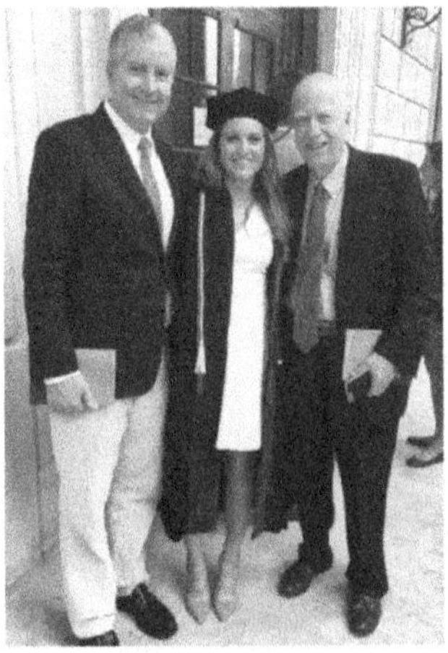

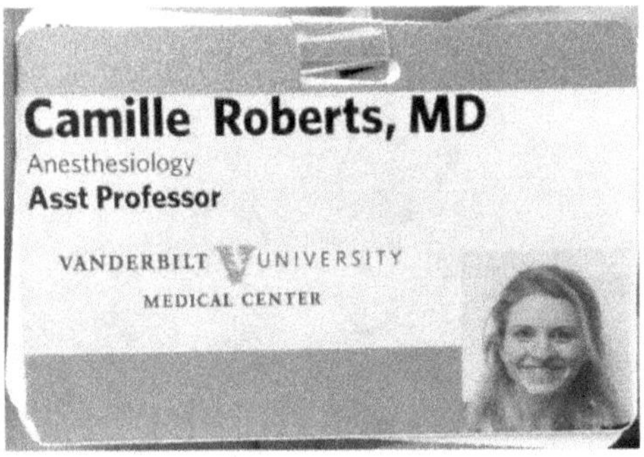

Figure 47. Carey Camille Roberts, center on left, a grandchild of WCR, graduated from Georgetown University School of Medicine and is now an anesthesiologist at Vanderbilt, a 4th generation physician.

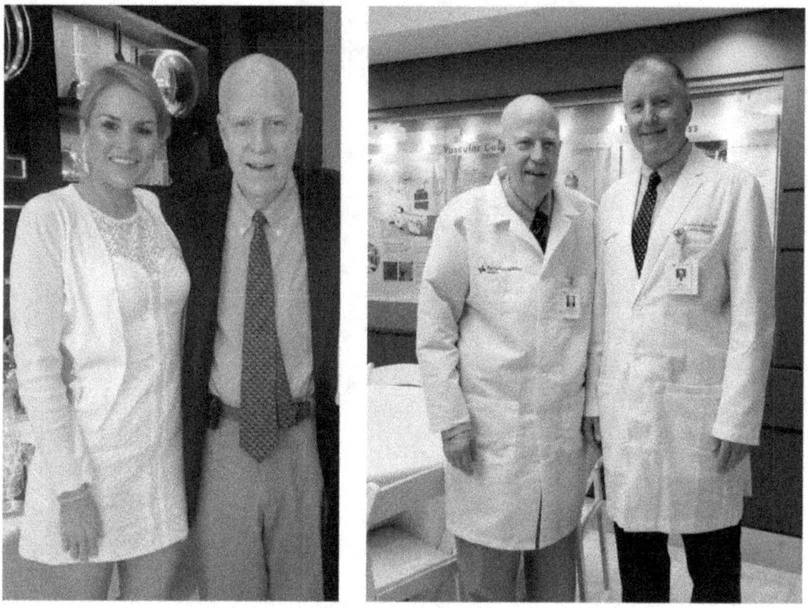

Figure 48. Left, WCR with his oldest grandchild, Amelia Roberts Knox. She lives in Dallas and has 3 children. Right, WCR with his second son, Charles, who moved to Dallas in 2018 and served as Chair of the Department of Cardiac Surgery.

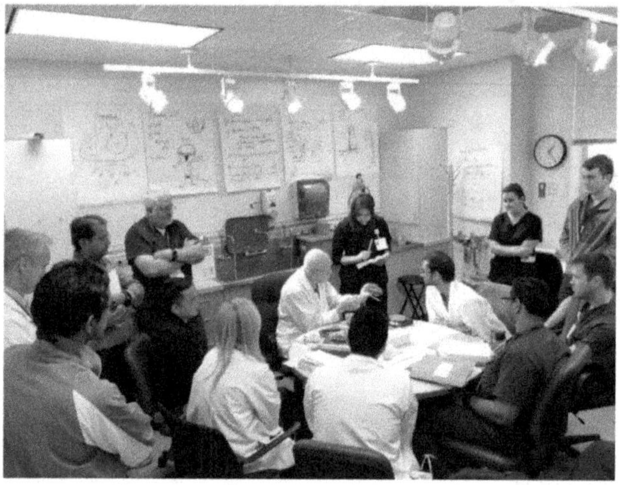

Figure 49. WCR held a weekly conference at BUMC in which he reviewed the cardiovascular specimens received from the autopsy suite or the operating room—hearts, valves, tumors, aortas, devices, etc. Under the direction of Dr. Peter McCullough (far left), the cardiology fellows routinely attended. This format remained consistent for 60 years (1964-2023).

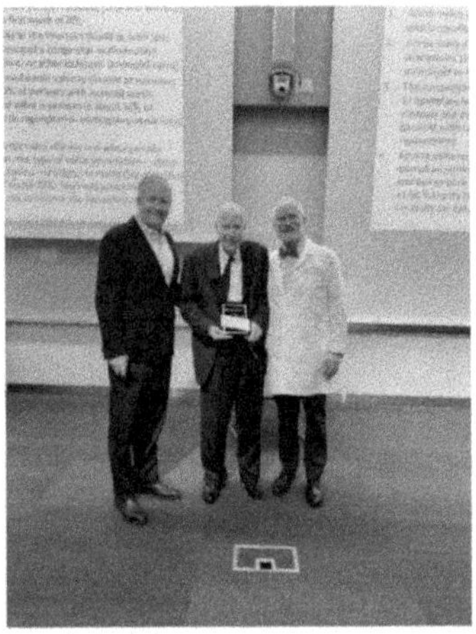

Figure 50. The last speaking engagement of WCR was in Austin, Texas, at the invitation of Dr. George Rogers of Dell Medical School in October 2022. At its inaugural grand rounds in cardiology, WCR spoke on aortic stenosis, a favorite subject over 6 decades. The number of "Presentations" recorded in his C.V. is 2363.

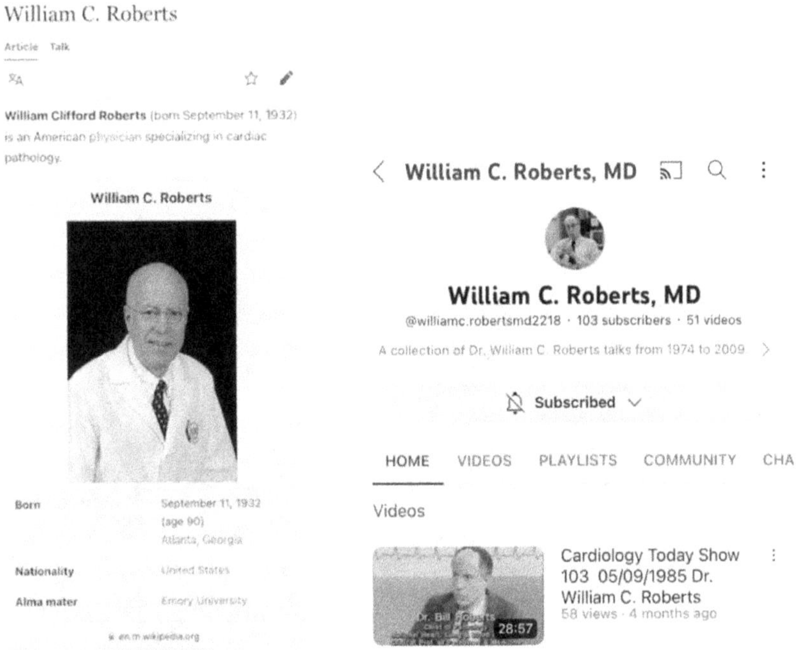

Figure 51. Left, a Wikipedia page was created in 2010 by a research fellow at Baylor. WCR's "influences" are listed as "Jesse Edwards, Glenn Morrow, and Eugene Braunwald." Right, 51 talks by WCR were preserved on tapes over the years and were uploaded to YouTube. His confidence at the podium and command of the subject matter is evident.

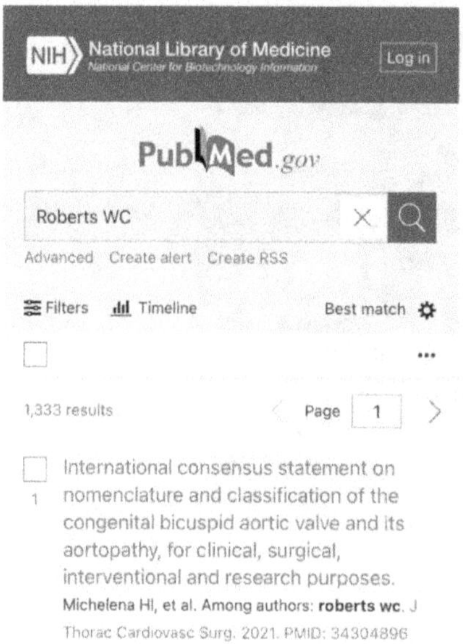

Title
1. Best publications
2. Aorta
3. Aortic regurgitation
4. Aortic stenosis (new TOC 9-9)
5. Aortic syphilis
6. Cardiac sarcoidosis
7. Cardiovascular cancer
8. Coronary artery bypass grafting
9. Coronary artery disease
10. Heart transplantation
11. Hypertrophic cardiomyopathy
121. Infectious endocarditis
13. Isolated coronary anomalies
14. Mitral stenosis
15. Mitral valve prolapse
16. Mitral valve regurgitation
17. Myocardial heart disease
18. Preventive cardiology
19. Primary and secondary lung disease
20. Prosthetic heart valves
21. Pulmonary hypertension
22. Usefulness of Measuring 12-lead QRS
23. Valvular heart disease
24. Miscellaneous

Figure 52. Left, Publications of WCR were 1,333 on January 8, 2023. It is interesting that WCR appears on a "Consensus Statement," because he generally opposed consensus guidelines, particularly in preventive cardiology. Right, WCR collected his individual publications in numerous books beginning in 2023 and these are available on Amazon.

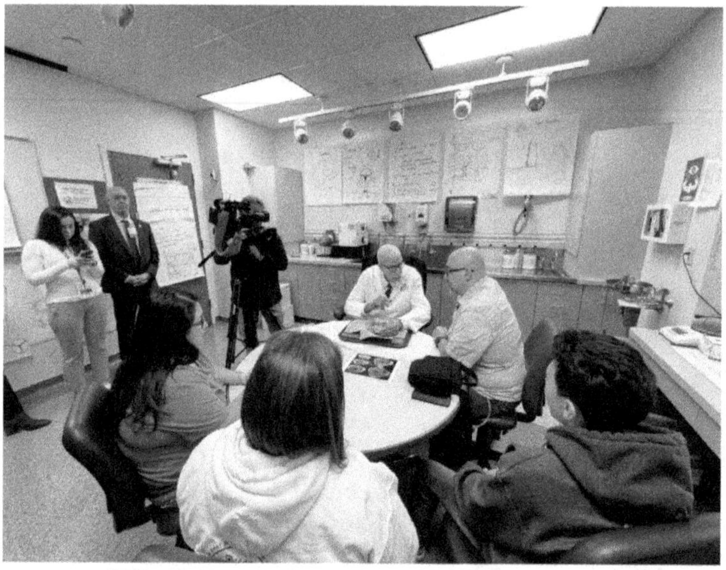

Figure 53. WCR began a program at BUMC called "Heart to Heart," for cardiac transplant recipients to see their own original heart. The patient and family members would come to his laboratory and WCR would examine their original heart, explaining the cause of the heart failure to the heart transplant recipient. These were very moving experiences for the patient and family who usually came for educational purposes. This program received considerable attention in the media. This program started by WCR at BUMC is the first of its kind, perhaps the first time in human history that a person has an opportunity to see and touch his or her heart.

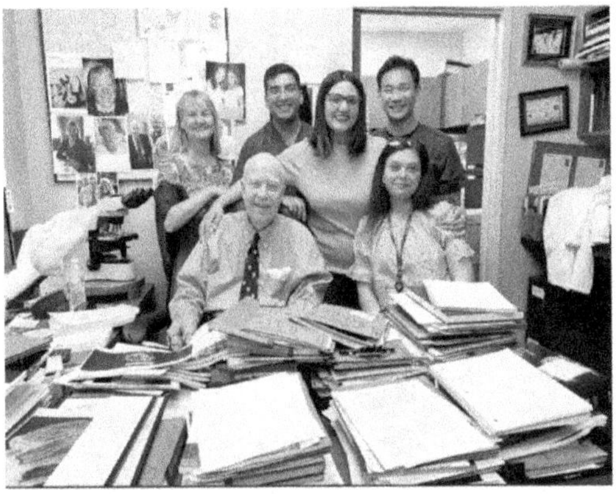

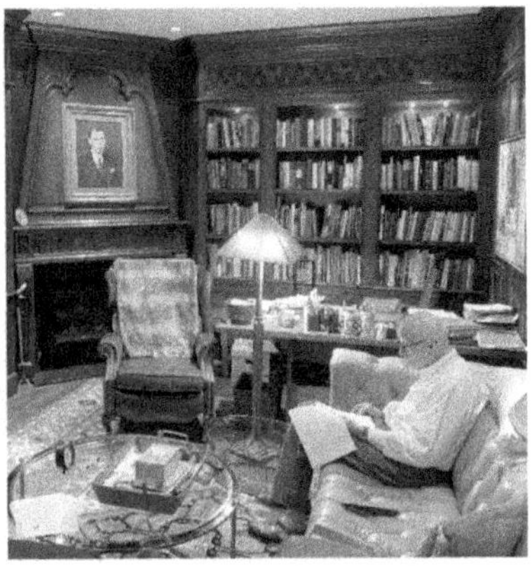

Figure 54. Throughout his 60 years as a laboratory chief, WCR had around him a team (left). His last team leader was Saba Ilyas, seated to his left. The desk of WCR was never clear at work or at home (above).

CLINICAL SIGNIFICANCE

- Physicians need to develop financial security so that their patient decisions are free of inappropriate financial reward.
- That requires becoming financially secure, which requires regular savings and appropriate spending.
- The best way to become financially secure is to invest in the stock market regularly over a long period of time.
- Buying and holding is not ideal, but it is better than frequent buying and selling.
- Stay out of debt.
- Stay healthy and live long. Good health is better than gold.

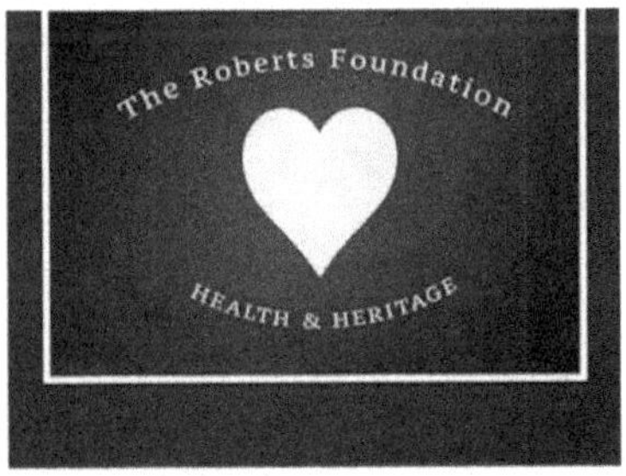

The Roberts Foundation Founded By
William C. Roberts, MD

Our Mission

The Roberts Foundation was founded by William C. Roberts, MD, in December 2018, with a mission to inspire scholarship and achievement in the fields of Health and American Heritage.

Figure 55. WCR was frugal with money and a long-term investor in stocks, especially railroads, oil and banks.[11] In addition, he was the "Generation One" donor to the Roberts Foundation (right).

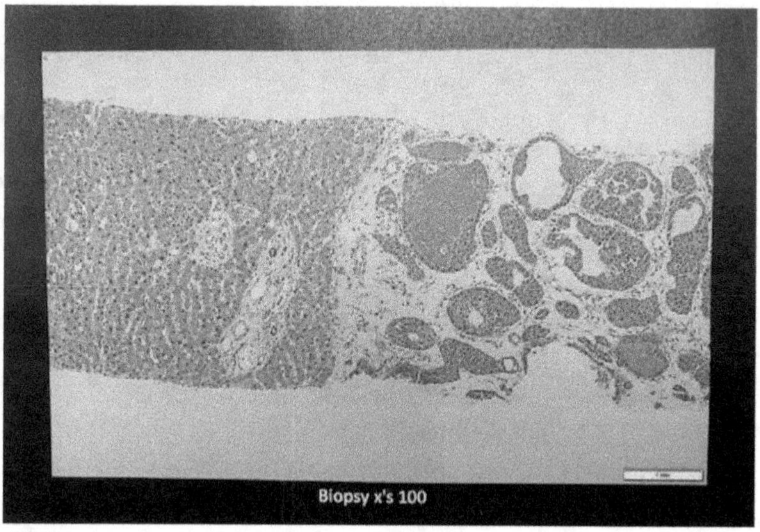

Figure 56. Percutaneous core biopsy of the liver of WCR showing, on the right, malignant metastatic renal cell carcinoma. Presently, WCR is undergoing treatment, and through it all, coming to work and processing the cardiovascular surgical and autopsy specimens at BUMC. He is beloved by his family and friends, and he is content with his 90 years on planet earth (CSR, February 19, 2023).

Declaration of interests

WCR is the father of the author.

1. Roberts WC, Fye WB. William Clifford Roberts, MD: an interview by W. Bruce Fye, MD. *Baylor Univ Med Cen Proceed* 2007;20:257–268.
2. Roberts WC, Roberts CS. William Clifford Roberts, MD: an interview by Charles Stewart Roberts, MD. *Am J Cardiol* 2007;100:338–390.
3. Roberts CS. The physician legacy of Stewart R. Roberts, MD (1878-1941), "The Osler of the South. *Am J Cardiol* 2022;162:191–196.
4. Roberts SR. *Pellagra: history, distribution, diagnosis, prognosis, treatment, etiology*. St. Louis: C. V. Mosby Company; 1912:272.
5. Roberts WC. Dr. Stewart R. Roberts' "An Ideal of Modern Medicine. *Ann Int Med* 1969;70:1016–1017.
6. editor. In: Roberts CS, ed. Selected articles and letters of Stewart R. Roberts, MD (1878-1941): the Osler of the South. Cambridge Scholars Publishing; 2022. p. 532.
7. Braunwald E, Ross RS, Morrow AG, Roberts WC. Differential diagnosis of mitral regurgitation in childhood; Clinical pathological conference at the National Institutes of Health. *Ann Int Med* 1961;54:1223–1242.
8. Maron BJ, Roberts WC. The father of septal myectomy for obstruction of HCM,who also had HCM. The unbelievable story. *J Am Coll Cardiol* 2016;67:2900–2903.
9. Roberts WC. Life lessons from modern day greats in cardiovascular disease. *Am J Cardiol* 2009;103:287–291.
10. Roberts WC. Tomlinson Fort of Milledgeville, Georgia. Physician and statesman. *J Hist Med Allied Sci* 1968;23:131–152.
11. Roberts WC. The importance of obtaining financial security. *Am J Med* 2020;133:1403–1405.

Roberts CS. WCR 90: Aspects of the Life and Work of William C. Roberts, MD. *Am J Cardiol.* 2023;195 Suppl 1:S2-S30. doi:10.1016/j.amjcard.2023.02.018

PROC (BAYL UNIV MED CENT)
2023;36(6):772–774

https://doi.org/10.1080/08998280.2023.2247946

Taylor & Francis
Taylor & Francis Group

Lessons from the life of William Harvey

Charles Stewart Roberts, MD

Department of Cardiac Surgery, Baylor University Medical Center, Dallas, Texas, USA

ABSTRACT
William Harvey (1578–1658) discovered that blood flows in a circle and described this new finding in a short book in 1628. He had superb educational opportunities but also faced great difficulties, which he met with personal and professional resilience. A study of his life is worthwhile. Presented here are 11 lessons drawn from Harvey's life and legacy.

KEYWORDS William Harvey; circulation

In his anatomy lectures in London in the year 1618, William Harvey (1578–1657) asserted that blood flows in a circle, challenging the authority of Galen.[1,2] Ten years later in 1628, Harvey published a short book in Latin, *De Motu Cordis* (*Figure 1*),[3] immortalizing him both in biology (*Figure 2*) and in medicine.[4,5] The study of a major medical figure can be instructive. The following are some lessons from the life of William Harvey.

1. *Understand that there are no shortcuts to knowledge*. The eldest of seven sons, Harvey was bred to learning in the late English Renaissance, like Shakespeare, part of an effort to raise the family status from yeoman to gentleman. His academic training was rigorous: 16 hours a day for 6 years at Cambridge University (1593–1599) and another 2 years at Padua University (1600–1602). Like Shakespeare, he banked a treasury of knowledge through slow, deliberate study. Harvey's education was broad, including both the humanities and the sciences. Scholars in that period were fluent in both and considered neither off limits. Like Shakespeare, Harvey also mastered disputation, a method of debate in which an understanding of traditional authorities and of the argument from each side was expected. As Zadie Smith wrote, "Our Shakespeare sees always both sides of a thing."[6] It was with a balanced background that Harvey inquired into the circulation.
2. *Go abroad*. Had there been no Padua, there would be no *De Motu Cordis*. Some educational experience abroad at the undergraduate, graduate, or postgraduate level widens the perspective. It was in Padua that Harvey was exposed to a tradition in anatomy that included Vesalius, Fallopius, and Fabricius. Realdo Colombo was one of the Paduan anatomists whose legacies influenced Harvey; Colombo discovered (or rediscovered) the pulmonary circuit. It was in Padua that Harvey first studied the valves in veins where that inquiry was a tradition. An Italian way of thinking was undoubtedly different than an English way of thinking in the year 1600, and this exposure no doubt influenced his views the rest of his life.
3. *Add a language*. Harvey was fluent in Latin, as most European scholars were, which he learned from Canterbury Grammar School. We may also assume that he achieved fluency in Italian while living in Padua. Harvey expressed himself simply and clearly in *De Motu Cordis*, inserting the word "circle" and its several derivative words (circulation, circuit, circuitous) 27 times, beginning in the famous chapter 8. Two-thirds of modern English words are from French (or Latin), owing to the Norman Invasion of 1066. English speakers would do well to learn a Latin language if only to enhance understanding of the English language and to improve communication.
4. *Seek a mentor*. Both of Harvey's books could be considered responses to books by Fabricius, his mentor in Padua, an anatomist for whom Harvey had tremendous respect. In 1603, Fabricius published a book on the venous valves arguing that their purpose was merely to

Corresponding author: Charles S. Roberts, MD, Department of Cardiac Surgery, Baylor University Medical Center, 621 North Hall Street, Suite 120, Dallas, TX 75226, USA (e-mail: charles.roberts@bswhealth.org)
The authors report no funding or conflicts of interest.
Presented as the Ronald C. Jones Lecture in Medical History to the Department of Surgery, Baylor University Medical Center, February 22, 2022.
Received March 29, 2023; Revised August 7, 2023; Accepted August 7, 2023.

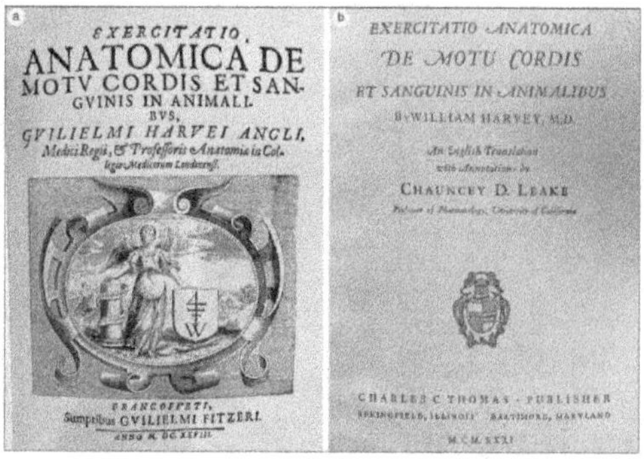

Figure 1. **(a)** Title page of Harvey's book, left, published in Latin in Frankfurt in 1628. **(b)** A translation by Chauncey D. Leake published in 1931.[3]

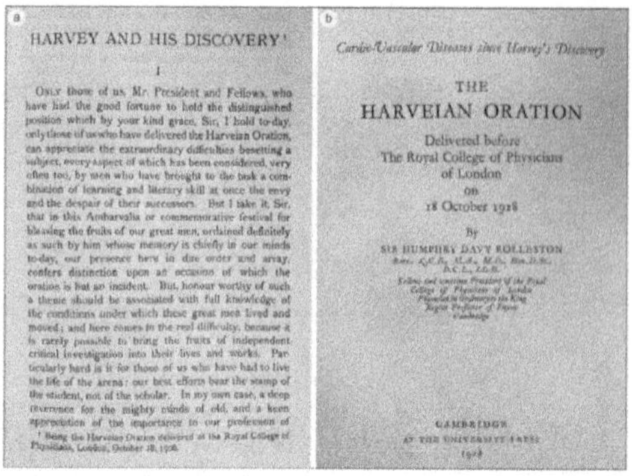

Figure 3. Two examples of the annual Harveian Oration: **(a)** one delivered by William Osler in 1906 and **(b)** one by Rolleston in 1928.

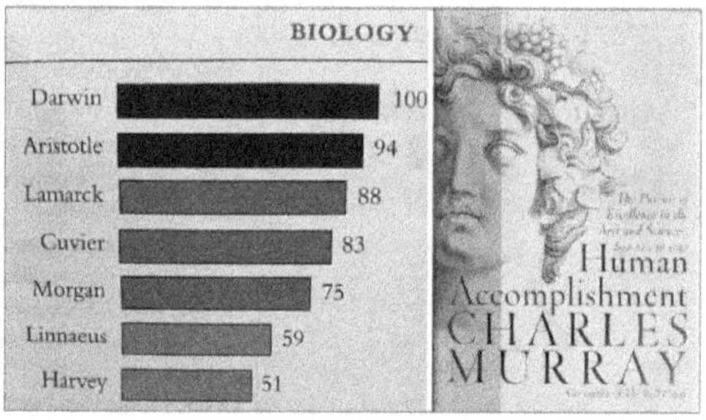

Figure 2. Harvey was ranked seventh in the category of biology by Charles Murray in his 2003 book, *Human Accomplishment*.[5]

limit the flow of blood from the liver to the extremities (centripetal flow). Harvey clearly took issue with this view and in *De Motu Cordis* made the case for centrifugal flow of blood from the extremities to the heart in the veins. Fabricius had also published a book on generation (reproduction) posthumously in 1616. Harvey's later book *On Generation* in 1651 is, in large part, a contrary response. Mentors may not only expand the mind, but also serve as a traditional authority against whom one may react creatively.

5. *Learn medical history.* References or citations in a manuscript are a clue to scholarship. Harvey cited 149 persons in his anatomy lecture notes and 17 previous authors in *De Motu Cordis.* Aristotle and Galen were cited the most among the "ancients," and Columbus and Fabricius among the "moderns." Harvey was also keenly aware of the arguments of his contemporaries, such as Caspar Hofmann of Altdorf and Jean Riolan of Paris, both ardent Galenists.
6. *Remember comparative anatomy.* Harvey considered Aristotle the supreme biologist. In his anatomy lecture notes, Harvey referred to the anatomy of more than 80 animal species. In *De Motu Cordis,* he described 37 animal species and his own experiments in several.[7] His 1628 book concerns the motion of the heart and blood *in animals.*
7. *Take on major subjects.* Harvey's two books were on entire systems: the circulatory system and the reproductive system. While every contribution is important on some level, it seems sensible to keep in mind an overall research goal that is broad and meaningful.
8. *Keep in mind that major research is lifelong.* Harvey was 50 in 1628 when his first book was published. He had lectured on anatomy for 12 years and carefully formulated his case. He was up against 15 centuries of Galenic tradition, in which arteries and veins were considered separate systems, where blood ebbed and flowed and was consumed in organs and tissues.
9. *Forebear disasters.* Every consequential life includes tragedies of various degrees. Harvey and his wife were not blessed with children. He failed to persuade numerous contemporaries of his "discovery," including Casper Hofmann in 1636 in a live demonstration at Altdorf University, and Jean Riolan in correspondence. His reputation suffered with his 1628 book and his practice declined. In the English Civil War, Harvey sided with the monarchy, and the Parliamentarians ransacked his London lodgings in 1642. His vast trove of unpublished research papers and his personal property were destroyed. After 6 years of Civil War, King Charles, in whose court Harvey served with deep loyalty, was beheaded in 1649. Harvey went into retirement with a brutal case of gout and died in 1657, at age 80, while Cromwell still ruled as Lord Protector, 3 years before the Restoration. Despite these difficulties, Harvey demonstrated both personal and professional resilience.
10. *Recognize that medical immortality is attained in publications.* Without *De Motu Cordis,* Harvey would be rarely mentioned. The unpublished writings destroyed in his lodgings during the English Civil War are lost to history. In the Great Fire of 1666, a decade after his

death, the College of Physicians building he funded, together with the medical library he donated and the statue made for him, burned to the ground in London. His book *De Motu Cordis*, however, continues to circulate four centuries later.

11. *Endow education*. Harvey left money in his will for the establishment of a "grammar school" in Folkstone, his hometown, which remains today (The Harvey Grammar School for Boys). The annual Harveian Oration (*Figure 3*) of the Royal College of Physicians, initially funded by Harvey, also endures as an event associated with great honor to the speaker. Educational endowments seem more durable than monuments, but perhaps neither are more lasting than publications.

Harvey has been admired and studied by many in the last 4 centuries, including Thomas H. Huxley, who wrote in 1878 that Harvey is "entitled, beyond dispute, to be regarded as the sole discoverer of the circulation of the blood, and the method of its propulsion by the heart."[8] Harvey died with "the great truth" he had discovered generally accepted by medical leaders. A study of the details of his life provides many lessons for future scholars.

ORCID

Charles Stewart Roberts http://orcid.org/0000-0003-1843-7844

1. O'Malley CD, Poynter FNL, Russell KF. *William Harvey. Lectures on the Whole of Anatomy. An Annotated Translation of* Prelectiones Anatomiae Universalis. Berkeley, CA: University of California Press; 1961.
2. Aird WC. Discovery of the cardiovascular system: from Galen to William Harvey. *J Thromb Haemost*. 2011;9(Suppl 1):118–129. doi: 10.1111/j.1538-7836.2011.04312.x.
3. Leake CD. *Exercitatio Anatomica de Motu Cordis et Sanguinis in Animalibus* [Anatomical Studies on the Motion of the Heart and Blood in Animals] *by William Harvey, M.D. An English Translation with Annotations*. 4th ed. Springfield, IL: Charles C. Thomas; 1958.
4. Wright T. *William Harvey. A Life in Circulation*. Oxford, UK: Oxford University Press; 2013.
5. Murray C. *Human Accomplishment. The Pursuit of Excellence in the Arts and Sciences, 800 B.C. to 1950*. New York: HarperCollins; 2003.
6. Smith Z. Speaking in tongues. *The New York Review of Books*. February 26, 2009.
7. Royal College of Physicians. *William Harvey and the Circulation of the Blood* (videotape). https://wellcomecollection.org/works/y683v77d. Accessed August 7, 2023.
8. Huxley TH. William Harvey, born April 1, 1587, died June 3, 1658. *Nature*. 1878;13(439):417–420.

Roberts CS. Lessons from the life of William Harvey. *Proc (Bayl Univ Med Cent)*. 2023;36(6):772-774. Published 2023 Aug 31. doi:10.1080/08998280.2023.2247946

31

William Clifford Roberts, MD [1932–2023]
A Remembrance

As a cardiac surgical associate at the NIH in Bethesda for 2 years, I attended my father's Monday conference regularly. There was a case of a healed traumatic aortic rupture. The fellow discovered that the patient was in a motor vehicle accident "several years before death." To this fellow, WCR said, "Write this case up and have it on my desk by Friday." He added, "It takes about as long to write a brief report as it does to write up the chart. Know the case precisely before going to the library to search the literature." He told the fellow to put the aorta in his pocket to remind him what it looked like. "This is a single task, a single mission." What to search for in the library? "Are there any cases of healed traumatic aneurysm of the descending thoracic aorta?" In 30 years, WCR had seen only 1 other, who died 7 days later, not 7 years. This was 1989, of course, before the ubiquitous use of CT scans.

The material for his case reports was this weekly conference in cardiovascular pathology over 6 decades. During these conferences, WCR would personally examine each surgical and autopsy cardiovascular specimen that was submitted—a heart or valve or aorta—and a chart would be created for each patient. He would typically examine each specimen as "an unknown." To him it was a provocative way to conduct the conference. He urged his students and residents and fellows to "remember one thing about each case." To him that was >600 "new things" a year. He believed that studying the case at hand was better than general reading.

In a personal review of his own publications, William Clifford Roberts, MD (WCR) listed 269 case reports out of a total of 1784 publications over a 60-year period, 1961–2022. This sheer number of case reports by one physician in cardiovascular disease is perhaps a record in the field..

As an editor in chief of 2 medical journals, he carefully considered the value of case reports:

> Usually, case reports have only 1 point, and information not pertinent to that point is unnecessary. Indeed, unnecessary words and nonessential details actually prevent clear focus on the patient. Thus, these "Brief Reports" must be brief—no more than 2 or 3 double-spaced typed pages with few references. Reports only 1 page long will be favored over those 3 pages long. Pertinent illustrations may be the dominant element in conveying the message...Brief Reports require clear thinking. Each word must count.

In nearly every case report of WCR, there is an illustration or photograph. WCR preferred "drawings not words." He would say, "There is nothing more important than absolutely perfect photographs." In his first 20 years at NIH, he spent every Tuesday and Thursday morning from 9am to noon with a photographer. He believed the subject should occupy "85% of the frame."

WCR graduated from Southern Methodist University (1954) and Emory University School of Medicine (1958), then had 6 years of residency training. For the next 60 years (1964-2023), he focused exclusively on cardiovascular pathology. The first 30 years were spent at NIH in Bethesda and the second 30 years at Baylor University Medical Center in Dallas. He held his weekly conference past 90 years of age.

My younger brother, John David Roberts, observed that WCR was "an intense scholar, but also a loving person. He had both qualities. He was loved for the person, not the accomplishments. One would never know he was a physician in daily interactions. He was satisfied to be unknown. Though in the Public Health Service for 30 years, he never wore the Navy uniform, even when it was recommended at NIH. As a father he required respect, which included "Yes Sir" and "No Sir." Manners were important to him, especially at the table for the evening meal, where each of his children was asked to express what he or she learned that day.

He will be remembered by his family not only for his contribution to the field of medicine, but for his hungry intellect, his indominable work ethic, his high standards, and his loyalty to loved ones.

Charles Stewart Roberts, MD
October 1, 2023

Roberts CS. William Clifford Roberts, MD (1932–2023): A remembrance [Preface]. In Roberts WC. *Case Reports in Cardiology*, Vol. 1-8. Routledge; 2023.

32

Editorial

Coronary Surgery as a Supra-Specialty

Coronary artery bypass grafting (CABG) is an elegant operation on the first 2 branches of the aorta. A PubMed search of "Coronary Bypass" lists 85,133 articles on May 3, 2024. It is perhaps the most studied operation in the history of surgery and remains the most common operation in cardiovascular surgery. Coronary surgery is evolving into a supra-specialty,[1–3] however, which is appropriate, I believe, for these following reasons:

(1) Technical skill: gentleness. Perhaps the most distinguishing feature of a coronary operation is the need to respect endothelium. Virchow's triad looms heavy in the mind of a coronary surgeon. Injury to endothelium puts grafts and native coronary arteries at risk of thrombosis. Nonexperts may rather thoughtlessly injure endothelium—by crushing conduit with forceps, by traumatizing the conduit on the field, or by careless preparation of the coronary target. The coronary surgeon only touches the adventitia of a conduit, which is treated with utmost gentleness. This is step one in coronary surgery.

(2) CABG: the choreography. The "underbelly" of the operation—opening, conduit harvest, cannulation, cardiopulmonary bypass, cardioplegia, decannulation, hemostasis, closure— is generally done "the same way every time." The vascular anastomoses, however, shift the operation to another level, where repetition and experience are crucial. A typical CABGx4 requires 7 anastomoses within a 90-minute time frame, the period during which the aorta is clamped, and the heart is stopped and preserved with cardioplegia. During these 90 minutes, most CABG operations can be performed on the still heart. Coronary surgeons have a stopwatch ticking in the mind during a CABG. The time on the heart-lung machine, and the time the heart is stopped (aorta cross-clamped) must be minimized, in general, for a good outcome. The technical skills required under this time constraint can be considerable. Coronary targets can be small, the conduit can be small, and the suture used is fine (6-0, 7-0, or 8-0 polypropylene—"The Blue Suture"), requiring high magnification loupes, just short of an operating microscope. Every anastomotic stitch counts in a CABG.

(3) The anastomosis: a perfection. The coronary anastomosis (Figure 1) requires first a complete understanding of the pertinent language—heel and toe orientation, whether open or closed, side-to-side or end-to-side, interrupted or continuous suture, toggling, and tying. Residents can emerge today from training programs, unfortunately, and not understand how to sew 2 blood vessels together. The number of CABG procedures required to complete a thoracic surgery training program has greatly decreased.[4] In the early days of CABG, there were masters, perhaps because they had to study and learn the operation from its origins. The stitches at the heel and toe must be finely placed, for example, compared to the body of the anastomosis. In addition, giving proper instructions to a first assistant during an anastomosis is an art in itself.

(4) Epicardial topography: the target. CABG is an epicardial operation. It is not "open heart" surgery in the sense that the chambers or aorta are not opened. It is an open chest, closed heart operation. In valvular operations, the heart is opened; in CABG, it is not. A mastery of epicardial coronary anatomy is necessary. The first 2 branches of the aorta have many variations—left or right dominance, surface or intramyocardial courses, and large and small branches. Knowing how to identify and prepare the coronary target on the surface of this 4-chambered muscle requires experience and expertise.

(5) Artery or vein: the conduit. Coronary surgeons, for the most part, have experience and knowledge of conduits —what, when, and where to use. Veins provide an excellent short-term but not long-term outcome. Patient longevity must be considered when choosing conduits. The younger patient, or one with a decade-plus expected longevity, deserves arterial conduits when feasible. The risk of mediastinitis, however, must be considered when contemplating the use of bilateral internal mammary arteries in the morbidly obese. The conduit harvest site itself is also important —the internal mammary artery bed, the leg, and the arm, when violated, deserve care.

(6) Complicated cases: the algorithms. A minority of CABG operations involve departures from usual protocols. A calcified aorta, for example, is a circumstance that requires a modification in technique—either a "pump-assisted" CABG is done without clamping the aorta, or an off-pump technique is used. Another circumstance is a heavily diseased target that requires an endarterectomy to construct an anastomosis. A third circumstance is concomitant valvular heart disease, usually aortic stenosis or mitral regurgitation, that may require treatment at the time of CABG. A fourth circumstance is severe heart failure. CABG in these patients requires thoughtful algorithms, such as whether to add mechanical circulatory support and in which phase of care. Intraoperative adaptability is necessary in all these circumstances and more.

(7) Coronary atherosclerosis: the disease. Coronary atherosclerosis, the most common cause of death in the Western World, is a disease that requires a lifetime of study. Like cancer, it requires expertise to manage, and the surgeon plays a role, not just intraoperatively. The language of atherosclerosis is different than the language of valvular heart disease or dysrhythmias, or even heart failure. A detailed history of coronary events is necessary to obtain in every patient—a history the surgeon should hear directly from the patient, not simply by reading a chart. A proper appointment with a preoperative patient probably requires 30 minutes.[5] Postoperatively, optimal medical therapy must be continued or initiated by the surgeon.

(8) Interventional cardiologists: the relationships. The coronary surgeon interacts primarily with interventional

Funding: none.

See page 42 for Declaration of Competing Interest.

https://doi.org/10.1016/j.amjcard.2024.05.006
www.ajconline.org

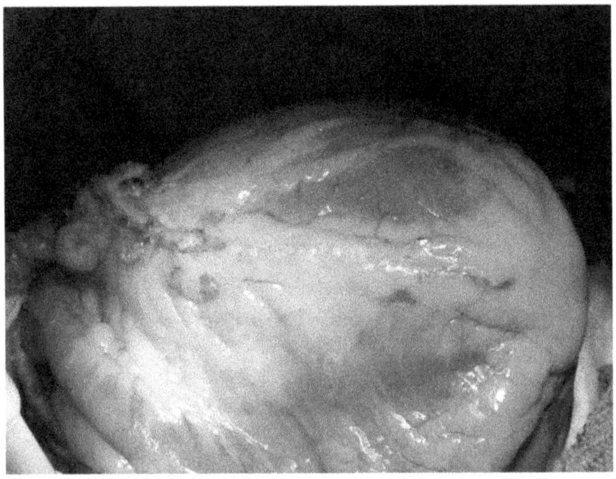

Figure 1. Left internal mammary artery sewn to the left anterior descending coronary artery.

cardiologists who have expertise in percutaneous coronary interventions. Both types of cardiovascular specialists generally understand when to recommend percutaneous coronary intervention, CABG, or optimal medical therapy only. Both specialists usually attend the same conferences, ideally a weekly cardiac catheterization conference and a weekly cardiac surgical conference to discuss patients. Other cardiology specialists are rarely involved in direct referrals for CABG.

(9) Phases of care: the team. Surgery is a discipline with 3 phases of care—preoperative evaluation, the operation, and postoperative care. Neglect of any of these 3 phases of care is detrimental to the patient and to the reputation of the surgeon. Coronary patients have special requirements in

Table 1
A Society of Thoracic Surgeons rating of 3-star reflects careful attention to all 3 phases of surgical care—preoperative, operative, and postoperative

Coronary Artery Bypass Grafting
Baylor University Medical Center
Society of Thoracic Surgeons Ranking
2018 - 2023 (11 Data Periods)

Harvest Date	STS Rating	Program Rank Percentile
12/31/2018	☆☆☆	Top 10th
6/30/2019	☆☆☆	Top 10th
12/31/2019	☆☆☆	Top 10th
6/30/2020	☆☆☆	Top 10th
12/31/2020	☆☆	10 - 90th
6/30/2021	☆☆☆	Top 20th
12/31/2021	☆☆☆	Top 20th
6/30/2022	☆☆☆	Top 20th
12/31/2022	☆☆☆	Top 20th
6/30/2023	☆☆☆	Top 20th
12/31/2023	☆☆☆	Top 20th

each phase of care. A monthly meeting to review protocols in all 3 phases of care is necessary to achieve excellence. Apart from colleagues in cardiology, physicians in anesthesia, critical care, nephrology, and hospital medicine play major roles in the care of CABG patients. Nurses, of course, are involved in virtually every aspect of each phase of care. Service-line input is necessary from all participants to optimize care.

(10) Postoperative data: the results. For every CABG operation, a 17-page data form is completed, if the institution participates in the Society of Thoracic Surgeons database, which nearly every program in the United States does. The Society of Thoracic Surgeons grades every program on a star scale—1-star means the bottom tenth percentile, 2-star means average at tenth to ninetieth percentile, and 3-star has meant the top tenth percentile in the past. The denominator changed recently from 1 to 3 years of data, and 3-star designation now represents the top twentieth percentile. Institutions are rather fixated on this program designation and perhaps rightly so. No better way has been developed to compare early postoperative results. The coronary surgeon, however, must think long-term, which is not measured in this scheme. A 3-star designation is a mark of a good team and service line (Table 1). All 3 phases of care play a role in the achievement of good outcomes.

To apply a utilitarian principle to the field of heart surgery, CABG has done the greatest good for the greatest number for the longest time. In my opinion, CABG is better done by those who do it often and well, by those who have a particular interest in atherosclerosis, and by those who understand the principle of gentleness in operative technique, particularly with respect to endothelium. It is a specialist operation within the domain of cardiovascular surgery.

Declaration of competing interest

The author has no competing interest to declare.

Charles Stewart Roberts, MD*
Department of Cardiac Surgery, Baylor University Medical Center, Baylor Scott & White, Dallas, Texas
*Corresponding author: Tel: 469-800-7760;
fax: 469-800-7770.
(Charles.Roberts@BSWHealth.org).

CRediT authorship contribution statement

Charles Stewart Roberts: Writing – review & editing, Writing – original draft.

1. Roberts CS. Cardiovascular surgery as a single specialty: the case to unify cardiac and vascular surgery. *J Thorac Cardiovasc Surg* 2008; 136:267–270.
2. Mack M, Taggart D. Coronary revascularization should be a subspecialty focus in cardiac surgery. *J Thorac Cardiovasc Surg* 2019; 157:945–947.
3. Mack MJ, Squiers JJ, Lytle BW, DiMaio JM, Mohr FW. Myocardial revascularization surgery: JACC historical breakthroughs in perspectives. *J Am Coll Cardiol* 2021;78:365–383.
4. Roberts CS, Bocanegra NR. Comparison of the first 100 coronary bypass patients of a supervised resident with his first 100 as an attending surgeon at the same institution. *Am J Surg* 1999;178:348–350.
5. Roberts CS. Counsel for the coronary surgeon. *Am Heart Hosp J* 2007;5:107–109.

Roberts CS. Coronary surgery as a supra-specialty. *Am J Cardiol.* 2024;223:40-42. doi:10.1016/j.amjcard.2024.05.006

Appendix A

Clarence S. Weldon, MD: An Interview by Charles S. Roberts, MD

Dr. Weldon (1929–2006) was Professor and Chief of Cardiothoracic Surgery at Washington University for 16 years, after training at Hopkins under Alfred Blalock, MD. Dr. Roberts (1960-) was a Junior Assistant Resident (2nd year) in Surgery at Barnes Hospital in St. Louis.

Several Division Chiefs and Department Chairs of Washington University School of Medicine (and Barnes Hospital) are mentioned in this interview:

Chief of Cardiothoracic Surgery	Chair of Department of Surgery
#1 Evarts A. Graham (1919-1951)	Evarts A. Graham (1919-1951)
#2 Thomas H. Burford (1951-1968)	Carl Moyer (1951-1965)
#3 Clarence S. Weldon (1968-1983)	Walter F. Ballinger II (1967-1978)
#4 James L. Cox (1983-1997)	Samuel A. Wells, Jr. (1981-1998)

Charles Stewart Roberts, MD: I am speaking with Clarence Weldon, MD, at his home in St. Louis on May 30, 1988.

Clarence S. Weldon, MD: Cardiac surgery is a lot of cutting and sewing. The only thing that really is comparable, I guess, is vascular surgery, which is a little bit comparable. But GI surgery is all kind of involved in a lot of medical treatment now. Neurosurgery isn't really surgery at all; I mean it's sort of sucking out the brain and looking at x-rays a lot but never has been much besides that. GU is fairly exciting I think. Orthopedic surgery I thought was going to be exciting 5 years ago when I thought they might do a lot with mechanical implants and so on, but I think that it is in the same doldrums it has been in for years and years.

Roberts: Did you consider any other field?

Weldon: I wouldn't go into medicine, but you're in medicine. If I were in medicine I wouldn't go into surgery; I would go into radiology or ophthalmology, although I don't know ophthalmology well enough to talk about it. The ophthalmologists have a marvelous thing; they don't have any internists. They are their own internists, which is a perfectly marvelous thing. You don't have people telling you what to do. Another sad thing about cardiac surgery, of course, is that all the excitement in it—the things that have been exciting in the past, aside from inventing operations and doing them—learning how to do good, safe, cardiopulmonary bypass has been solved. Nobody's even working on it anymore. I mean, the companies work on it to improve their equipment, and so on.

Diagnostics, which was terribly exciting, has been completely taken away from surgeons by cardiologists. We won't even have cath labs after a while. It will all be done by echo and various kinds of imaging. Surgeons are going to be out of it—I mean just way out of it—so that you will have to fill prescriptions, fill surgical prescriptions. The ophthalmologists don't have that, you see—they don't have anybody trying to steal everything from them. They're their own internists, so that makes a particularly exciting field. It's an awfully good way to make money.

They make a lot of money. I never did, but that's because I have always been an academic surgeon. I was an academic surgeon in the days when academic surgeons didn't make money. They do now. They must—Cox [James L. Cox, 1942-, Chief of Cardiothoracic Surgery at Washington University, 1983-1997] just bought a house for $1.2 million. They must make money. But I didn't make a lot of money, and the private practice of cardiac surgery really came sort of in the middle of my career. It wasn't even available when I began.

Roberts: It was strictly academic cardiac surgery then?

Weldon: Yes. There were a couple of anomalies, but they were very, very few and far between. Even at Baylor, DeBakey and Cooley, and so on—that was full-time. Two of the anomalies were Burford [Thomas L. Burford, 1907-1977] and Ferguson [Thomas B. Ferguson, 1923-2013], who went into private practice by virtue of the fact that the medical school exploded, and there was a big fight between the medical school and the hospital. In the middle of that fight, Burford announced that he was going into private practice. They couldn't have gotten another cardiac surgeon to come here at that time if they had paid him 10 million dollars, because the place was in such chaos.

Roberts: When you came in 1968 ...

Weldon: By that time, it had been solved. This was back in '62 or '63, and the medical school was in such chaos that there was some question about whether it was going to survive. Edgar Queeny came in and demanded that the place be run like a business, closed the clinics and built the hospital with a restaurant and a swimming pool on top of it, doctors' offices—virtually tried to convert it into a private hospital with no regard at all for what was happening to the university or the medical school. Closed the clinics, said they didn't make money. Closed them. They were on hospital property. Everybody resigned. The dean resigned, everybody resigned.

Roberts: And this was about 1962?

Weldon: '61, '62, '63, around there. Everybody who could do anything else resigned. There wasn't anybody here. That was when Carl Moyer [Chair of Surgery, 1951-1965] resigned. And that's when Burford said, "I am going part time." That is when he invited Ferguson back to join him. Ferguson was in private practice in Florida. But they were terribly anomalous. Everybody else in the country who was doing cardiac surgery in the sixties was in an academic full-time job. There wasn't anybody charging fees for it except Burford and maybe Alton Ochsner or somebody. By that time, the Ochsner Clinic had been built, I think, and the Mayo Clinic, the Cleveland Clinic, a few private hospitals were involved in it, but you couldn't get a job doing private practice.

And it wasn't really until coronary artery bypass surgery started, which was in '70, '68, '69, beginning, but '70 really, by the time people learned to do angiograms. There was sort of one doctor in the country who knew how to do angiograms of the coronary circulation—Mason Sones [1918-1985] at the Cleveland Clinic—and by the time he taught other people to do it, it was 1970. Well with that, then private practice jobs opened up in great numbers and have multiplied ever since, so that now the overwhelming number of people who do cardiac surgery are in private practice, and of course they make enormous amounts of money. I mean they charge, what, $5,000 per operation, 2 or 3 operations a week, that's $15,000 a week times 50 weeks in a year—how much is that? It's a million and a half dollars or something like that, you see?

In the meantime, academic places have had to compete for surgeons by offering higher salaries, and that's what's happened now. And I am sure that the school is paying a lot more. I came here as head of the division at $30,000 a year, and by the time Walter Balinger [Chair of Surgery, 1967-1978] got canned, I was making $75,000. I think they pay something like half a million dollars now. Not me, but you know, Cox and a few other people make an awful lot of money now. So you can make a lot of money in this profession; you can do that.

Roberts: You were head of the division for 15 years?

Weldon: 16 years [1968-1983]

Roberts: How was it when you came here?

Weldon: Well, Burford was a strange man. He was, on the face of it, an egomaniac—actually, rather insecure. Awfully disagreeable, not many people liked him. Very handsome. Incredibly handsome. Movie-star handsome and that sort of ... that sort of ... uh ... he was always combing his hair. Seriously. He had always been like that, and that sort of colored his personality, I think. You know, I mean it does color people's personality. People who are very good looking are told that they are good looking from the time they are children. And it colors their personality. And it did his, I think. And he was big with the ladies. He was something of a womanizer. He married early and had a wretched marriage. He married again and was married until he died, and they were wretchedly unhappy in the final years of their marriage. She was a scrub nurse. Beautiful woman. Louise Burford. Still beautiful. Beautiful at 70 or 75, or whatever she is now. Very beautiful. But that marriage was like a battleground. It was just awful. I mean, they despised each other at the end of the marriage, just despised each other. Said so. And he was having some kind of an affair with his secretary. I don't know how much of an affair it was, but he was giving her money and taking money from Louise and the kids and giving it to this secretary. Took drugs in the form of paregoric. I can't imagine anyone taking paregoric for pleasure, but he did. Smoked incessantly. More than I do. Incessantly. I mean, chain-smoked right until he died.

He was a very dashing young surgeon. Very dashing. He had gone to North Africa, really right out of his training during the war, and the rules at that time were that gunshot wounds to the chest were to be left alone, just as the rules that vascular wounds in the Korean War were to be left alone. And, just like Frank Spencer in the Korean War, Tom Burford said, "Fuck you," and opened the chest and took the blood clots out. And of course it was a tremendous revolution. I mean, this was a time, this was in the '40s, when people were still futzing around about which way you could get into the chest and which way you couldn't. And he had been here with Graham [Evarts A. Graham 1883-1957], you know, so he just opened the chest and took the blood clots out and cured those soldier boys.

Roberts: He was a star.

Weldon: That's right, and there were a lot of people there who saw this good-looking boy doing this, and I went to visit (I'm trying to think of his name). I went to visit a surgeon in Scotland once who was big—instrumental in early mitral valve surgery. He had invented an instrument to dilate the mitral valve. I can't think of his name. At any rate, he told me he went down there and visited them during the war. He was with the British, and he went down there to Africa and he said, "I saw this young fellow Burford opening these chests and taking the blood clots out," and he said, "I was so impressed, I came home and said, 'I want to be just like Tom Burford.'" Then he told me that he came to St. Louis later to visit him and the man had changed so much, he couldn't believe it was the same person.

Anyway, Burford really never did much else that amounted to anything. I mean, he was the chief of surgery, of thoracic surgery, at Barnes, and he did all right in that capacity, but he developed a nasty personality. Whether it had to do with his woman troubles, or whether his career didn't advance the way he wanted it to—anyway, he became very malignant and nasty. Known as "Black Tom Burford," with some reason.

He did a couple of things all right. I mean, he was big in early repair of coarctation in infants, but not much. He didn't get much done. He did everything, but he didn't do it any better than anybody else. He wasn't very inventive; and when the heart surgery business came along, he was a little on the old side. Not terribly, but a little bit, and then he was sort of fiftyish or late forties, and you know it was a young man's business. It was something for the people who were just getting out of the lab.

I mean, Dr. Blalock [Alfred Blalock, 1899-1964; Surgeon-in-Chief at Hopkins, 1941-1964] stepped aside and never did an open-heart case, and we used to beg him to do one. We would say, "Come in and sew an open-heart case, and you ought to do an open-heart operation. You started the whole thing, you know; do an ASD. We'll have it all ready for you. All you have to do is sew it up." "No," he said, "I don't want to have anything to do with it. I didn't develop it. I don't want to have anything to do with it."

Well, it was just the opposite of Burford, you see; I mean, he was the "big cheese" and so he was going to get in it tooth and nail, and he was going to do it. But he was not trained to do it. He wouldn't go away and watch other people. He just decided, you know, that if this was surgery, then there was nobody better on earth to do it than he was, since he was obviously the best thoracic surgeon in the entire world, and therefore he ought to. And the carnage was enormous. I mean, everybody died. They blamed everybody. They blamed Roper, blamed Ferguson. Finally, Roper [Charles L. Roper, 1925-2015] drew away from him, wouldn't have anything to do with him, went off and started doing the thoracic surgery.

Roberts: Did Roper start out doing cardiac and thoracic surgery?

Weldon: Hearts. Hearts. Yes, hearts. Roper did the first successful mitral valve replacement that was ever done at Barnes. The others had all died. Well then, I came in 1968. Walter Ballinger came in 1967.

Roberts: Did he recruit you?

Weldon: Yes, he was at Hopkins briefly and knew me there. And there was a search here. They offered the job to Mallone, who turned it down. They offered the job to Najarian, who turned it down, and I think Walter may have been their third choice. I think that is possible. Walter came out and they got a rule through saying that Burford could still continue as head of thoracic surgery only if he returned full time, that there was none of this business about being in private practice and running a division. You could be in private practice and work at the hospital, but you couldn't be in private practice and run a division. Well, by this time he was making lots of MOOLAH, you see. I mean, he charged for dead patients as much as the live ones. So he said, "No."

So Walter offered the job to Paul Ebert, who turned it down, and then to me. And I took the job with an unbelievable amount of innocence. I mean, it's inconceivable to me that any human being, let alone me, could have been as innocent about job seeking as I was. But I was, as I have often been in my life, unhappy about my situation. I was at Hopkins, and for a year, I did all of the heart surgery because everybody had gone. Frank Spencer had gone, Henry Bahnson had gone, Dave Sabiston had gone. The guy who was next in charge was a fellow named Bob Gertner, and he died shortly thereafter of acute alcoholism, having been an unknown alcoholic from the age of 12. Absolutely the most brilliant person I have ever encountered in surgery.

Roberts: What was his name?

Weldon: Bob Gertner. No question about it. His father ran a string of movie theaters in Baltimore. No question about it, Bob Gertner was the brightest man I have ever encountered in heart surgery. He was a teenage alcoholic. He went through prep school, college, medical school, then the residency training program at Hopkins, and was on the staff for 7 years before anybody discovered it. In the twilight of his life, he was drinking straight grain alcohol out of a Coke bottle. Got cirrhosis of the liver, did his own paracentesis, hit a big vein, and bled to death intra-abdominally. Bright, just as bright as any human being could be. The man was a genius.

Roberts: So it was you and him doing cardiac surgery.

Weldon: So for a year I did cardiac surgery at Hopkins. And I really wasn't very well equipped to do it. I mean, it was just thrown at me. And we had a lot of misfortunes and so on. So finally, I said to George Zuidema [Surgeon-in-Chief at Hopkins, 1964-1984], "Look, I'll do this, but I've got to have a little bit more preparation." And so I took off and went out to Mayo Clinic and stood there and watched Dwight McGoon and John Kirklin operate for 3 weeks. Never took my eyes off them for 3 weeks.

Then I came back and started doing it without too much trouble. But then they decided that they wanted a scientist. They didn't want me, they wanted a scientist, you see. So they hired Vincent Gott [Chief of Cardiac Surgery at Hopkins, 1965-1992], who was the sweetest man in the world. He really was. And he had been working in a laboratory and had developed some kind of stuff that you smear on plastic or metal and so on to prevent clots. And everybody thought this was the answer for everything, because you could smear this stuff on everything and nothing would clot. The stuff never worked. But you know, it got Vince the job.

When Vince arrived, I had to teach him how to do heart surgery. He didn't know. But he was terribly kind and terribly patient and put up with me, you know, and learned and is now a very good heart surgeon. But I essentially spent a year and a half teaching Vincent Gott how to work. I mean, he didn't know how to do anything when he got there, and what we were doing was congenital hearts and valves. We weren't doing coronaries, of course.

But you know, I saw the handwriting on the wall. I mean, that was not going to be my job. It was Vince's job, and so I was very, very, very eager to get out of there. I got offered some things that I didn't want.

Roberts: What were you offered?

Weldon: Well, I was offered a job in New York at Montefiore, I think. Henry Bahnson offered me a job at Pittsburgh, but you see, it wasn't his job. He was head of surgery and cardiac surgery, but it was to come work with him. I made a terrible mistake. It would have been an ideal job. I should have taken it. But it didn't sound like much to me at the time. There was another job offer in New Haven at a Yale affiliate hospital; it wasn't very good.

So when Walter [Ballinger] offered me this job, I jumped at it. And I came here really without knowing what was going on here. As I say, unbelievable innocence. I met Tom Burford—I'll never forget. I met him at the AATS meeting in Los Angeles. Had lunch with him. He brought Ferguson along with him who didn't say a word. Tom Burford, in the typical Tom Burford way, said to me, "You can come to Barnes if you want to, son, but we'll destroy you. Ferguson and I, we'll destroy you." It was just a sort of challenge to me, but that's what they did in the end.

And Burford and I, when I came, he wouldn't talk to me, but then I organized this lecturer thing, you see, and maybe, (I thought) you bastard, I'll kill you with kindness. I had his portrait painted, and I got it hung down there next to all the biggies down around the auditorium, and I got the lecturer. I got some people in town to give enough money so we could get it started. There wasn't a lot of money, but .... And then we became very good friends. I mean, that's the kind of guy he was. I mean, you could win him over that easily. We became very good friends, and he turned on Ferguson and Roper. He hated them, especially Ferguson. Just despised him just before he died.

Roberts: Why?

Weldon: He didn't like Ferguson and he used to complain to me about him all the time. Of course Ferguson writes his obit now and writes articles about what a great man and the whole thing. That's the way people are, see? Anyway, this was a nice job for me for about 10 years until they fired Walter.

Roberts: What year was he fired? [1978]

Weldon: It seems to me about 4 years before I was [1983], so that was 8 years ago, 7 or 8 years ago. Walter got a bad deal. He did all the right things, you know. Actually, he has quite a distinguished record here. I mean, he has several other people he brought along that head departments. John Collins at Stanford, Jaffe in New York, Leslie Wise somewhere in New York. There are 3 or 4 people who head departments. Sam Wells hasn't put anybody in a department yet. He probably will, but he hasn't. Anderson here. He had a very good laboratory.

I mean, they started all this business, Walter started all this business about islet cell transplantation and it is still going on. I mean I am not aware of anything that Wells does except put parathyroids in the arm. Jesus, they did that in the last century. So, you know, I mean Walter did all the right things, being the head of a department. He was terribly disagreeable in the job. He was very ... he made everybody angry. Everybody. He made the dean angry and the vice-chancellor angry, and the other department heads angry.

He really didn't have any friends, and then he made a fatal error. It couldn't have been simpler, but he made a fatal error. He operated on the wife of an ammunition manufacturer who gave a lot of money to Washington University to ease their conscience. At any rate, she had a liposarcoma and Walter operated on it and cut down and found the benign lipoma which always lies on top of a liposarcoma, removed it (the big lipoma), and told her she was all right. She wasn't. She had liposarcoma. She had a fatal disease. I mean, there isn't anything anybody could do about it. Nothing, you see. So she went down to MD Anderson, and they put her on a bunch of meds, you know, and nearly killed her. I mean, it didn't do any good. You know, it doesn't do any good. They put her on all kinds of funny drugs, and it didn't do any good, but she died of a liposarcoma.

Well, you see, the family were very upset, and if that family is upset, then Washington University is upset; and Bill Danforth [William H. Danforth, Chancellor of Washington University, 1971-1995], who didn't know anything about this kind of thing, was furious, you know, and essentially this sort of treacherous man vowed to destroy Walter Ballinger at that moment. I am serious. Not a lot of people know this, but it is true. Because he had operated improperly, according to Danforth, on this donor.

Then Walter really got in trouble. He had this ... George Zuidema [at Hopkins] hired this woman who had been a nurse at Hopkins to be his business manager. I forget what her proper name was. Anyway, Walter thought this was just neat, you see, and he did everything the way George did, so he hired a business manager, and he hired this lady to do the same thing. I mean, if you suggested to Walter that perhaps she ought to do something slightly different from the way she was doing it, he went into a tirade. I mean, he just let her do whatever she wanted. I mean, he thought she was wonderful. Well, the woman was a crook. She was a crook. She was stealing money, and she was stealing it by putting all of her relatives on the payroll when they weren't there. They were getting paychecks. And then there was this rumor that went around that Walter had been on the take. Absolutely untrue. Absolutely untrue. But apparently unbeknownst to Walter, she had done some things which she thought would be nice to sort of worm herself into his good graces. Only he didn't know it, like she was paying part of his bill at the country club or some such nonsense like that. Anyway, this rumor went around that Walter was on the take. He wasn't. I'm sure.

I mean, he just got railroaded the whole way through the thing. The guys didn't like him. Kipnis didn't like him, Paul Lacey didn't like him, the biggies in the school didn't like him. Bill Danforth didn't like him because of the operation on the donor, you see, so Walter responded to this by virtually losing his mind. I mean, he just became awful. I really thought he was losing his mind. He started writing letters to people saying what he was going to do.

The whole place was in disarray. It was a terrible mess. Well, they solved all this by firing Walter. He divorced his wife, and he went off and became a born-again Christian. He did. Saved him, I think. He was like my ex-wife. She was into Catholicism. Powerful stuff. Anyway, they gave him a sabbatical for 2 years, and then he came back and has been sort of gentlemanly since. Every once in a while, the old Walter creeps through, but he has been sort of gentlemanly ever since. He has a nice new wife, a younger girl, very rich. And he seems to be at ease with himself.

Then they appointed Bill Fair, who was a urologist, as head of the department, temporary chief of the department. But Bill Fair, first of all, didn't know how to do the job, didn't want to do the job, and sort of didn't do the job, except he would attend the meetings he had to. So during this period of time, we drew completely away from general surgery.

It was during this period of time we built 2200 and the new operating rooms and the ICU. We just sort of separated ourselves completely. And then a number of other things happened during that period. One was that John Connors, whom I had put over at the Jewish Hospital, was suddenly imbued with a sense of enormous importance. I mean, he somehow got the idea that he was the premier heart surgeon in the world. Seriously, he began making all sorts of astronomical demands, and so on, one of which was more money. And so I discovered quite by accident one day that the Jewish Hospital, now Jewish Hospital pays Jewish Hospital people. That doesn't come out of Washington University money, but they are Washington University appointees. But they had upped Connor's salary to $250,000 per year. This was while I was making $75,000.

So I went over to the Dean. I really behaved badly, but I went over to the Dean and just screamed and hollered and said "It's not going to be this way" and made everybody mad. Everybody. All over money, you see. The second thing that happened was that the coronary artery surgery business started to grow; and Ferguson, who had been doing nothing, started to get busy doing coronary arteries. All of a sudden, I had Connors on one side of me making $250,000, and Tom Ferguson making $1,000,000 and not putting a penny into the division.

During this time, what Ferguson had done while not operating was political work. Work for the societies and so on. Couldn't get enough of that because he didn't have any work to do there. I mean, I was doing all the heart surgery. Well then, you know, this paid off. He got to be president of the STS and then got to be president of the AATS and then editor of the journal, and so on, all because of the work he had got done. Honestly, I mean he had really worked very hard for those organizations during that period of time.

Well, suddenly, he was the most important heart surgeon in the country, you see. Started making irrational demands, you know. Connors, on one side of me, was my own guy, you see; I put him over there. Connors was demanding more and more money and more and more autonomy, and Ferguson on this side, was making more and more money and getting more and more positions and stuff. Ferguson started making demands. He wanted his own resident. I said, "F you, you're not going to get your own resident." He wanted his own operating room all the time. I said, "No, no, no." He said, "I'll go to the Board of Trustees." I said, "Go to the Board of Trustees. If you don't know where they are, I'll take you there." See. Feeling fairly confident at this time.

All of the time this was going on, there was a search for a new chairman of surgery. They kept parading heart surgeons in at me without ever talking to me about it. Never said anything. Suddenly I would discover on my desk that I had an appointment to see Nick Kouchoukos. Had an appointment to see Andy Wechsler. Heart surgeons that I knew were suddenly coming in to be chief of surgery. Nobody, the Dean, ever called me.

Roberts: Who was behind it?

Weldon: Committee. The committee was picking these people. Sam Wells, but he was not a heart surgeon, you see. I liked him. I thought he was great because the rest of them were heart surgeons, you see. Well, they offered Wells the job. He turned it down. Then they offered it to Kouchoukos. He turned it down. Then they offered it to Andy Wechsler. He turned it down. Then they offered it to Wells again, and he took it. I don't know why; they did something.

In the meantime, Ferguson kept making more and more demands, and finally we were having a difficult schedule down there one day, and I told a resident, "You delay Dr. Ferguson's case a half hour and put me in there and let me follow in the next room. That will work out better; we'll get everything done that way." He came downstairs, thought his case had been started—typical business, you see. His case hadn't been started, so he stormed out of the operating room. This was almost exactly the time that Sam Wells had accepted the job, you see. So I went back upstairs. Ferguson came storming into my office, almost broke the door down. Came into my office and said, "I will destroy you. I will remove you from this job. I will destroy you."

Whereupon he got on the airplane and made 5 or 6 trips to Durham, explaining to Wells what needed to be done. He needed to bring someone else in here. It is a bad situation, so on, so on, so on. Wells was here a year and a half, I guess, and I thought he was indifferent to me. Not especially cool, but indifferent. But he's sort of like that with everybody. That's just kind of the way he is. Never had the slightest suspicion that he was displeased about anything. Never. I mean, he was complimentary about things. I never had the slightest idea. Meeting Ferguson in his office all the time, I mean, I'd have to wait if I went up to see him until Ferguson came back out. You would think that they were brothers who had just found each other or something. That kind of pissed me off, you know.

For 4 years, Chuck, I was mad. Angry. Angry about Connors, about the school, about Ferguson, angry about parading heart surgeons through. Angry about everything. Brought the anger home. My marriage dissolved; no question that that played a very real role in it. Meantime, my wife was getting more and more important in the university. You know, couldn't say enough marvelous things about Sam Guze, the Dean, you see. He was my enemy and her boss, and the whole situation was incredible.

So about 3 months before the end of the year, I went up and asked to see Wells. Went up to see Wells and said, "I came up to tell you that I am going to appoint Ron Leidencross," and he said, "No, you're not." I said, "Why not?" He said, "Because I'm replacing you and I'm replacing you with Jim Cox. He will be here tomorrow." And Jim Cox arrived for his first visit the next day after Wells told me that. And then he accepted the job, and you know the rest.

What has happened since then is that there really has been very little effort to accommodate me in the department. I mean, really sort of quite the contrary. I was sort of immediately eliminated from all departmental activities, but allowed to continue to operate; taken off everything. I mean, not even consulted about anything. Not even the Burford lecture, which I started. Not even consulted about that.

Now, this went along pretty well for 3 years, and now Cox is ready to make bigger changes in the department. He is going to make it a lot like it is at Duke. I mean, he wants to have a lot of surgeons, so they hired young Ferguson, who was part of the deal, by the way. I mean, he worked for Cox at Duke. That is one of the reasons why Ferguson was angling to get Cox to come here. He wants to have a lot of people, and there are only so many patients, you know. There are fewer patients now than when I was running it. And I have a fair share of them still.

So they're picking at me, you know, about operating time, giving me a junior resident each time I operate or for most of the time, putting me on that angioplasty screwup schedule most of the time so that I had hard cases. Made a special fuss when one of my patients died about, you know, not quite working up to snuff anymore because I'm getting a little old, and that sort of thing. There's been all of this going on. Perfectly obvious. I'm not stupid, you know.

What they would like for me to do is to leave, which would free up things for young Ferguson and the other young guy. Took congenital heart surgery by fiat. Just removed me from that, despite the fact that this is what I did. I mean, if I was known for anything, I was known as a congenital heart surgeon. Took me out of that altogether. Put Spray over there. See, that is a controlled practice. You can do with it what you want. No privately practicing doctors involved in that.

So, in response to all this pressure, they are getting exactly what they want. I am quitting at the end of this month [age 60] just because, you know, it's a most unpleasant and uncomfortable situation. If I stay here, I will become a fool or an object of derision, neither of which I want to become. So that is that.

Now, having bored you with all that, let's talk about your career. You want to become a heart surgeon. You're sure you want to be an academic heart surgeon. If you're quite sure you want to be an academic heart surgeon, you have to learn to get your teeth in people's back. I was never very good at that.

You know, I was terribly much under the influence of Alfred Blalock, like everybody was who trained with him. He was an incredibly alluring man, and you know, I sort of wanted to be like he was. I didn't want to be the most famous surgeon in the land, but I wanted to be a teacher and have a laboratory and all that S that was big in those days.

But I was never really much interested in power, you know; and at this place, and I think at most places now, the power struggle is enormous. And people—that's what people are interested in, and they get their teeth in people's back, and I was never very good at that. I was awfully good at complaining, awfully good at raising hell, and awfully good at making people mad, but I was never very good at politically achieving ends. I wasn't very good at that. It is a sort of power struggle, you know.

Whispering about people is not my forte, you know. If I thought that somebody was a S, I said, "You are a S." You see, whispering about people was not my forte. I have never been very good at that. But there are an awful lot of people who are very good at whispering. And they accomplish a great deal by whispering. That works very, very well.

Now, I would think that if you want to be a heart surgeon for some reason or another, I would think that this is probably going to be a very good place to train. I think that Cox has made some very good moves. He hasn't really got the residency training program into a mature state yet. He inherited some people that I appointed who were not very pleasant. You know, they were my appointees, and they were not entirely loyal to him. He went through that for 2 years. But I think that it is just a question of time. He had a debacle this year. I mean, he fired one resident, so he had one senior resident and two junior residents. The two junior residents were acting as senior residents, so that needs some maturity, but that will come.

The appointments, by and large, are okay. I think Bolman is quite good and is running the transplantation program very effectively. The problem with transplantation is that that is about what you can do with it unless they get grafts from monkeys or something. That's about what you can do with it. I mean, the curve is flattening on the number of operations being done. His (Cox's) own interest thus far hasn't taught anybody. I mean, he does it all himself so far. Now, that is going to change, too. He will teach other people, and his resident, I guess, will be able to go out and do WPW (Wolff – Parkinson --White) surgery. They'll have as much hold on coronary artery surgery and valve surgery as anybody else. It is just a question of what happens to that.

I think that congenital heart surgery is a mistake. I mean, it is a disaster area. It always has been. It didn't matter to me, because I really didn't care what Goldring knew or Alex Hartman. I could operate on the patients and report the surgical results because it didn't matter. It matters a little bit more now, since that has been done, and what you have to do now is study patients and so on. It is a terrible gang they got over there, you know, what's his name, who runs it. Anyway, they only got 2 cardiologists, and they are both bad. And it's a nothing outfit, nothing, so it will never compete with Boston Children's or Chicago Children's or Toronto or Los Angeles.

They got this surgeon that came down to Louisville, from Paul Ebert's place, going gangbusters. I mean, he has done 30 switch operations and 50 heart transplants in neonates or something, just going gangbusters. They are treading water over here, and I don't think Cox understands that area. I don't think he realizes how bad it is…And I don't expect much there, but as far as training goes, there is enough material to train there, unless you specifically want to be a congenital heart surgeon, and then you would go somewhere else anyway. Have to go to Great Ormond Street; it's like going to Mecca, you see. You have to do that…

Roberts: Where did you learn congenital? Did you learn it here or at Hopkins?

Weldon: I was self-trained. I was at Hopkins. In that era, I was. I came up with everybody else. I mean, I was doing congenital heart surgery, the same kind of stuff they were doing at Great Ormond Street. Never had many patients, but I was one of the people who worked out some of the things for congenital heart surgery.

Roberts: Who taught you the most in congenital heart surgery?

Weldon: Henry Bahnson taught me how to operate. No question. He was sort of a second-in-command at Hopkins when I was there and when I was training. And he was the most active surgeon. Dr. Blalock was at the twilight of his career.

Roberts: Did you operate very much with Blalock?

Weldon: Yeah, sure, but not as much as I did with Hank. I mean, we were doing open heart surgery when I was training. Not doing it very well, but we were doing it. And Hank was doing all of that. Hank and Frank Spencer. A little bit David Sabiston—not much, a little bit, not very good. But Dr. Blalock was just doing closed operations, coarcts and ducts, and he also did some general surgery.

Roberts: What were your 2 years at NIH like with Glenn Morrow?

Weldon: Glenn finished the residency when I was a senior medical student, or a junior medical student, I guess, and Glenn went to the NIH directly after his residency, so Glenn was at the NIH for about ... He didn't go there first. First, he went first to the Public Health Hospital in Baltimore. He was there for 2 years, and then they opened the clinical center

He must have been at the clinical center 3 years, when I went down there. The first year he was down there, Jerry Kay was there with him and then Alex Haller, and then Bob Gertner, and then "Bricks" Baker, and then me—so there were 4 years before me. Only 3 of those were clinical fellows. The clinical fellowship program was established 3 years before. Jerry Kay was not a clinical fellow. He was part of the staff down there. But I think that as far as this place goes to train, I don't think that there is probably any place that is any better to train, and Cox is young. That is the real advantage.

I mean, one terrible mistake you can make is to go, to start a program where the guy who's running it isn't going to be finishing it when you finish. That is a dreadful mistake. Get off to, say, Sabiston's program only to discover that they got a new chief halfway through your training. Because of that, it might be good, but it also can be a dreadful disaster, and almost all those first years for anybody are very uncomfortable. And they were uncomfortable for me.

My first couple of years were just terrible for me. I inherited some people that Burford had hanging on, and it was just chaos and everybody is mad because you've come and the camp is divided. Some people want to be awfully friendly, and some people hate you for coming, and so on. Cox had the same thing. When he came, there were people who were mad that he was coming and replacing me. There were people who were so happy that somebody was replacing me that they didn't know what to do. He inherited people I had appointed. He had the same trouble.

Dave Sabiston, when he went to Duke, had a terrible time. I mean, there were people who were lined up on one wall rooting for Will Sealy, people who were on the other wall rooting against Will Sealy. Just chaos for about 3 years. The same thing happened with Dr. Blalock when he came to Hopkins, you know; he had 3 years of pure hell. So the last thing you want to do is get into a program where you do not have any suspicion at all that they are going to change leaders in the middle of your training period, because that's very, very bad. So it is just a mistake to start out with somebody who hasn't got enough years left to finish you. Don't, whatever you do, make that mistake. Now that's not true with Cox. He's only 40 or 41 or so, so you've got plenty of time. You've got 20 or 25 years, unless somebody gets him. This place will eat you up and spit you out pretty fast. No question about that. So I think it is a good training program to get into.

Roberts: When you were a chief at Hopkins, who was the other chief resident?

Weldon: A guy named Nathaniel Perriman Collins. He was a marvelous surgeon. A marvelous surgeon and an awfully nice guy. Quick, agile, everything you want to be. He left Hopkins angry about something. Angry because he had not been asked to stay, I think. I had been. He wasn't. I think that may have been the reason, but it may have been some other reason. Anyway, he left, and he left forever. He went into private practice in Houston, Texas, where all the biggies were. Has a very big practice down there, I understand. Does general surgery, and somebody told me that at the last reunion he did return to Hopkins with a lot of forgiveness for the place. Got reports that Perry had been back. He was married to a woman whose father was the biggest guy, whatever you call them, in the Southern Baptist movement. He was head of the congress or whatever it is...she was always going around telling people about how evil it was to smoke or drink. These were in the days when everybody who was anybody smoked and drank. I mean, you had to be some kind of a nut not to, you see. And public prayers and all that stuff. And he was married to her, and she didn't like Hopkins.... Whether that had anything to do with it or not, I don't know. The report came back that she died of breast cancer, but apparently it wasn't true. Apparently she showed up at Hopkins right by his side, somebody told me. So Millie Brawley, who was there, Bob Brawley's wife, went up and said, "Miriam?" And Miriam said, "Yes, Millie, how are you?" And Millie said, "Miriam, I thought you were dead." There was a report that she had died of breast cancer, but apparently she had not.

Roberts: You knew Charles Hatcher?

Weldon: I did know him, sure. He was the resident before me. Charlie is a very bright fellow. He is very bright. You know, there are not that many people in medicine who are very bright. There really aren't. I mean, they are a pedestrian lot, by and large. I have never encountered brains that have really knocked me out in the entire profession. Glenn was a bright fellow, but screwy in a way. Charlie was bright. A good surgeon. He was a good surgeon.

Roberts: Didn't he operate on Blalock?

except to meet with you at the end of the year, like we do, to tell you what was going to happen—and even then, he wasn't very friendly. He said to me, "Well, what do you think you want to do?"—you know, the same, all very routine, like they do. Anyway, I would go through that, sure I was going to get fired every year, and then finally, you recognize when you're in the track. I mean, when you get 6 months on the plastic service, you know pretty well that you are in the track.

At any rate, then when I got on the heart service, it was like the 5 years in between had never existed. It was the same thing. We would sit in his office and talk about ... Anyway, I was embarrassed by this time. I later discovered that he did this with all his residents. He would go into his office and say, "Oh, what am I going to do about Dandy? They want to throw him out of school." Well, I had no idea what to do about Dandy, so you just sort of sit there, so you say, "Dr. Blalock, tell me a little more and maybe I can solve this problem for you." Anyway, from then on we were very good friends. And we were good friends until he died [1964].

I was on the staff, he had appointed me to the staff [1963]. I was on the staff for one year before he retired [1964, age 64]. And Hank had gone by that time, but David Sabiston was still there. Dave and I were on staff there together, and then George Zuidema came [1964] and David left.

Roberts: How did you and Sabiston get along?

Weldon: Almost the same thing. I mean, Dave imitates Dr. Blalock as much as he can imitate him.... But Dave Sabiston and I were on staff for a year together, and I thought he was my best friend. I mean, he was constantly in my office complaining about this and complaining about that and gossiping about this person and gossiping about that person. He would say, "Come here a minute," you see, call me into his office and say, "Did you hear so and so about so and so?" That kind of guy, you see. The minute he got the job at Duke, he wouldn't even talk to me at national meetings, he wouldn't recognize me, still doesn't. He spoke only to people who counted then, to Dr. Francis Moore ("Ah, there's Dr. Francis Moore. I have to speak to him."). That's the kind of guy he is.... He speaks only to people who he thinks might further his interests...

Roberts: What was your relationship with Glenn Morrow [1922-1982, Chief of Surgery at Heart Institute of NIH, 1953-1982]?

Weldon: Glenn, first of all, was awfully friendly with me. We were good friends. We really were, always, right up to the time he died, we were good friends. I mean, there wasn't that much difference in our ages. We were very good friends, I mean we did a lot of things together, we went places together, and I was at his house often to eat, and his kids were little, and we were very good friends. He was the best man at my wedding. And we worked *together* more than I worked *for him* at that time. I mean, he was trying very hard to get open heart surgery started and having a lot of trouble doing it.

Roberts: You had completed an internship?

Weldon: That didn't matter, you know. I was what he had. Me and Waldhausen, and he had good people: John Ross, Ted Cooper, and Waldhausen and me. We were the people he had, and he depended on us a lot. It all changed later. He became sort of professorial, and people called him "Dr. Morrow" and so on. But I never called him Dr. Morrow. I mean, we sort of worked *with him.*

What we were trying very hard to do in those 2 years was to get the heart-lung machine working so that he could operate on people, and we did. We did get it working. We got it working in a very dramatic way. I mean, he had this guy Melrose there who had a heart-lung machine. Melrose of the Melrose technique of putting potassium in the heart. Dennis Melrose was there. He was an ENT doctor who decided he wanted to get into the heart surgery business. Not as a heart surgeon, but he did with this Melrose technique. He was bright, but a J, an awful J. And Dennis had this heart-lung machine which had everything the matter with it.

Glenn had put a lot of money into it. He had his people working on it there at the lab building, you know. I mean, the engineers were making all kinds of servo mechanisms and all that baloney, you see, that didn't amount to anything. He had the wrong idea with it, and he insisted on operating on people with it, and they died. Every one of them died. Thirty-five people died in a row. Thirty-five people. Bang. Bang. Bang. Bang. Bang. Thirty-five people. Then Glenn would go home and get drunk. If they didn't die at the operation, they would die that night.

It was full of air and pieces of lint and God knows what, but it wasn't much different anywhere else. At any rate, then Glenn would go home and have about 6 martinis, and you know, I don't know how Phyllis ever lived with him. I mean, he would just get so drunk it was just incredible and appear the next morning. If you called him, he couldn't talk to you. Couldn't talk to you.

Anyway, finally Waldhausen and I went marching in. Waldhausen and I had a little powwow, and we had to do something about this, it was very bad. So we went marching into his office and said, "Glenn, we came to talk to you." We said, "This thing isn't working and it ain't never going to work. You can't go on killing people like this. It's getting bad and it will get in the newspaper after a while." "Well, what am I going to do, we ...." I said, "What we're going to do is that this one that they have in Cleveland is supposed to be working. We're going to go out there and see about it and see if it does, in fact, work."

So some little tiny outfit in Cleveland called Penco Corporation was making this heart-lung machine for the Cleveland Clinic, and Waldhausen and I went out there and spent two weeks, I think, and I saw the worst surgery I have ever seen in my life at the Cleveland Clinic, but a good heart-lung machine. GX and WX were there, and they were two of the biggest klutzes I ever saw in my life. They used to ligate all the bleeders in the chest, and they'd put the stitch in and then they would tie it around one side of the clamp. Not around one side and then around the other—just around one, and I figured they got a 50/50 chance of getting the bleeder. It was just terrible surgery.

We went to see the guy who owned this little company and told him what we wanted, and he made a pump for us and we brought it back to the NIH, and Waldhausen and I went to the lab and did ... this is *unbelievable.* We operated on 20 dogs with an hour bypass through a median sternotomy in the dog, sat there at night and drained blood out of their chests, stayed up with the damn dogs all night. Nineteen of the 20 dogs survived the operation. You couldn't do that today. You really couldn't. I mean, it's hard to get dogs to survive a cardiopulmonary bypass.

Roberts: Did you report that?

Weldon: No. At any rate, then we started using the pump and people started living, and I used to run the pump.

Roberts: While you were at NIH?

Weldon: Yeah, I ran it whenever, because I mean we had used it in the lab. John and I used to run it. And so you know, Glenn was grateful, and he was the sort of man who was not above being grateful. And he was grateful, and he continued to be friendly with me, and there was some question about.... Henry Bahnson was opposed to my coming back from NIH. He and Glenn didn't get along. Henry Bahnson was opposed to my coming back. He wanted somebody else. I don't know who it was he wanted, but there was somebody else.

Roberts: You had only done one year at Hopkins?

Weldon: Just an internship. And I offended Hank somehow, or maybe not, maybe there was just somebody there that he was championing. At any rate, he spoke against me and for somebody else. I later discovered this. I wish I never had, because I adore Henry Bahnson, and he and I are very good friends now. Really, very good friends now. I mean, he has been much honored in retirement. Now I get invited to everything that happens. But at that time, he was opposed to my coming back, and Glenn came and made a trip from Bethesda to see Dr. Blalock.

Glenn and I remained close friends. I sort of drew away from him in the last years. It was like, I couldn't stand it. He was so sick, and you know, I just couldn't stand seeing that. There were a lot of people who ran down there, you know, but I didn't, I mean I couldn't stand it. I'm not that kind of guy. He didn't know whether they were coming or not, he was all stroked and stuff; and they had a big memorial for him and I didn't go. I just ...

Roberts: He admired you a lot, as my father said. He must have spoken of you.

Weldon: He may have; I don't know. Well now, what are you going to do with aortic valves?

Roberts: What angle do you suggest?

Weldon: Well, you know Dick [Richard E. Clark, d2014, Chief of Surgery Branch, Heart Institute, NIH, 1983-1990] has an awful lot of experience with analyzing valves and stuff. I hired Dick here with the promise that he was going to have a biological valve, not a biological valve, a valve made of artificial materials that simulated the biological structure. That's what we talked about before I hired him. He had finished the program with Charlottesville and then spent 2 years in the Navy at Bethesda, and I hired him out of the Navy program. He was satisfying Army duty. He was in the Navy 2 years, so he was 2 years past his residency, and when I hired him that's one of the things he was going to do. He was very much interested in fabrics and structural design. He is a trained engineer, you see, and electron microscopy, surface microscopy, and all that malarkey, and he had a lot of connections with engineers and computer people and so on, and he set up a very big program when he got here, and it did involve all those people—I mean, it was a multi-big hotdog thing.

I mean, we had everybody involved that you could involve. We had the computer experts and we had structural engineers and sound engineers and engineers up the gazoo, and the object of this was that we were going to structurally analyze the native aortic valve and how it worked, and then it was going to be simulated by weaving the fibers of the fabric in the same way that the collagen fibers existed in the aortic valves. There were a lot of studies on how the collagen fibers are in the aortic valve leaflets and how they move, and all kinds of studies he did, but he never came up with anything that worked, that could even be implanted very well in a dog. I mean, he came up with something and showed it to me, and I said, "That's it? That ain't gonna work." I mean, it was awfully crude.

Well then Dick got sidetracked. First of all, he was unhappy. He just never made it here as a clinical surgeon. He wasn't ever a very good clinical surgeon, and the word got around that he was a lot worse than he was. It was an awful place for whispering. And there were a couple of unfortunate things. I told him to go do a ductus one day, and he went over there and ligated the pulmonary artery instead of the ductus. Phil Dodge called me over there and said, "I only want to ask you one question. Could you have done this?" And I said, "Phil, honestly, no." You know, I don't know how he did that. I don't understand how he could have ligated the pulmonary artery instead of the ductus.

Well then he would do things like someone would send him a patient, and it would be something like lung cancer and they would want the patient operated on. Dick would go up and he would go over the chart in great detail, and he would make calculations and he would write this long note about it, and then he would summarize everything by saying that the patient's workup had been totally inadequate and the following things needed to be done to complete the workup. Well, you know there are very few people who want to hear that S. Very few. And very few of them have patients to refer. So he was dead. People told me, "I will send you a patient but if you send them to Clark, it will be the last one you ever get." Meanwhile, I had a bunch of private surgeons down the hall who were trying to get everything they could. Roper and Ferguson. I mean, it was a terrible mess. So Dick got pissed, you know, and he was always complaining, and he came and complained that I'm not promoting his career—and it was true, I wasn't.

Roberts: What were you expected to do?

Weldon: Give him cases. He wanted to do the TETS [tetrology of Fallot], he wanted to do the triple valve replacements, but he wasn't any good. He really just couldn't operate very well. He would get all tied in knots in the middle of the operation, and it would be disaster after disaster. You know, he is okay, but he shouldn't have been trying to do the things he was doing. I mean, he was just one of those people who should have got in it at a little lower level of expertise.

But then his lab work took... he sort of gave up on this aortic valve, you know, and it was really was a multi-institutional ... I mean the organizational background of that aortic valve study would have boggled your mind. I mean, it involved 13 institutions and half a dozen engineering institutions in the country and all the very best people, I mean it really did.

But he gave up on that and jumped on this cardioplegia S, you know. He got in on this calcium blocker, see. He was going to study that up one side and down the other. But then his work was a little.... I mean, he would make clinical studies on people who had 10 drips running, and they would make claims about what had happened. Well, he couldn't tell what had happened, no matter what. It was like those patients over there with 10 drips running, and he'd give a little nifedipine and say something happened. You can't do that, you know.

And then he became more and more disgruntled, and he was involved in all of this that was going on. My unhappiness, sort of the feud that developed between Ferguson and me, and he was trying to cozy up to Ferguson because Ferguson was president of this and president of that. I was never trying to cozy up to Ferguson. My response to Ferguson was different. But not Dick's. Dick wanted to kind of cozy up to him and he would do things. He'd tell him one thing and tell me the other, and it just got very bad. And then he made it clear that he wanted to leave after Cox came. He was here for a year with Cox, and then the job at the NIH, you couldn't give to anybody. It was such a bad job.

Roberts: There was no money?

Weldon: Money? $60,000 a year or something like that, something outrageous. I mean, you know I was paying Dick $150,000 for doing nothing, but Dick is rich. His father died and he is rich. He wasn't rich before his mother died (his father had sent the money to his mother). And when his mother died, he was rich. And then he could afford to take that job. I mean the only other person they were considering was Blakemore. I think he is a sort of a has-been surgeon in Toledo. And they really couldn't have given that job to anybody, it pays so little.

Roberts: I would think that for a young person, it would be a good job, though.

Weldon: Yes, they ought to abandon it. I mean, there isn't really any reason to have a clinical center down there. I'm not suggesting that they should abandon the laboratories. They shouldn't have a clinical heart center. I mean, that's ludicrous. That served a purpose down there when they were trying to start open-heart surgery. There was a lot of wherewithal down there to try to put together a heart-lung machine. It wouldn't do any good to put together a heart-lung machine and ask Clark if he wanted to try it out. There was some reason to have a clinical center there. Furthermore, people were working out the pathophysiology of heart disease. Cardiologists, Braunwald and all that crowd, were very busy down there.

But now there is nothing down there. I mean, they got a bunch of Greeks and then Glenn [Morrow] had this Greek connection. I mean, over there they gave him a Pompidou medal or something because he operated on some Greek woman with an ASD or something. He went over there, and they gave him the Pompidou medal and ... not Pompidou—what's the guy's name over there, the Greek—not Pompidou, something like that. At any rate, they gave him a medal, and from then on, this bunch of Greeks would come to the NIH to get operated on. Well, they would get operated on free with taxpayers' money. I mean, once that plane load started, you couldn't stop it. That is still what Dick does. I mean, that is who they operate on down there. Greeks. I mean, that ought to be stopped. They ought to close that. Not the labs, but the clinical center. Ain't nobody doing any important clinical work down there at all. I mean, they don't even have a board-certified surgeon. They've got Dick, who doesn't operate, I think. Then they got this other guy, what's his name ...

Roberts: McIntosh and Mike Jones.

Weldon: McIntosh, who has no boards. And then who else they got?

Roberts: Mike Jones. He's in the lab almost all the time.

Weldon: But there's no reason why they should be doing coronary artery bypass surgery at the NIH. I mean, there isn't. It strikes me that if you want to study the structure of bicuspid aortic valves and try to work out the natural history of how they calcify and when they calcify, I mean we really don't know. I mean, they all calcify, but what about their anatomy and structural arrangement leads to earlier calcification than otherwise? I mean, if you've got all this data, you ought to be able to figure that out, and that would be very valuable information. Furthermore, if you want to submit them to any kind of analysis about the way the fibers run and .... going all the time in the lab, you know, and he could tell you all about how much flow and what the profile of flow is.

Roberts: The bicuspid aortic valve would be interesting to study.

Weldon: Well, I think that would be a very interesting thing to do. To take a bicuspid valve and try to figure out what arrangement leads to what kind of turbulence pattern, and what kind of turbulence pattern leads to calcification, and is it turbulence that causes calcification, or is there some other structural abnormality in the valve that predisposes to calcification. No one has the slightest idea why bicuspid aortic valves calcify, but they all do. Tricuspid ones do, too, but it takes infinitely longer. I mean, you have to be 70 or 80 before your tricuspid valve calcifies, whereas your bicuspid valve will calcify when you're 40.

Now the street noise is that it does it because of turbulence, but that may or may not be so. The reason why people say that is because a ductus calcifies, but a ductus is a really different kind of structure. You get calcium in areas of turbulence. Not always—you don't get it in pulmonary valves very often, but whether it has something to do with flow or whether it's got the structural abnormality, collagen fibers are arranged differently, or the surface endothelium is arranged differently, or something. I think that is an excellent study. But I think it would involve setting up mock circuits, and I think it would involve dissecting these valves, decalcifying valves and, you know, trying to get some information about their skeletons, fiber arrangements, and then the anatomy of the valve as it exists. Early ones that calcify at 20, are they different from the ones that calcify at 40? Or different from the ones that calcify at 60? Is there some clue to why they did that? It's an excellent idea, I think. But I can't imagine any better help than Dick, because he did all that stuff.

Roberts: I did not know that Dr. Clark's focus was valves.

Weldon: For 10 years. On the aortic valve, specifically. For 10 years, Dick did nothing but work on the aortic valve. You ought to get hold of his bibliography. He wrote a lot, too. He published a lot of stuff, you know, on the fiber arrangement.

Roberts: Do you mind if I ask you what paper you liked the best of your own writings. I noticed that you wrote the first couple as a medical student.

Weldon: I started that stuff when I was down about thrombosis being caused by electricity. We had this elaborate theory. It was very popular for a while. Other people worked on it for a while. Doesn't have anything to do with it. I am sure it is a biochemical phenomenon. But we had this idea that when you injured the epithelium, there was a change that we could demonstrate in the electrical potential, of course. The idea and its positivity. It becomes more positive, and the platelets carry a negative charge and they are more attracted, a bioelectricity. I am sure it is not so. I am sure it is a biochemical phenomenon, but we did a lot of stuff. I had this little apparatus that I used to put platelets in, and then I would suspend the platelets in various blood plasma-proteins, solutions of plasma-proteins, and measure the electrophoresis apparatus, electrophoresis apparatus 25 years ago, and watch through the microscope and watch the migrations of the platelets in an electric field and then change the protein and see what it would do and work out sort of what happened. You get a curve with a charge on the platelet changes in response to the number of proteins in the blood, and so that was the kind of stuff I was doing when I was in medical school, and we were trying to make clots in the lab, setting up potentials across coronary arteries.

Roberts: Creating thrombus.

Weldon: In fact, I was very interested in it and interested in the vascular clot.

Roberts: One paper I would especially like to get a reprint of.

Weldon: You better come in a hurry. I'm going to throw everything away.

Roberts: It's the one on surgery in world history.

Weldon: That's the AOA lecture I gave. It was just a kind of cutesy-pie lecture. It had to do with people who had operations and survived the operation. It had to do with Rishner's bouginage of his urethra, which is a marvelous story, and I told this in a very dramatic way. He was at Langdock and he couldn't urinate, and they said he was going to die. They got this young surgeon who came out and made a thing of wax and mastic, beeswax and mastic, and dipped it into it like a candle until it got more and more on it, and he passed it into the urethra of Rishner while two of his courtiers held him standing up. He was standing up and they held him, and they passed the catheter and withdrew it, and the cardinal urinated two liters of urine, or five liters of urine, I forgot what, and they put it on display and they showed it to everybody. He had a perineal abscess, which was the cause of the problem. He didn't have prostatism. He had a perineal abscess, and he later died of the perineal abscess, but 20 years later. He died of sepsis.

And then I talked about Louis XV, who had an anal fissure operated on, and that is a very dramatic story, too. You see, Madame what-was-her-name, his mistress, was very much involved, and they operated on him and had to cut it 4 times, and they did it without general anesthetic. And then I talked about the attempted assassination of President Garfield, and he died of sepsis, but it took him 6 months to die. It was a very dramatic speech.

Roberts: Where was he shot?

Weldon: Shot in the abdomen. The wound injured the splenic artery, so he developed a splenic artery aneurysm, but the bullet went in and missed the pancreas and then went down in the retroperitoneum and he got a big abscess in the groin, but he died of sepsis. He didn't really injure anything. He just died of pus. But it was all about the doctors coming in, and I knew the names of all the doctors who came in, and they probed the wound with their fingers and stuck instruments in it, and so on. It was a very dramatic speech about how he wanted to go to Ohio, and they said he couldn't, so he went to New Jersey and died in a cottage there.

And I talked about the President who had his jaw removed on a yacht. He had sarcoma of the palate, and they took out his jaw, and it is a very dramatic story, too, because a repeal of the Sherman Anti-Trust laws was about to be done, and the President had to appear. So they made him an artificial jaw, which he wore long enough to preside over Congress. Nobody knew he had had his jaw taken out. It was all done in secret. John Erdman from Columbia University did the operation. It was Grover Cleveland.

Let's see what else is in that talk. I forgot. I talked about Krupskaya's thyroidectomy. Nadia Krupskaya was Lenin's wife, and she got Grave's disease and exophthalmos and was operated on by Kocker. I reviewed the correspondence between Lenin and his brother. Lenin's brother was a doctor, and he wrote to his brother about K's condition, asking what should be done. Finally Alexander Yulenoff, Vladimir Yulenoff's brother, who was the doctor, recommended that she go to Berlin and be operated on by Kocker, and Kocker did a thyroidectomy. She lived for many, many years and was responsible for the Moscow purge trials of Kamenev and Zinovyev [1936-1938].

I reviewed all that Soviet history, and I talked about the gunshot wound Lenin had. He was shot by Fanny Kaplan, an anarchist. A German anarchist shot Lenin in the neck, and they explored it and removed the bullet. It was lying right next to the carotid artery, and there was some other stuff in there. Anyway, it was a very dramatic speech.

End Note

During my 2 years at Barnes Hospital in St. Louis [1998-1990], I had the privilege of working with several of the surgeons mentioned in this interview. I first assisted Dr. Roper one morning on a very challenging lobectomy through a redo thoracotomy. He was a superb general thoracic surgeon. Dr. Ferguson was always gracious when I took care of his patients in the ICU. It was indeed also a privilege to interact with Dr. Cox who was, and continues to be, at all times, friendly and supportive. Years later, he wrote a letter of recommendation for me to join the Cosmos Club in Washington, DC. I assisted Dr. Ballinger, a distinguished gentleman, on many inguinal hernia repairs. He gave me an inscribed copy of his book on trauma. I had the privilege of second assisting Dr. Wells on several thyroidectomy and parathyroidectomy operations. He was meticulous, in and out of the operating room.

My first interaction with Dr. Weldon was memorable. I came in to close the leg incision during a coronary bypass operation. He looked down at me closing the leg, from his surgeon position, and said, "And what position in this august body do you hold?" "Intern, sir," could be the only response.

Dr. Weldon and I stayed in contact briefly after the interview, and our mutual departure from St. Louis. My wife, Pamela, and I met him in at the Waldorf Hotel in New York City for Sunday brunch one weekend, traveling from Bethesda. He was a kind of Renaissance man, authentic and kind to a trainee 32 years younger. His 18 years in retirement from surgery (1988-2006), I hope, were happy. This interview stayed in manuscript form for 37 years. It shows the periodic political challenges that perhaps every heart surgeon faces in a long career.

—Charles S. Roberts, MD
June 8, 2025

Weldon CS, Roberts CS. Clarence S. Weldon, MD: An Interview by Charles S. Roberts, MD. May 30, 1988 (previously unpublished).

Appendix B

WILLIAM CLIFFORD ROBERTS, MD: An Interview by Charles Stewart Roberts, MD

William Clifford Roberts, MD, and Charles Stewart Roberts, MD

A Half-Century in the Cardiovascular Arena

Over the last decade, several physicians have encouraged me to interview my father for publication. For one reason or another, I failed to comply with these requests until recently, when we both attended a medical meeting aboard a ship in the Mediterranean. The men and the opportunity had finally met.

Having also pursued a medical career in cardiovascular disease, I am well acquainted with the medical work of my father. We lived under the same roof for my first 18 years of life, so I know his work habits and many of his strongly held medical opinions. The summer before departing for college, I worked in his laboratory at the National Institutes of Health and completed a project with him. It involved measuring the sizes of coronary arteries in patients with differing heart weights to learn if coronary size was proportional to cardiac mass. Ten years later, I returned to the National Heart, Lung, and Blood Institute as a Clinical Associate in the Surgery Branch, which was down the hall from my father's Pathology Branch. I made a point to attend his weekly conferences during those 2 years, and learned a great deal. We also spent many Saturdays together completing manuscripts.

My father has interviewed 125 people for publication, and now the tables are turned. He has been in medicine for a half-century and has contributed significantly in the field of cardiovascular disease. Over the last 25 years, I have had occasion to observe him at his desk in Bethesda and later in Dallas poring over manuscripts submitted to *The American Journal of Cardiology*. He will not enjoy a weekend until he is up to date on the manuscripts. I am surprised that he took the time to allow me to interview him, and hope the readership, and those friends who requested this interview, will not be disappointed.

Charles Stewart Roberts, MD
Chairman, Section of Thoracic and
Cardiovascular Surgery
The Heart and Vascular Center
Winchester Medical Center
Valley Health System
Winchester, Virginia

Charles Stewart Roberts, MD (hereafter **Charles**): *Today is October 24, 2006, and I am seated with my father, Dr. William C. Roberts (hereafter **William**) (Figure 1), in the Connoisseur Room of the Crystal Serenity ship in Sorrento, Italy. We are both attending the 15th International Cardiovascular Symposium hosted by Dr. Mahfouz el Shahawy of Sarasota, Florida. Dad, this is not your first medical meeting on a cruise?*

William: Correct. It is my fifth.

Charles: *Have you enjoyed it?*

William: I've loved it.

Charles: *How many talks did you give on this cruise?*

William: Three.

Charles: *What were they on?*

William: Preventing and arresting atherosclerosis; systemic hypertension, the magnitude of the problem and the importance of lowering an elevated pressure; and how coronary artery disease causes heart failure and how heart failure can be prevented in patients with coronary artery disease.

Charles: *Let's talk about your parents and their families. In what year were you born and where?*

William: I was born on September 11, 1932, at Emory University Hospital, which was then Emory University, Georgia, but is now Atlanta, Georgia.

Charles: *You are 74 years of age.*

William: Correct.

Charles: *What were the circumstances of your immediate family at the time of your birth? Where were you living?*

William: When I was born my mother, father and older brother (Stewart Ralph Roberts, Jr), who is only 11 months older than I am, were living at 1300 Ponce de Leon Avenue in a very nice house that my father had lived in for many years. It was about 2 miles from Emory University Hospital.

Charles: *How old were your parents at the time of your birth?*

William: My father was 54, and my mother was 26 (Figures 2 and 3).

Charles: *When did your family move to the farm in Stone Mountain, Georgia?*

William: I think it was 1935. My father had very high blood pressure. He knew that he was not going to survive long enough to see his youngsters grow up. As a consequence, he thought it would be a good idea, according to my mother, to move the family to a farm, a good place for young boys to grow up and also a place that could produce income to live (from milk and produce). I think he considered farming a good activity and good discipline for young boys (Figures 4 and 5).

Charles: *Your father, Stewart Ralph Roberts, died when you were 8 years old. Do you have any memories of your father?*

William: Unfortunately, few. I remember going hunting one afternoon with my father, my brother, and our neighbor, Tim Hudman. That's about all I remember. My brother, Stewart, being 11 months older and being the Junior, placed him in a bit more favored position than me, an understandable circumstance, and he remembers more about my father than I do. He went on a few train trips with my father, who traveled to see patients and to attend meetings. I have thought a bit about why I have so few memories of my father, and yet I was 8 when he died. The answer probably results in a large part from my father's severe heart attack (acute myocardial infarction) in 1937 when I was 4 years

0002-9149/07/$ – see front matter
doi:10.1016/j.amjcard.2007.04.009

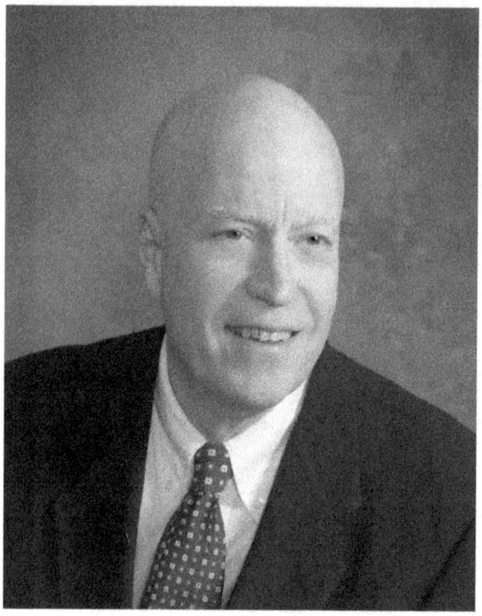

Figure 1. WCR in 2007 at age 74.

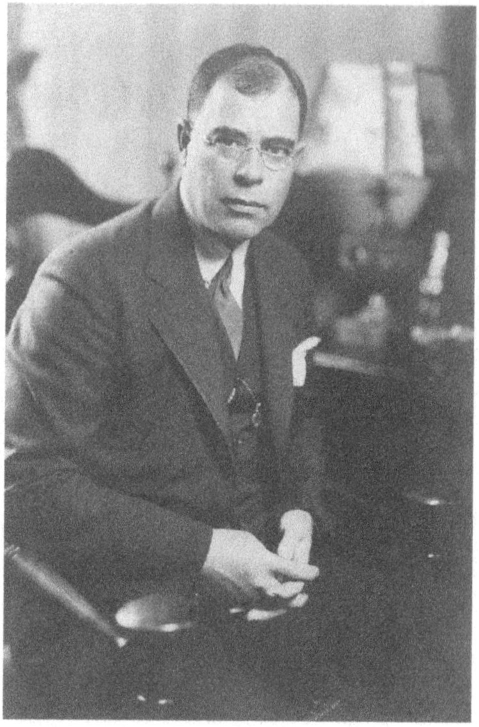

Figure 2. Stewart Ralph Roberts, MD, when he was approximately 54 years of age at the time WCR was born.

old. He was left with severe and progressive heart failure (ischemic cardiomyopathy). After recuperating for nearly a year at home (standard therapy at that time), he returned to his practice despite obvious heart failure. The usual therapy for acute myocardial infarction in 1937 included hospitalization for 1 month at complete bed rest, then home in bed for 2 months, then movement about the house for 3 months, and from 7 to 12 months gradual increase in out-of-the home activities. Because he had been president of the American Heart Association (1933 to 1934), he knew the standard therapy for acute myocardial infarction and so did his partners. His partners paid him $500 a month during the year he was out. Although my father went back to work in 1938 and worked until a second heart attack in April 1941, he went to bed as soon as he got home from work. I think my mother probably protected him from my brother and me so that he could rest, and that "protection" probably accounts in part for my poor memory of him.

About 20 years ago, my mother related the story passed to her about my father's visiting a patient, and by the time my father had climbed the steps to enter the house he was so short of breath he could barely talk to the woman's husband.

Charles: *There was a fire at the farm house at some point?*

William: Yes. My father died on April 14, 1941, and some months thereafter the house burned to the ground. We had gone to Emory Methodist Church, and then to my maternal grandmother's house on Tenth Street in Atlanta to have lunch. We soon got a call that our house was burning. We drove immediately back to the farm which was probably 12 miles away, and stopped at the fire station in Avondale and asked if they could come put out the fire. The fireman said that our house wasn't in their territory. When we arrived at the farm a lot of cars were parked in the long driveway. The house was in flames. Some of the neighbors, who had seen the flames from the road, broke into the house, and threw some books out the windows and saved some furniture downstairs but nothing from upstairs. We watched it burn to the ground. No firemen came to help. Today, our farm is entirely houses. About 20 years ago, while visiting Atlanta, I drove to Redan Road to see what that farm area looked liked. I couldn't identify one relic that I had known as a kid. The farmland (118 acres) had been replaced with numerous houses.

Charles: *What happened then?*

William: We moved to Atlanta. Bill Neal, my mother's brother-in-law who was married to her sister Charlotte, had just volunteered for the Army. They had put their house, located at 16 Woodcrest Avenue, a couple of blocks off of Peachtree Road near Brookwood Hills railroad station, up for sale, and my mother bought it from them for $6,000. The next month, Bill Neal was ruled ineligible for the service (some foot deformity), and the Neals bought a larger house.

Charles: *Your mother lived in that home for how many years?*

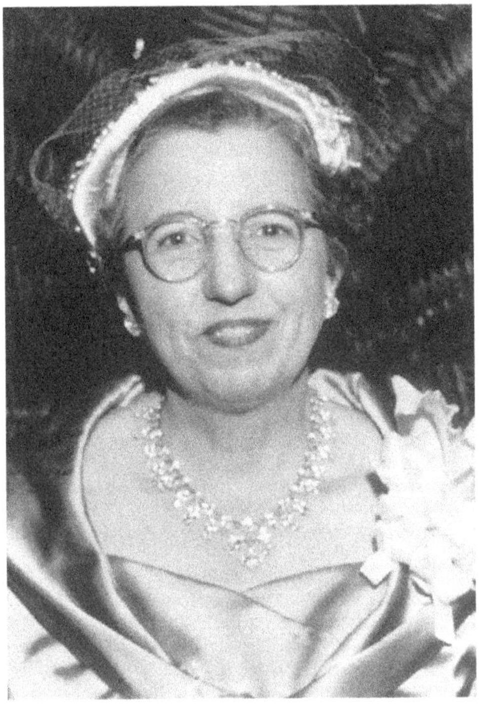

Figure 3. Ruby Holbrook Roberts, WCR's mother, in 1957 at the time of her oldest son's wedding when she was 53 years old.

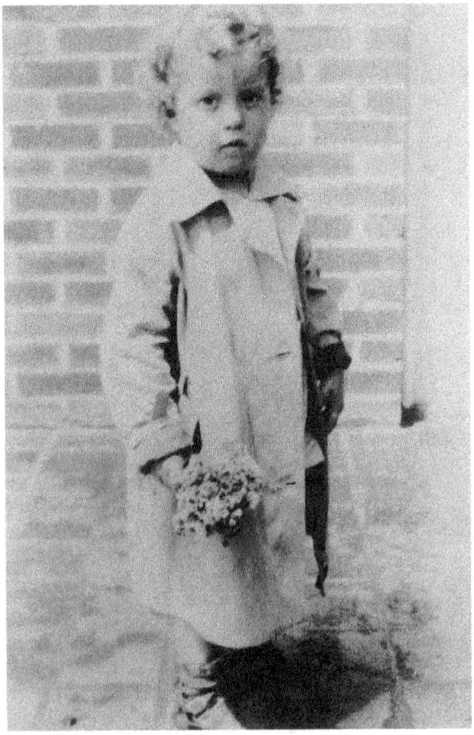

Figure 4. WCR as a little boy.

William: For 46 years (1942 to 1987). She then moved in with her sister, Sarah, to a nursing home. I left home for college in 1950, and my brother a year earlier, so she lived alone for nearly 40 years.

Charles: *Talk about your mother.*

William: My mother was born in 1903 and died in 1994 at age 91. She was healthy all her life until age 84, when she had a stroke (possibly secondary to atrial fibrillation). Her voice changed a bit after that, and she became progressively weaker. Until 1987 she had been very active. My mother was very kind, sweet, pleasing, nonjudgmental, nondemanding; she never felt sorry for herself, and she usually had a smile on her face.

Charles: *She was from a big family?*

William: Yes. She was 1 of 11 siblings (10 girls) and 3 half-siblings (2 girls). My mother's name was Ruby Viola Holbrook. Her father had been married previously and was left with 3 offspring when his first wife died. My mother's father died at age 45. His last child was Charlotte, and he died just before Charlotte was born. My mother's father was a carpenter who built some of the fancy furniture in the Pullman Railroad cars. He apparently had a number of episodes of pulmonary insufficiency as an adult. My father, according to my mother, thought he had tuberculosis. That makes sense, because at least 3 of my mother's sisters also had tuberculosis, which was fairly common in Atlanta and other places in 1910 or so.

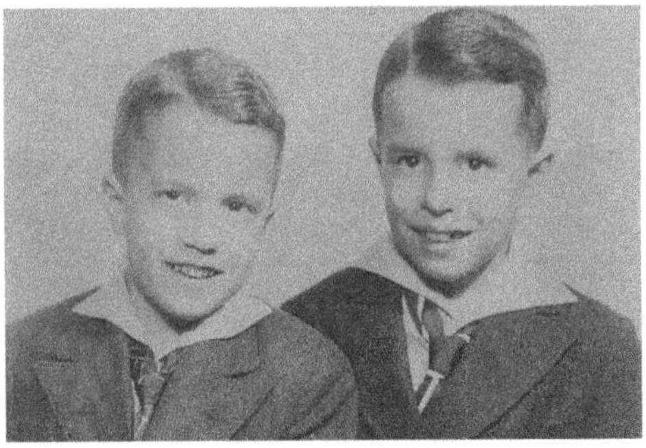

Figure 5. WCR *(left)* and his brother, Stewart Ralph Roberts, Jr, probably about 1940 when both were in grammar school.

Charles: *Was your mother close to her siblings?*

William: Yes, very close. All her siblings worked hard. Mother was particularly fond of Vivian, a half-sister, who they called "sister," and who worked for a bank. Sister managed the family's financial affairs after their father died.

Sister was very smart. (Today almost certainly she would have been an officer in the bank, but in those times women were not permitted to go very far in business.) Of those 12 sisters, including the 2 half sisters, 8 married. The single aunts lived their lives in Atlanta. We all got together at Easter, Thanksgiving, and Christmas. Although all of the sisters worked hard, they never appeared unhappy or depressed. They never expected too much out of life. If somebody passed away, they were saddened but each considered death and illness a part of life. My mother worked exceedingly hard. Only the last 3 sisters were able to go to college. The first 9 had to go to work as soon as they finished high school. In the early 20th century, there were only 3 high schools in Atlanta: Commercial High which emphasized typing and shorthand—very practical things — and Girls High and Boys High. My mother and her sisters all went to Commercial High School. Late in her life, she told me that she was very sorry that she didn't have the money to go to college, for if she had she would have gone to Agnes Scott College in Decatur, Georgia, and majored in English.

My mother was a very dear lady. We were quite close. On a typical day, she worked from about 8 A.M. to 5:30 P.M. Then she would come home and fix dinner. (Most kids in the neighborhood ate earlier than we did. I always wanted to eat earlier, so that I could go out and play with them.) My mother, brother, and I would have dinner together, and then I usually would rinse and stack the dishes. Then my mother and I would usually talk some in the living room. She had her own business (Medical Placement and Mailing Service) and didn't really have anybody to talk to about business problems. She would talk to me about them. I enjoyed that and I got the impression after awhile that she sort of liked what I had to say. In a way, these discussions were a bit of a confidence builder for me. I never remember my brother participating in those conversations. Visitors to our house were usually my mother's single sisters and her female friends. Thus, my brother and I grew up in a very female-oriented environment. Because none of the single sisters or my mother had gone to college, the conversations were not especially inspiring. Two married sisters also lived in Atlanta, but my brother and I saw the 2 uncles only on the 3 holiday feasts (mentioned earlier). My mother tended to put men on a pedestal, since she grew up in a female environment. My mother always referred to my father as "Dr. Roberts." I doubt if she ever called him "Stewart." As far as I know, my mother had only one date after my father died. At work, she was liked by her male business contacts. She dealt with men as with other women in a very relaxed manner. My father and mother were married only 11 years, and she was only 37 when he died.

Charles: *What was her career path?*

William: After graduating from high school, she got a job with the telephone company (AT&T). From there she went to another company (I don't remember the company's name). Then she saw an advertisement in the newspaper that there was a position open in a physician's office on Juniper Street, near the corner of Fifth Street. She lived on Tenth Street. That appealed to her, because she could walk the 5 blocks to work. That job offer was from her future husband. She went to work in his office at age 24. He was twice her age. His office building, formerly a residential house, was initially called "The Roberts Clinic" and later "The Roberts Memorial Clinic." There, my father saw his private patients. She became his secretary. When he would see patients in the examining room, she would accompany him. He would dictate his findings, and she recorded his dictation in shorthand. As a consequence, she was with him a good bit. In the early mornings, my father visited his patients in Emory University Hospital, and then he would drive to the Juniper Street office later in the morning. My mother would type the dictations from the previous day before he got to the office. She told me that when she walked to work those 5 blocks, she would whistle and somebody told her one time that she was a happy girl. I got my whistling habit from my mother. Later, she became a hummer, and she would walk around the house humming.

My mother assisted my father with his manuscripts. She would go out to his house, have dinner with him and his first wife, and then he would dictate some of his medical manuscripts. Afterwards, she retuned home and the next morning type the manuscript. Thus, she got to see how he lived in the Ponce de Leon house, which I visited about 20 years ago. I knocked on the door and 2 Delta Airline pilots greeted me and graciously showed me around. It is still a beautiful house. They showed me a plaque in the basement with the Roberts name on it.

I think it was a mistake to move to the farm. My brother doesn't agree with me, but the move was in the midst of the Depression. The farm was costly. They built a house, bought cows, eventually bought ponies for my brother and me, and paid and boarded an overseer and his family. The farm drained them of money. The entire period (11 years of marriage) they were heavily in debt. My father divorced his first wife in 1928 and borrowed about $25,000, a lot of money at that time, to fund her alimony. (There were no children from the first marriage.) My mother called his first wife a "social" one. She apparently spent several months each year in Florida. Her name was Louise Welch. I regret that I never met her. Although he had divorced his first wife, he didn't propose to my mother for a number of months. As a result, she moved to New York City. After some months, he came to New York, proposed to her, and they got married there in December 1929. The great market crash had occurred in October 1929 and as a result that $25,000 my father foolishly borrowed and sunk into stocks became worthless paper. He had that debt to pay back the rest of his life, plus borrowing for the farm and equipping it. Then in 1937, he had a heart attack and couldn't see patients for a year. I think once he got back to work in 1938, he didn't have the physical capacity to see as many patients as he had previously. When he died in April 1941, my mother was left with a good bit of debt. Although she was married to a prominent physician, she was in debt the entire marriage and she paid the debt back by 1946.

After 1946, she formed her own business called the Medical Placement and Mailing Service. It consisted of herself, 1 other full-time employee, and a part-time (often me) employee to handle the mailing services. She would place secretaries and nurses in physicians' offices. Occasionally, she would place a physician with an insurance company. Initially, her fee for placing a secretary or nurse in a physician's office was only $25. It was hard to make a living on that. Eventually, that increased to half the first month's salary. Generally, the physicians would pay the fee. The other part of the business was a mailing service. She would send out announcements of meetings for physicians. Some physicians, particularly surgeons, who would do various operations, would ask her to send out 1,000 or so of their reprints to their referring doctors. She had a couple of mailing machines. The stencils of typed addresses would be placed into the mailing machine, and then by hitting the foot pedal the name would be printed on the envelope or on the back of programs so that they could be folded, sealed, and mailed. To keep the mailing lists up to date (because physicians moved, retired, or died) nearly every night during my growing up my mother would be in her bedroom typing the physician addresses. I was the mailing part of that office operation off and on for a long time. Her office was located initially in my father's former office building on Juniper Street at 5th Street. She was on the second floor, and the physicians were on the first floor.

Charles: *When did she retire?*

William: In the late 1970s. Somebody walked into her office, and said, "I'll give you $75,000 for this business." She said, "Ok." They gave her $75,000 and then the new owners closed the business. I never quite understood, but it was a godsend. That was the most she had ever made. In retrospect, I think she would have been better off if she had stayed with the insurance company. Keeping her mailing service up-to-date was a constant effort.

Growing up we had only 1 vacation, a trip to New York City including Coney Island. She took 1 of her lady friends, Sarah Vickery, and my brother and me. She did not work on Saturday or Sunday, but she worked Monday through Friday and every night. She never felt sorry for herself. She never complained about working. She cooked our meals. We usually had no household help. Most of the housecleaning was done by my brother and me on Sundays. We'd go to church, return home, clean the house, and then go out to play.

Charles: *Was your mother protective of you or were you independent?*

William: To be frank, I thought my mother knew relatively little about boys and understandably so. She grew up in an all-female family, and she had 3 boys. She had had very little experience with boys. Only 1 of her married sisters had a son. There was only 1 male cousin in the whole family aside from my brother and me. Our youngest brother, Ross Holbrook Roberts, was severely mentally retarded. He was born in 1935 and died nearly 25 years later. My father apparently couldn't believe that he had a retarded son. My mother identified the situation earlier than he did. At age 5, he was sent to a private home for these type kids. My mother later told me that sending him away was the hardest thing she ever had to do.

Charles: *This was the Stewart House Training School in Frankfurt, Kentucky?*

William: Yes.

Charles: *Did she send Ross away after your father had died?*

William: No. It was before. It was a joint decision, probably in 1939 or 1940. I'm sure my father said they had to send him to a private home. After my father died, there was not enough money to keep him in the private institution. He was transferred to a public home in Augusta, Georgia (Gracewood Training School), where he lived until he died in 1960. My mother went to see him about once a year. Putting him in a home away from home clearly was the right thing to do, since he was very mentally retarded.

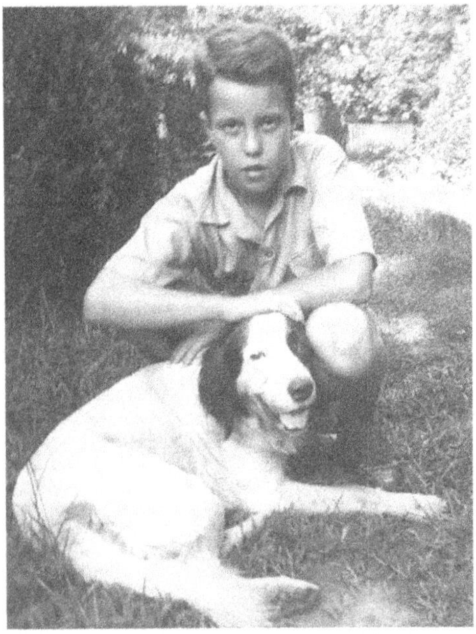

Figure 6. WCR with Rex, their birddog, probably about 1940.

Charles: *Did you ever meet him?*

William: Yes. I went down to Augusta a few times with my mother. I never liked it. The very mentally undeveloped just wasn't a pretty sight.

Charles: *What were your mother's expectations of you growing up? You mentioned your independence earlier?*

William: When we moved to Atlanta, my brother Stewart was in the sixth grade, and I was in the fifth grade at Spring Street Grammar School (Figure 6). I liked it. It wasn't far from home. My brother was put in a class with Ms. Adams, and the other sixth grade teacher was Ms. Clifton. Ms. Adams was a disaster, and Stewart just couldn't stand her. When I entered the sixth grade, I was put in Ms. Adams class also. Stewart told me later that he was mad at mother for permitting that. I tried to keep up with what Ms. Clifton's class was doing. The downside of being in Ms. Adams class was when I entered O'Keefe Junior High School, I was placed in a class with relatively poorly performing students. The school had 7 or 8 seventh grade classes: class 72 was the smart students, 73 the next smartest, and I was about 78 or 79 when entering junior high school. By the eighth grade, I had worked up to about 85 (range 82 to 90), and by the ninth grade, I was about 93.

My brother and I were essentially independent from the time we came to Atlanta. We had bicycles and rode them everywhere and anywhere. Stewart and I bought our own clothes. When bringing home a report card, I don't ever remember a discussion about our grades, whether good or bad. There was no external pressure to do well. I took a typing class in the eleventh grade fortunately. Before that my mother would often type a paper I had written.

Charles: *Was religion important in your home?*

William: Yes, until I went away to college. I went to First Presbyterian Sunday school. My mother would pick me up afterwards and then we would drive to St. Mark's Methodist Church for the 11:00 A.M. service. St. Mark's Church was on Fifth Street, close to my father's office. My mother was always a religious person. Although I don't recall ever seeing her reading the Bible, she certainly believed in God. She never cursed or drank alcohol or smoked. She was always good to her fellow men and women. She had no element of arrogance. She was a very humble. The First Presbyterian Church for me was important for both social and intellectual development, because each Sunday evening there was a service conducted entirely by and for the young people. I gave a few talks at those services, the first I had ever given. I worked on those talks, and I enjoyed that activity. My brother didn't participate in the Presbyterian services, and he often did not go to St. Mark's Church for the 11:00 A.M. service.

Charles: *Did you read the Bible yourself?*

William: I did some, but I am not a good student of the Bible. When I did, it was usually the New Testament, not the Old Testament.

Charles: *Did you pray?*

William: Yes, every night before I went to sleep.

Charles: *Did you memorize any passages or prayers from the Bible?*

William: Some: The Lord's Prayer, the 23rd Psalm, and the Apostle's Creed. The standard ones I knew.

Charles: *You would describe your religious home environment as neither fundamentalist nor secular but somewhere in-between?*

William: Yes. As a youngster I always thought of myself as being very religious. I tried to be a good boy. Although some of my high school friends would curse like crazy, I refrained from cursing until I was in my 40s, and I limited the words to *damn* and *hell*. One other thing about independence. I think that my personality was such that I thrived on it. I loved not having somebody have a clamp on me. I was a *free* kid. I avoided cigarette smoking, and alcohol drinking (until I was 27), which was probably good, because I went through college and medical school never having to experience a hangover or depleted energy from drinking alcohol. And I didn't have a lot of money. My mother gave me $100, if I wouldn't smoke until I was 21. A lot of boys and girls my age smoked. Fortunately, I did not.

I had a paper route from the time that I was in the eighth grade until I was a senior in high school. I had the best paper route in the area. It consisted of 2 large apartments, 2 blocks apart, the houses on Peachtree Road in between, and 2 other streets. I could throw the route in 45 minutes. When I was busy somewhere else, another fellow would throw the route for me, and I would pay him. Several boys wanted my paper route.

Charles: *This was the Atlanta Journal/Constitution?*

William: At that time, it was only the *Atlanta Journal*, the afternoon paper. The *Constitution* was the morning paper. They eventually merged. I always had money in my pocket because of the paper route.

Charles: *Did you have any other jobs?*

William: In high school, I had a job during my junior year at the YMCA right after school until 6:00 P.M. I farmed out my paper route that entire year except for the weekends. I didn't particularly like getting up on Sunday morning to throw those papers, but it was worth it. The man who hired me was George Abbott, who became a mentor and for awhile a substitute father. He was a great guy. He hailed from Boston. He was head of the YMCA in Atlanta. Sometimes after work, he'd take me to dinner. He had gone to Harvard and thought I should go to Harvard, but I thought I wasn't that good a student. He wrote to them, and I took some test to see if I was bright enough, and it came back saying that if I would go to a prep school for a year after high school that maybe then they would consider me a candidate for Harvard. My family didn't have the Harvard kind of money, and I wanted to get on with it. Nevertheless, I was flattered that he even considered me a potential candidate. He also was the basketball coach at the YMCA. I loved playing basketball. I wasn't good enough to make the high school team, but we had a YMCA league and I played in it. I was a late developer. When I got my driver's license at age 16, I was 65 inches tall and weighed 110 lbs. Those numbers were on my first driver's license. During my junior and senior year in high school and my freshman year in college I grew 7 inches in height.

Charles: *When you stopped developing, what were your dimensions?*

William: When I went off to college, I think I was 70 inches tall and 145 lbs. I lifted weighs a lot my senior year in high school. My usual weight through the years has been 165 lbs, but presently I am 175. I am 6 feet tall.

Charles: *What about Henry Grady High School?*

William: I liked it very much. I was in the first class of Henry Grady High School. Previously, that high school had been Boys High. As Atlanta grew, some of the previous junior highs were converted into high schools. Henry Grady High School was co-ed. This was 1947, right after the end of World War II. Grady didn't have enough classrooms to accommodate all the students, so there were wooden shacks outside the main building. Henry Grady was on 10th Street, a 1/2 mile from where my maternal grandmother had lived.

Charles: *Atlanta was a segregated community?*

William: Correct. The old Grady High was an all-white school. I went to my 55th high school reunion in 2005. Henry Grady High School had expanded. It's beautiful. It went from all white to all black and now about 50–50 black–white. I wish I had been an athlete in high school, because so many of my friends were athletes. But I wasn't. Football and basketball and track were big sports there.

Charles: *Who were your classmates at Henry Grady High School?*

William: One of my friends was Jid Thompson. (He subsequently changed his name to Jed.) He was a half-back on the football team, captain of the track team, and made better grades than I did. All the girls liked him. Once in a physics class, I bet him that I would make a better grade on the next test than he did, and I did. Another friend was Frank Taylor, who lived down the street. He smoked and drank too early and his academic output diminished, which was a shame, because he was really very bright. There were a lot of bright students at Grady High School. A good number in the Jewish community went to school there. I had an algebra teacher in the tenth grade who told me that I was pretty good at math. I loved that teacher. That was a major intellectual boost for me, because it really made me work in algebra and math after that. I didn't want to disappoint her.

Charles: *Did you have a counselor to talk to about college or did you talk to your mother about college?*

William: No, neither.

Charles: *Did you talk to anybody about college?*

William: No. I applied to Southern Methodist University (SMU) entirely because of hearing about it through its football team. Doak Walker had been a 3-year All American and Kyle Rote, a 2-year all-American. In retrospect, I wanted to go to a college away from home, to a co-ed school, and to one located in a city about the size of Atlanta. I applied to SMU and was accepted almost immediately.

Charles: *Did you apply to Emory or any other places?*

William: No. Only SMU. My mother accepted my desire to go to SMU, which was 850 miles from Atlanta. I knew my being that far away was going to be a major shakeup for her, because she would be home by herself. Although I thought going a long way away to college was selfish of me, I think I realized that I needed this type of change, and I sensed that my mother also thought it would be good for me. I liked the idea of Texas. I had never traveled, except for the trip to New York City and a summer camp once in North Carolina. When going off to SMU, I didn't know a soul there, but I liked that type of opportunity.

Charles: *Did anybody from Henry Grady High School go to SMU?*

William: No, not when I went, but the second semester of my freshman year one of my high school friends, Bill Chesnut, moved with his family to Fort Worth. He called me and asked how I liked SMU? I told him I thought it was great. So he came to SMU beginning the second semester, and we roomed together. He also pledged Phi Delta Theta fraternity. My roommate the first semester was a fellow from Athens, Greece, who had been a fencing champion there. He was a very handsome fellow and all the girls loved him. It was like living with Babe Ruth. Lots of nights he wasn't there!

Charles: *Compare Georgia and Texas in 1950?*

William: For 6 years, I had ushered on Saturday afternoons at the Georgia Tech football home games in Atlanta, showing people their seats. I got to see all the home games free. When I went to SMU, their first opponent was Georgia Tech. Georgia Tech kicked off to SMU and SMU brought it back to the 30-yard line. I was sitting on the 30-yard line at the other end of the field. It was single-wing formation then. They hiked the ball to Kyle Rote, and he took off through right tackle. He was coming right at me. I had to make up my mind in that instant whether I wanted him to be tackled by Georgia Tech or wanted him to go all the way. He went all the way, 70 yards on that first play. I liked SMU.

I didn't have a car, and I was far from sophisticated. Texas was a great experience. SMU at the time had a reputation of being a college for rich kids, but that was not entirely true. The tuition was quite reasonable then. I worked periodically on Saturdays, selling price-reduction coupons at shopping centers, e.g. half-off oil change, etc. I learned I was pretty good at that. A fellow would pick up about 5 of us college kids, and we'd go to the shopping centers. If a coupon sold for $1.00, the seller could keep half of that. I made a good bit of spending money doing that. I was the top seller usually every Saturday.

Charles: *Who paid for your college?*

William: My mother did. My father had left some money for college, and so I was not required to work for tuition or books. I lived in a dormitory, and it was inexpensive compared to today. I also worked during summers and saved money from that. In medical school, I worked as an extern at Crawford Long Hospital during my junior year and at Emory Hospital during my senior year. It was good training.

Charles: *What did you study in college?*

William: I went to college thinking I was going to be a businessman, even though I knew little about business. I majored in English. An English major at SMU could get English-course credits in certain history classes. I took more history classes than I did English classes. I found the Shakespeare class a bit difficult. The Shakespeare tests consisted of describing scenes when various Shakespeare phrases were presented. I found the girls to be quite good at that. I wasn't very good at that. By the time I became a junior, I decided I wanted to go to medical school. I studied hard in college. Proportional to the amount of time I spent studying, I should have made better grades than I did. I got to be a better student as time went on in college. By the time I hit medical school, I was more sophisticated about studying than I had been in college.

Charles: *What about your fraternity, Phi Delta Theta?*

William: I had been in a fraternity since the ninth grade in high school. Fraternities were popular in high schools in Atlanta at the time. By college, I was a little tired of that stuff, but it was a group and I thought being in a group was important. I went through rush and I liked 3 fraternities—KA, SAE, and Phi Delta Theta. Many of the Phi Delts had grown up in Dallas, went to Highland Park High School, and I decided that that was the fraternity I wanted to be in. When the pledges were dished out, however, I didn't get an invitation to join Phi Delta Theta, but I did get invitations from the other 2 fraternities. I decided to wait it out and see what would happen. Sure enough, by the third week in the freshman year, I got a bid and joined Phi Delta Theta. We had 23 in my pledge class, about 10 of whom still live in Dallas. It is a fairly close group. (I've been very derelict since I've been in Dallas in not doing my share of socializing with that group, but I'm still quite busy, and it is difficult for me.) I was impressed with SMU, particularly the students from Highland Park High School. These were sophisticated fellows. They had done well in high school. *George Hurt* (whose nickname was "Happy"), for example, had been a 3 or 4 letter sports star in high school, made all As, came to SMU and still made all As. He got into medical school after 3 years and was #1 in his class at Southwestern, and #1 by far, one of his classmates later told me. He never left Dallas and did all his training in Dallas. *Malcolm Bowers,* who studied extremely hard, came to SMU on a football

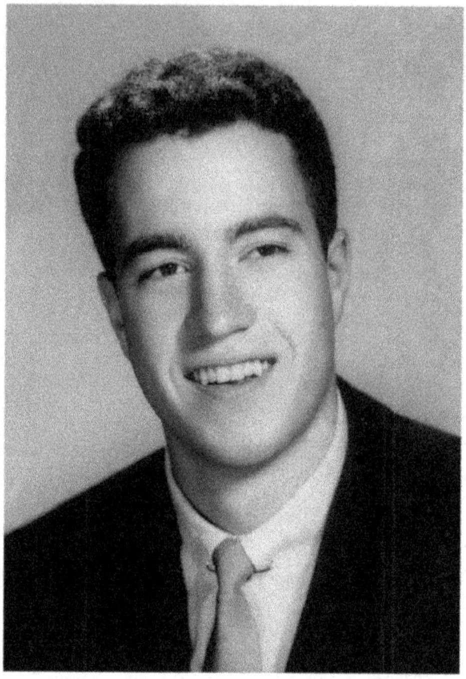

Figure 7. WCR as a junior in college at Southern Methodist University.

scholarship as a quarterback. He also made straight As in college and went to Yale Medical School, became a psychiatrist, and is on the Yale faculty. *Dave Weakley* and I had some classes together. He wore glasses and carried his books like a girl. When spring came, I didn't see him anymore. I asked, "Where's Dave?" It turned out he was a track star. He was a 200-yard and 400-yard high hurdle champ in the Southwest Conference for 4 years. He had never mentioned his track exploits to me. He went to Columbia University Medical School and became an ophthalmologist and practiced in Dallas. SMU had some super students. These kids were from far more sophisticated families than me. They had traveled some, and were much better off financially. I was very naïve when I entered college.

Charles: *Were you aware of the family connection you had to SMU when you enrolled there? Robert Stewart Hyer from Oxford, Georgia, was SMU's first president.*

William: I learned about that after I had been in college for about a month (Figure 7). My mother told me that Dr. Hyer would have been proud. Also, after pledging at the fraternity, I asked why I had not received an invitation to pledge earlier. They said they didn't know anything about me. When I told my mother that I had pledged Phi Delta Theta, she indicated that my father's sister's husband in Macon, Georgia, would be proud of me, because he had been president of the Phi Delta Theta alumni in Georgia. I thought: "Where was he when I needed him?"

Charles: *Were you aware of your father's fraternity?*

William: I was. He was a KA. I almost became a KA, but the Phi Delta Theta group felt more comfortable to me. SMU had a reputation of being a party school when I went there, but there was absolutely no alcohol drinking on campus. None! If you had a beer in a fraternity house and the administration learned of it, the fraternity was banned from rushing the next year. As a consequence, most fraternity parties were in hotels in the city, not on campus.

Charles: *Are you loyal to SMU?*

William: Yes. SMU helped get me into medical school. I also feel an incredible loyalty to Emory University for accepting me into medical school. I gave SMU a large donation in 2005.

Charles: *Are you proud that your daughter went to SMU?*

William: Yes. I'm going to do right by Emory in the near future. Emory made me who I am professionally. No doubt about it. After my freshman year at SMU, the Korean War broke out and several of my classmates volunteered. It seemed that the earlier I could get out of college, the better. So I went to Emory University in Atlanta the summer between my freshman and sophomore years. I studied like a maniac for those 3 classes and made 3 As. My brother, Stewart, was impressed. Those 3 As that summer probably helped my getting into the Emory School of Medicine. My father's influence also helped enormously I'm sure.

Charles: *What other summer jobs did you have during college?*

William: After graduating from high school, I got a job as a proof chaser for *The Atlanta Journal/Constitution*. That job had a major influence on me. A proof chaser takes the dirty ink proofs (galleys) to the various advertising agencies around town. Walking around town during June, July, and August was hot and sweaty work. Walking into the very sophisticated advertising offices all dirty from the ink and sweaty from the heat was a striking contrast to their polished dress. By the time I got to college, I pledged to myself to study hard because I didn't want to be a proof chaser all my life. The summer after my sophomore year in college, I got a job driving a truck hauling gravel for paving roads in Atlanta, but after a couple of weeks the union went on strike and I was unemployed. I went to the Georgia Employment Office and they had listed a job as a clerk typist at the Lockheed Aircraft Plant in Marietta. I was told that the job could be mine if I proved that I could type >45 words per minute. (I had taken a typing class in high school.) I went home and practiced that weekend and typed 48 words per minute in the test and got the job. It was a great job. The summer after my junior year, I worked as a counselor at a camp in St. Mary's, Minnesota. (A college mate had been a summer counselor there for years, and he told me about the opportunity. My mother approved.) It was a wonderful experience. In addition to counseling a cabin of boys, I read a tennis book so I could teach the tennis classes. I used to make up bedtime stories of taking a canoe through the Okefenokee Swamps in South Georgia at night with snakes hanging down from the tree branches and alligators viewing us from the water. Although the kids would have nightmares, they pleaded for another story nearly every night. In my senior year in college, I applied to be a Rybe Bush picker with the US Forest Service in Idaho. I had been told that Rybe bush pickers were called upon to fight summer forest fires (and there were always forest fires), and the pay was double or triple overtime and therefore the summer work could be very profitable. But, by the time college ended the Forest Service had not notified me. Somehow I got a job in the wheat fields in the Panhandle of Texas. After a week or so, it started raining (even in Texas) and I had to work around the farm. (There is never slack time on a farm.) Then, all of a sudden, I got a letter from the Forest Service indicating that the Rybe Bush picker job was available for me. I hitchhiked to Idaho and picked Rybe bushes for the summer. I lived in a tent for 2 months. When I entered medical school, I weighed 184 lbs, the most I'd ever weighed. It was a very good experience. After a month or so in medical school, I was back to my usual weight of 160 to 165 pounds. After my freshman year in medical school, I bought some good grass cutting equipment, including a motorized edger and did that work until the second year classes started. I made a lot of money that summer before getting married on August 20, 1955.

Charles: *So after 4 years at SMU, you went to Emory Medical School. Let's talk about your father (Figure 2). What was your father's family background?*

William: He was born in Oxford, Georgia, located about 40 miles east of Atlanta, on October 2, 1878, and he grew up there. He died on April 14, 1941. His father was James William Roberts (1852 to 1917), who initially was a Methodist minister, then president of a college (Wesleyan College, Macon, Georgia), and then a real estate agent in Atlanta.

Charles: *Your paternal grandfather had 3 careers?*

William: Yes. You and Cliff (William Clifford Roberts, Jr.) have found that a number of his sermons were published in *The Atlanta Constitution*.

Charles: *Did your father speak of his father? Or do you remember?*

William: I never remember his speaking of his father, who died before my mother had met her future husband, my father, and my mother never mentioned him to me.

Charles: *Your father was alive only during your first 8 years of life?*

William: Correct. He had a heart attack (acute myocardial infarction) in 1937, 4 years before he died, and he had chronic heart failure thereafter (ischemic cardiomyopathy). Because of considerable dyspnea during those last 4 years, he went to bed as soon as he got home from work, also during weekends, according to a letter in your book,[1] and I suspect my mother kept my brother and me away from him so he could rest. I also suspect that he was not a "hands-on" daddy. Thus, unfortunately I must have had little contact with him during his last 4 years.

Charles: *You have indicated that you have very few memories of your father. Did your mother speak about your father to you?*

William: Yes, but only if I questioned her about him.

Charles: *Did any others speak to you about your father after he died?*

William: After I was grown, if I met someone who I happened to find out knew my father, I always asked them what they remembered about him.

Charles: *Did you know your father's siblings?*

William: Yes. Four of them. My father was the oldest, then Warren, Charles, Helen, and James. I did not know the half-brother, Forest, or the half-sister, Eileen. I was unaware of the 2 half siblings until you boys came along. I never met either of them. Warren was a lawyer who married a wealthy lady. They lived in Macon, Georgia. It was always a thrill to go to Macon, Georgia, to see the Warren Roberts's family. His wife was lovely. They had 5 kids, 1 of whom became a neurosurgeon, 1 an Episcopal minister, 1 a professor of history (at Tulane University in New Orleans) and 2 delightful daughters, 1 of whom was a Phi Beta Kappa in college. Warren was charming and absolutely dominated the conversation in the room he was in, but in a very pleasant way. He dressed immaculately, always wore a beautiful suit with a starched shirt. He smoked cigars. I was always enormously impressed by him. James, a general surgeon, was very popular apparently among his professional colleagues. His wife, Maude, was 5 years older than he. They had no children. They lived on Juniper Street, just up the street from my father's office. James, who had good training in surgery (Grady Hospital, Barnes Hospital, and the Mayo Clinic), was 76 inches tall, and my father apparently loved him dearly. According to my mother, he was a bit lazy, preferring playing bridge to operating, but he was an excellent surgeon. In 1938, he had sudden hemoptysis, was found to have cancer of the lung, and died within a couple of months. My mother said that his death devastated my father. My father and his brother, Warren, apparently had some differences. His brother, Charles, also was a charming man. He lived in Macon in a small house down the hill on College Street from the mansion on top of the hill where Warren lived. He was in the hardware business and had 1 son, Charles Jr.

Charles: *Your first cousin, Lamar Roberts, son of Warren Roberts, went to medical school?*

William: Yes, he went to the University of Texas at Austin to college and to Duke University for medical school. Then he went to Montreal for his neurosurgical training.

Charles: *What professional accomplishments did Lamar Roberts attain?*

William: He left Montreal to be head of neurosurgery at the University of Florida in Gainesville and was there for most of his career. When he was in Montreal, Canada, he wrote a book, *Speech and Brain Mechanisms*[2] with his mentor, Wilder Penfield, who after Harvey Cushing and maybe Walter Dandy, was the most prominent neurosurgeon in North America.

Charles: *Did your father travel nationally or internationally?*

William: My mother indicated that he was afraid of airplanes and never flew, and he died in 1941 before air travel became so common. He did a good bit of traveling on trains for medical meetings and patient consultations. The founder of the Coca-Cola Bottling Company and the founder of the Retail Credit Company (later Equifax) and several other prominent men were patients of his. My mother told me that my father traveled to Miami, Florida, on several occasions 1 year to see a patient there. After a year, the patient asked my father how much he owed him. My father apparently said, "$3,000." The man said that was insufficient since he had traveled to Miami several times that year on the train, that there were the travel expenses and office expenses, etc., back in Atlanta. My father apparently said that $3,000 was adequate. My father never received a penny! He also traveled abroad to study pellagra in 1912 in preparation for his book on pellagra.[3] In December 1927 to February 1927, he was in Europe, mainly Edinburgh and Vienna, where he purchased many old and new medical books.[1] His US travels were usually east of the Mississippi. I learned after moving to Dallas, however, that my father had spoken once to the Texas Medical Association in Dallas. My father, who was quite religious, took care of many preachers in the Atlanta area and others in the South, and they were never charged. He also took care of a number of physicians and their families and, of course at that time physicians did not charge to take care of members of other physicians' families.

Charles: *What was your father's academic position?*

William: A little background: he was born in Oxford, Georgia, on October 2, 1878. (His first child, Stewart Ralph Roberts, Jr., was also born on his birthday, October 2, fifty-three years later, and he, according to my mother was overjoyed.) He graduated from medical school in 1900, when he was 21 years old. (At that time very few physicians went to college or finished college. One could go to medical school right out of high school.) Thus, he graduated from medical school in 1900 and from college (Emory at Oxford) in 1902. After a year teaching biology at Emory College in Oxford, he went to Chicago and got a master's degree in zoology. His master's dissertation was entitled "A comparison of the cervical and brachial plexuses in certain reptiles."

Charles: *After Chicago he came back to Atlanta and went into practice?*

William: He, I believe, returned to Oxford, but after a few months moved to Atlanta, where he lived the next 45 years. In 1905, there was no such thing as "full-time" clinical faculty in a medical school. (Flexner's report on how terrible medical schools were in the USA did not appear until 1910.) Medical school clinical faculties were unpaid volunteers. That's how it was his entire life. He never received a nickel from Emory Medical School despite being on its or its predecessor's faculty for over 35 years.

Charles: *Emory University was established in 1915, having originated as Emory College at Oxford, Georgia. Your father became Professor of Clinical Medicine in 1915. Describe his academic life as far as you know it.*

William: He had a faculty position at Atlanta College of Medicine from the time he moved to Atlanta in 1905. He taught medical students and house officers his entire professional life. As you indicated, Emory University started in Atlanta in 1915 and its medical school merged with the Atlanta College of Medicine the following year. Emory Hospital was finished about 1920. For its first decade or so, it was purely a community hospital. The major teaching of medical students was done at the public hospital, Grady Memorial Hospital, in downtown Atlanta. According to a letter received from a former Emory Hospital house officer in internal medicine, my father apparently rounded on his private patients with 1 or more house officers and then accompanied them to see their public or charity patients[1]; conducted 2 ward clinics, 1 hour each, with 7 students throughout the year; and during 4 of the 12 months spent an additional 3 hours weekly each year with senior students, and gave some lectures to the full medical school classes.

Charles: *Your father was professor of clinical medicine at Emory's medical school from 1916 until 1941, teaching often but part-time, while maintaining a busy private practice?*

William: That's correct. The first permanent clinical faculty member in the department of internal medicine at Emory started in 1941 after his death. That was Eugene Stead, who was paid $600 a month.[4]

Charles: *Was your father a specialist or a generalist?*

William: He was a generalist for the first 20 years of his professional career. In 1926, the American Heart Association was formed, and the organization simultaneously started the *American Heart Journal*, their official journal, the title of which, however, was owned by the publisher (Mosby), not the American Heart Association. My father was on its editorial board for many years. In 1933 or 1934, he was President of the American Heart Association. He was known as a heart specialist in the 1920s and 1930s because he had an electrocardiogram (3 leads) in his office, and he saw many heart patients. He may have been the first cardiologist in the South—certainly he was in Georgia (Figure 8). He wrote a number of articles on heart disease from 1915 to 1940. In 1937, when he had his first heart attack (acute myocardial infarction), the only heart medicines available were digitalis, morphine, nitroglycerin, aminophylline, and sedatives like phenobarbital. Therapy for heart disease at that time was extremely limited. There was no treatment for valvular heart disease, congenital heart disease, cardiomyopathies, systemic hypertension, and no recognition that some systemic diseases, like systemic lupus erythematosus, sarcoidosis, rheumatoid arthritis, etc., could on occasion also affect the heart. There were no drugs to treat high blood pressure until the 1950s.

Charles: *Did you study his writing?*

William: Yes, a good number of them. He collected medical books. He was a student of the history of medicine. When our house was on fire, some passerbyers ran into the house and threw some of his collected books out of opened doors and windows. My mother gave most of his saved medical books to the library of Emory's medical school. When I became a medical student at Emory in 1954, I went to the section where his books were located. There weren't a lot, but it was pointed out to me by a librarian that some of his reprints were in the library. I went through the reprints and was allowed to take any where there was more than 1. Additionally, I made a list of all his publications by going through the Index Medicus. I made copies of the ones where reprints were not available. I came up with about 95 of his articles. Charles, I believe later you found that I had missed finding 10 or so of his publications in medical journals.

Charles: *What were the subjects of his publications?*

William: The topics varied. He wrote a lot about pellagra, the 4 D's—dermatitis, diarrhea, dementia and death. He was quite interested in pellagra and in 1914 published a book on the topic[3] (Figure 9). He spent some time in Italy studying pellagra, which apparently, at that time, was even

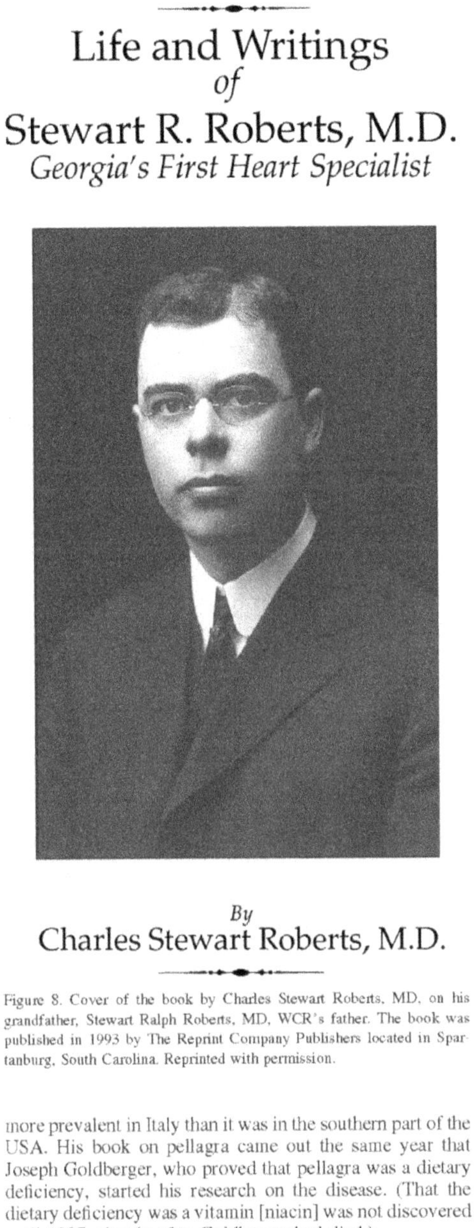

Figure 8. Cover of the book by Charles Stewart Roberts, MD, on his grandfather, Stewart Ralph Roberts, MD, WCR's father. The book was published in 1993 by The Reprint Company Publishers located in Spartanburg, South Carolina. Reprinted with permission.

more prevalent in Italy than it was in the southern part of the USA. His book on pellagra came out the same year that Joseph Goldberger, who proved that pellagra was a dietary deficiency, started his research on the disease. (That the dietary deficiency was a vitamin [niacin] was not discovered until 1937, shortly after Goldberger had died.)

Charles: *What did your father's book say?*

William: He speculated on a lot of different potential causes of pellagra. My father believed that pellagra was a dietary problem—that something was missing in the diet—

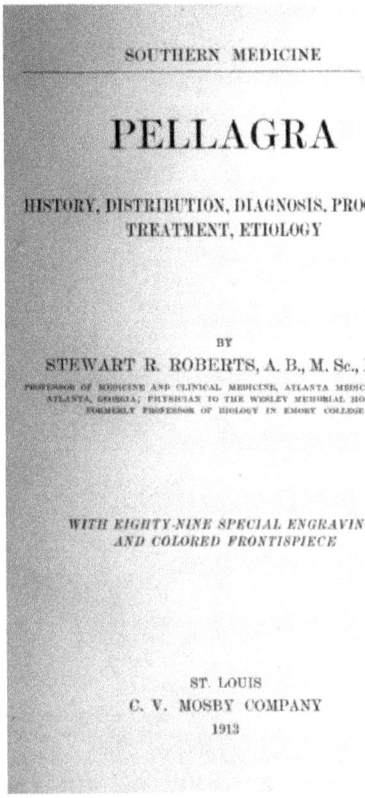

SOUTHERN MEDICINE

PELLAGRA

HISTORY, DISTRIBUTION, DIAGNOSIS, PROGNOSIS, TREATMENT, ETIOLOGY

BY

STEWART R. ROBERTS, A. B., M. Sc., M. D.

PROFESSOR OF MEDICINE AND CLINICAL MEDICINE, ATLANTA MEDICAL COLLEGE, ATLANTA, GEORGIA; PHYSICIAN TO THE WESLEY MEMORIAL HOSPITAL; FORMERLY PROFESSOR OF BIOLOGY IN EMORY COLLEGE

WITH EIGHTY-NINE SPECIAL ENGRAVINGS AND COLORED FRONTISPIECE

ST. LOUIS
C. V. MOSBY COMPANY
1913

Figure 9. Title page of the book, Pellagra, by Stewart Ralph Roberts, MD, WCR's father. The book was published in 1913 when Stewart Ralph Roberts was 34 years of age. On the undercover of this book WCR's father wrote the following: "To my second son, William Clifford Roberts, at seven years and 4 months. I hope he may love books, read and write much—Sunday, January 7, 1940." Reprinted with permission.

but there also was speculation that it might be an infectious disease. The people who had pellagra were mainly the rural poor. The cure of pellagra may be the beginning of atherosclerosis in the South, because the cure was to eat products of cows: their muscle (beef), milk, butter and cheese. Those who ate these products did not get pellagra and those with pellagra who ate these bovine products were cured of the disease.

Charles: *You collected your father's reprints and had them bound in 2 volumes. Were there any particular writings that you admired or that you do admire?*

William: I learned that he was a superb writer. I gave a talk recently on high blood pressure, and distributed a reprint of my father's article on high blood pressure written in 1936.[5] One of the enrollees came up to me afterwards and said, "Your father writes a lot better than you do," which is true. He was a wonderful writer. He wrote the Emory Creed for the college[6,7] (Figure 10). He was very loyal to Emory,

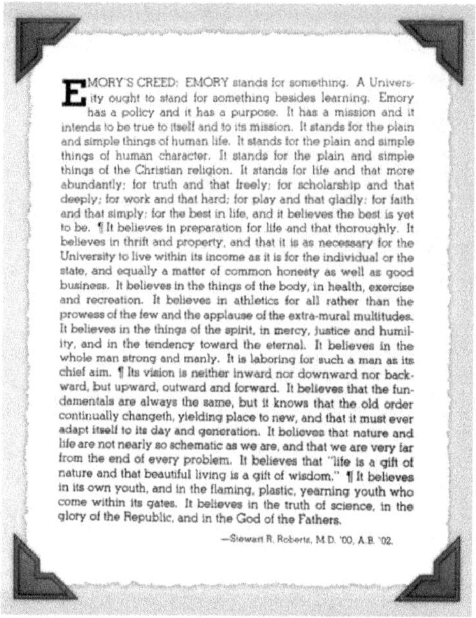

EMORY'S CREED: EMORY stands for something. A University ought to stand for something besides learning. Emory has a policy and it has a purpose. It has a mission and it intends to be true to itself and to its mission. It stands for the plain and simple things of human life. It stands for the plain and simple things of human character. It stands for the plain and simple things of the Christian religion. It stands for life and that more abundantly; for truth and that freely; for scholarship and that deeply; for work and that hard; for play and that gladly; for faith and that simply; for the best in life, and it believes the best is yet to be. ¶ It believes in preparation for life and that thoroughly. It believes in thrift and property, and that it is as necessary for the University to live within its income as it is for the individual or the state, and equally a matter of common honesty as well as good business. It believes in the things of the body, in health, exercise and recreation. It believes in athletics for all rather than the prowess of the few and the applause of the extra-mural multitudes. It believes in the things of the spirit, in mercy, justice and humility, and in the tendency toward the eternal. It believes in the whole man strong and manly. It is laboring for such a man as its chief aim. ¶ Its vision is neither inward nor downward nor backward, but upward, outward and forward. It believes that the fundamentals are always the same, but it knows that the old order continually changeth, yielding place to new, and that it must ever adapt itself to its day and generation. It believes that nature and life are not nearly so schematic as we are, and that we are very far from the end of every problem. It believes that "life is a gift of nature and that beautiful living is a gift of wisdom." ¶ It believes in its own youth, and in the flaming, plastic, yearning youth who come within its gates. It believes in the truth of science, in the glory of the Republic, and in the God of the Fathers.

—Stewart R. Roberts, M.D. '00, A.B. '02.

Figure 10. The Emory Creed, written by WCR's father and published in 1927 in the *Emory Magazine*, when he was 48 years of age (see reference 6 following the interview; published with permission).

and was on the board of trustees for a number of years. He also wrote "An Ideal of Modern Medicine,"[8] which has been republished in the *Annals of Internal Medicine*[9] (Figure 11). It is a moving piece. He wrote on some gastrointestinal conditions that simulate heart disease, angina pectoris, and some nervous disorders which affect our health and how our nervous system may affect our responses to various conditions. He wrote just over 100 articles; all but 5 or 6 were single authored. In the early 1930s with Roy R. Kracke, who was chairman of the pathology department at Emory, he wrote several articles on agranulocytosis and granulopenia, and they were published in prominent journals at the time, *JAMA* and *Annals of Internal Medicine.*[1] They were important studies. Dr. Kracke, a native Alabamian, later moved to the University of Alabama in Birmingham as chairman of the department of pathology there. They were good friends, according to my mother.

Charles: *I understand that he traveled a bit for speaking engagements?*

William: Yes, he apparently was a very good speaker. I would have loved to have heard him. Eugene Stead wrote me that my father was the best speaker by far at Emory during his time there as a medical student. He told me that he remembered his lectures 60 years later. Stead talked briefly about my father's lecture on pellagra. "It was absolutely spell-binding," he indicated. That was the time that speeches were written out. There were no slides, no Power Point. I guess in classroom lectures that he used a chalkboard, but the spoken word was the major thing—not like today when some presenters look at slides on the screen rather than at the audience. His speaking almost certainly made some of his publications easier. When he would go to Kentucky, for example, and give a talk in Frankfurt, Louisville or Lexington, his presentation might be published in the *Kentucky Medical Association Journal*. The fact that he had written it out for the speech made that process a bit easier I'm sure.

Charles: *What sort of legacies from the family standpoint did your father leave in your view, tangible or intangible?*

William: My father had a tremendous impact on me. His publications inspired me to simulate him. When I arrived at NIH in 1959, and realized the opportunity to publish, my heart leaped. No question my father gave me that hunger and thirst to leave a paper trail. I've always considered the coming up with an idea and packaging it for publication to be the greatest challenge and the greatest fun. Researchers have to have thick skin—getting manuscripts through scientific directors, editors, editorial boards. The successful researcher has to be persistent, resourceful, creative, and confident. Every researcher is fighting for editorial pages. Success in this arena is thrilling and most rewarding. Success, however, requires continuing improvement.

Charles: *One last question about your father. You have already lived 13 years longer than your father. What do you suppose he would have wished to accomplish further had he lived past the age of 61?*

William: I think he would have been a better father. I think he would have guided my brother and me and made us a lot more sophisticated early on. Growing up in a naïve environs required much catching up later. There would have been more talking around the dinner table on current events, history, questions asked. I don't mean to be critical of my mother, but I don't ever recall her asking me a single question. I grew up in an innocent world. I was always happy, but oblivious to the more sophisticated life.

Charles: *What do you think your father would have wanted to accomplish professionally if he had survived past 61?*

William: I think that he would have been enormously pleased with the idea of being a full-time faculty member on salary. He grew up in an era where that was impossible. I think he would have disagreed with Osler on that point. I think he would have thrived in a full-time faculty type situation. He would have been a good mentor. I suspect he was a pretty tough guy. His edges were probably sharper than ideal. Some of it was purposeful. My mother told me that sometimes he would walk into a cocktail party, somebody would offer him a cocktail, and he would say, "No thank you!" loud enough for everyone in the room to hear him. I suspect that he loved a new idea or concept. I think he was rigid in some things but probably very flexible in others. His articles on emotional reaction to illness show a great deal of sensitivity as to why we do what we do. I think he was a good judge of human character.

Charles: *Was he a biologist in the sense that he believed in the views of Darwin and Huxley?*

William: Surely he was. Absolutely! Nevertheless, he was a very religious man: he believed in Jesus Christ, the Bible, the church; preachers were his friends. Whether he

An Ideal of Modern Medicine

WHENEVER and wherever my work, by day or night, in peace or war, on land or sea, in laboratory or office, home or hospital, class room or open field, may I be patient, poised and thorough; loyal to science and to men, unselfish in labor and pure in life. May I hold that science is better than gold and men than greed, that service is proportionate to preparation, and reward to labor. May I use drugs only when indicated, diagnose before I treat or operate, clean before I deliver, use my laboratory, preserve a sense of proportion, respect but not worship my own opinion, seek consultation often, be slow to judgment and cautious in word and deed, and mingle in mind and touch with medical men. In the laboratory may I keep my records, in clinical cases my histories, and between them and me preserve the accuracy of truth. May I be strong with the weak, righteous with the wicked, wise with the foolish, honest with myself and kind to all men. May I avoid professional comparisons and sensitiveness, speak well of those of the household of medical faith, shun jealousy and eschew envy, follow progress, beware lest the demands of life chill my enthusiasm for study and knowledge, play sometimes and wander when I may. May I take injustice gracefully, disappointment easily, fight disease cheerfully, death hopefully, believe victory and defeat equally a part of the larger plan, and rise from both fresh for repeated conflicts. May I remember that I am heir to the same diseases as my patients, must meet the same death, pass with them beyond the River, and may I go with a smile.

ATLANTA
JANUARY 1916

STEWART R. ROBERTS

Figure 11. An Ideal of Modern Medicine written by WCR's father and published in 1916 when SRR was 37 years of age.

would have been such a religious man today is another thing. When I was growing up, I too was quite religious.

Charles: *Let's move on to medical school. Did you apply to other medical schools in addition to Emory?*

William: Yes. To one other medical school—Tulane. It's possible that there was something wrong with my application, but I never heard from them.

Charles: *Was medical school 2 years in the classroom and 2 years on the ward?*

William: Yes.

Charles: *Did you enjoy the first 2 years?*

William: Yes and no. I was not a good chemistry student. I never quite figured out how chemistry worked. I made reasonable grades. I was not married that first year, and dated my future wife too much. I enjoyed gross anatomy immensely. I did all the dissecting among the 4 students on our cadaver. (The other 3 later went into surgery, interestingly.) They apparently liked my doing the dissecting. I enjoyed pathology and the second year classes. When in medical school it never occurred to me that I would end up spending so much time in pathology.

Charles: *The last 2 years I assume you spent a lot of time at Grady Memorial Hospital?*

William: Yes. Your mother and I were married after my first year of medical school. It was easier for me from then on. I did better the second year than I did the first year.

During the second year I enjoyed pharmacology, pathology, bacteriology, and physical diagnosis. There were only 66 students in my class, including one woman. We were divided into groups of 8 students for the junior and senior years.

Charles: *Were there any teachers the first 2 years who were particularly memorable?*

William: One, Dr. Evangeline Papageorge, in chemistry. I thought she was an elegant lady. (She subsequently became one of the deans.) I remember her telling the class, "You are privileged. When you get to Grady Hospital be sure to polish your white shoes. Show respect for the individuals less fortunate than you." I've never forgotten that. I was also very impressed by the chairman of the department of chemistry. Although chemistry was hard for me, the chemistry faculty was superb. In the second year, Walter Sheldon, chairman of the department of pathology, was a very impressive teacher. Abner Golden also was good. (He later became head of pathology at Georgetown in Washington, DC, and after that at the medical school in Louisville, Kentucky.)

Charles: *Did anybody talk about heart disease your first 2 years?*

William: No, not as I remember.

Charles: *Did you make the transition to the wards easily?*

William: Absolutely. I enjoyed physical diagnosis. I found the ward services extremely exciting. I loved the wards.

Charles: *Did you gravitate towards surgery or medicine during your second 2 years of medical school?*

William: I absolutely loved surgery. It was almost like the anatomy class. I was with a group of 8—none of whom liked surgery. Three of those 8 became radiologists. As a consequence, I got to scrub on operations that were really theirs. All the housestaff in surgery knew that I was going into surgery because I just loved it. It was one of those things of not following one's instincts, which is not a good thing to do. Then, later in the junior year, I worked under Dr. J. Willis Hurst, who impressed me enormously. Although I loved surgery, I was not too impressed with the surgery faculty at the time. J.D. Martin was a superb surgeon, but I had no contact with him. I was sort of fascinated by the heart surgeon, but I had no contact with him. I was enormously fond of Elliott Scarborough, an oncology surgeon. So, instinctively, I felt good with my hands. But I couldn't let go of my father's being an internist and the enormous influence of J. Willis Hurst and W. Bruce Logue. I just didn't have the confidence at the time to do what my instincts were telling me to do. But certainly I have no complaints. I have been a lucky man.

Charles: *Tell about your relationship with Willis Hurst?*

William: Willis Hurst was stationed at the Emory Clinic connected to Emory Hospital in 1957. He took medical students on 3-week rotations. He made things come alive. During the 3 weeks I was with him, he was offered the chairmanship of the department of medicine at Emory, and even though I was just a little medical student, he discussed with me the positives and negatives of that position. He went to see Eugene Stead at Duke and Paul Beeson at Yale to get their views, because both had been Emory chairmen. When he returned from those visits, he told me a bit about them. In that 3-week period, I sort of bonded with Willis Hurst. He had a strong influence on me. If I had gone into surgery, I felt that I would have disappointed him.

It is interesting how people get into various specialties, some pure happenstance or somebody's influence. Proctor Harvey talked about Helen Taussig. Helen's father told her, "Go where you are wanted." I think that is an important principle. I sensed as an intern in medicine at The Boston City Hospital, and as an assistant resident in medicine at The Johns Hopkins Hospital, that to be a really good internist took plenty of smarts. I realized that I could be a good subspecialist–cardiologist— and a good surgeon, but I could not be a really superb generalist—there was simply too much that one needed to know. To be a masterful internist is a tremendous challenge.

Charles: *Did you do any externship outside the Emory system?*

William: After my sophomore year in medical school, I got a job at Crawford Long Hospital, which subsequently came under the Emory umbrella. I was an extern that summer, which was essentially like an internship, because they didn't have a full housestaff then. I was happy to get the job because I thought I would really learn something that summer and be a bit ahead when the junior year started. All of the other house officers were foreigners. The only course I had had was physical examination before that summer. It was a wonderful experience and then I kept it up during the junior year, working every fourth night. Sometime during that junior year I switched from Crawford Long to Emory Hospital, because they needed externs at night. They didn't fill their housestaff then.

The very first day of the junior year of medical school, I entered an elevator at Grady Memorial Hospital and on the elevator was Lyle Stone, just beginning his senior year in medical school. I inquired what he had done during the summer, and he told me he had an externship at Walter Reed Army Hospital in Washington, DC. I followed him off the elevator and asked him how he had gotten the job at Walter Reed. He told me, and I applied that night for the next summer. By spring I hadn't heard whether I was going to get the job or not, and so I applied for an externship at Emory Hospital and got it. Then, about 2 months later, almost summertime, I was notified that I had been accepted at Walter Reed. Fortunately, I was relieved from the Emory Hospital externship and Carey (my wife of 2 years) and I headed to Washington, DC, and Walter Reed Hospital. It was the break of my life. Meeting Lyle Stone on that elevator absolutely changed my life! When I got to Walter Reed, they asked me which service I wanted to be on. I replied, "What are my options?" Thoracic and Cardiac Surgery was mentioned, and I said, "I'll take it." The head of thoracic surgery at Walter Reed in 1957 was Hugh Blake. The only "cardiac" surgery they were doing at the time was suture obliteration (closure) of patent ductus arteriosus and resection of coarctation of the aorta. That was it. But Hugh Blake went out to the National Institutes of Health (NIH) to see Glenn Morrow periodically, and he occasionally would take me with him. Hugh Blake and I hit it off. I had never heard of NIH. Hugh Blake introduced me to NIH. I met Glenn Morrow at the time, but he did not remember the occasion or me. I learned that one could go to NIH and fulfill one's military obligation. That summer at Walter Reed was an eye opener for me. When I came back to Emory, I applied to NIH.

Charles: *When in medical school did you apply to NIH?*

William: I applied in my senior year. At that time, you didn't have to make commitments 2 years ahead of time. I applied for internships during the spring of my senior year. I got the externship job back at Emory Hospital when beginning my senior year, and I loved it. Willis Hurst was chairman of the department of internal medicine by then, and I adored him. The summer after Walter Reed, I visited Columbia, New Haven, and Boston. I walked into these hospitals wearing a tie, khaki pants, and no jacket. I walked into the office of the chairman of medicine with no appointment. That was how naïve I was. I told them I wanted an internship the next year. In a couple of the hospitals, house officers showed me around. In New Haven, Paul Beeson, who was chairman of medicine, showed me around for an hour. He asked me what grade I had made in pathology. He asked me a few questions about Emory, because he had been chairman there for 6 years. He was an incredible guy. In surgery I scrubbed every day and loved it. The housestaff at Grady Hospital let me scrub in on virtually every case I could. One surgery houseofficer let me do a hemorrhoidectomy.

Charles: *What did you make in surgery?*

William: Straight As! My grades improved each year. I finished 14th in a class of 66 in medical school. I found that out later, because I needed to know my standing. I applied to these fancy places, but I didn't get into any of them.

Charles: *Was there a match?*

William: There was some kind of match, because I remember being awakened around 6:30 A.M. by Tom Ferguson, who called me up on the day of the match. He was the chief of surgery at Grady and Professor of Surgery at Emory and asked: "Do you want an internship in surgery?" I thought, "That's a bad sign. I did not get matched!" I don't recall what I told him, but I went to Willis Hurst and he started calling hospitals for me. He got me a job at The Boston City Hospital (BCH). Ferguson wanted me. Boston accepted me. That is a very important difference. The BCH, politically, however, was a good move, because it probably helped me get into NIH.

Charles: *You were about to leave Atlanta for life. Before we go on, I noticed that you went to Henry Grady High School and were educated a bit at Grady Memorial Hospital. Who was Henry Grady?*

William: Henry Grady was the editor of the *Atlanta Constitution*. After the Civil War, he was the one, who, in essence, said: "Look Southerners, we lost the Civil War. We've got to accept that fact, we've got to become Americans. We've got to eliminate slavery in our minds. We've got to get along with black people and be true Americans and outgrow our Southern heritage."

Charles: *Talk about Boston. You started there in July 1958.*

William: I was thrilled to get there. Carey, in retrospect, I think, would have preferred my taking the surgical internship at Grady Memorial Hospital, because she had never lived outside of Atlanta. I had had those 4 years in Dallas, so I was used to being away from home. She lived at home during college. Moving to Boston was a big deal for her, but she was a good trooper. Although I admired Willis Hurst and Bruce Logue and some of the other faculty at Emory, I thought I needed to get on my own. Maybe I enjoyed that independence at SMU—not locked into anything. Maybe I thought the same thing about Boston. I found the BCH to be a mess. There were a lot of interesting patients; cirrhosis was everywhere. Patients commonly would come in with pneumonia and then by day 3 have delirium tremens. We strapped these patients down. I thought that I would have learned more at Grady, but the prestige of the BCH and Boston I think forwarded by career. I was taken by Dr. D. Denny Brown, who was head of neurology. He had neurology rounds every Saturday morning and demonstrated the physical findings in patients. (At Emory my training in neurology was miniscule.) I was fascinated by Dr. Brown's picking up the pertinent physical signs and making neurological diagnoses mainly from them, not from any fancy chemistry test. I enjoyed that very much. I saw quite a few patients with cardiovascular syphilis and/or central nervous system syphilis, things I had not seen before. I enjoyed it. I also went over to the Peter Bent Brigham Hospital (now Brigham and Women's Hospital) to visit my friend from college, Larry Embree, who was a first-year resident in internal medicine. (He had gone to medical school after 3 years of college, so he was 1 year ahead of me.) I enjoyed that experience. I attended a conference by Sam Levine. We had a patient at the BCH who we thought had low serum magnesium levels. I went over to the Brigham at 2:00 A.M. with his serum, and they ran the magnesium levels and it was about 1. I returned to BCH and gave the patient magnesium and he did well. That was fun. I spent 1 month on the tuberculosis ward at BCH. That was interesting. The staff physician who ran the TB ward always wore a mask. He had run the TB ward for 30 years and his PPD skin test was negative. I had never been in a TB hospital before. During that month, we often had time off in the afternoons, and Carey and I picked up sailing on the Charles River. We went sailing several afternoons that month. Cliff was born December 10, 1958, so Carey was pregnant when we got to Boston.

When we started looking for a place to live, BCH personnel told us about public housing, which we were hesitant about. We found an apartment in Brookline that cost around $90 a month. The wife of one of the surgery residents at the Brigham Hospital lived in the same place, so she and Carey became soul mates during their pregnancies. I made $100 a month—10 times as much as interns the previous year. The rent was $90 a month, and my mother sent us $50 a month. We left Boston debt-free. I ate virtually every meal at BCH that year. Our expenses were trace. It was a good year, but I was glad to go to Bethesda, Maryland.

After 1 joint medical-surgical conference where I presented a patient, John J. Burns, who was chief of the Boston University Surgery Service came up to me after the conference and asked what I was going to do the next year. I told him that I was going to NIH. He said that he was going to offer me a surgery residency. I was flattered and appreciative.

Charles: *Did you have any debt at age 26 going to Boston?*

William: No, none.

Charles: *When did you begin to think about the next year? Your internship was straight medicine?*

William: Yes, it was. Every house officer had to have 2 years in the military service at that time, either interrupting house officership or at least immediately afterwards. I had heard about NIH from Hugh Blake, who I mentioned earlier. I applied for the Clinical Associateship in the National Heart Institute (NHI) (later changed to National Heart, Lung, and Blood Institute) and also the Research Associateship. I hadn't written a single manuscript when I applied. I met with Robert Berliner, who passed on me.

Charles: *Who was he?*

William: He was the scientific director of the intramural program of the NHI. That was probably September or October 1958. He sloughed me off. Seven years later (1966), he gave me my entire laboratory: every full-time position I ever needed and every square foot I ever needed. If I had reminded him that he had turned me down 7 years earlier, he may not have given me that laboratory and those positions.

Charles: *When did the Clinical Center, the NIH hospital, open?*

William: In 1953. The original property was a private estate in Bethesda, Maryland. The National Naval Medical Center was built during Franklin Roosevelt's administration, and it was directly across the Rockville Pike from the NIH campus. The property was given to the Federal Government specifically for development of a medical research center. Construction started in the 1930s with 5 buildings. The Clinical Center was unique in that patients' rooms and research laboratories were on the same floor. The idea was that the research findings could be transferred immediately to the patients. Patient care was free, but patients had to have particular diseases or conditions that were being investigated to get admitted. If they died, they had to agree to an autopsy. It was an ideal research center.

I didn't get a clinical or research associateship in the NHI, but I heard that the pathology department had a residency program which also fulfilled the military obligation, and that 1 of the 2 or 3 years could be applied toward either a medical residency or a surgery residency. I applied for the pathology residency, which was actually located in the National Cancer Institute, but it was the pathology department at the time for all the institutes involved in the Clinical Center. There were 2 first-year residency positions open when I applied. I was told that I was the first alternate. I asked how often an alternate had gotten the job. They said never! Nevertheless, several days later I got a call that one of the accepted residents had pulled out, so I was in. On June 30, 1959, at about 6:00 P.M., Carey, Cliff, and I left Boston and the medical internship at BCH and drove to Bethesda, Maryland, arriving about 4:00 A.M. The Bethesda motels were full, so we got a room in a hotel near the White House. After about an hour's sleep, I went to NIH, arriving about 7:15 A.M. at the pathology department. No one was there. Nevertheless, getting there before the other residents allowed me to acquire the best desk, which I kept for the next 3 years.

Charles: *Describe those 3 years in the National Cancer Institute.*

William: As mentioned, the pathology department of the Clinical Center was located in the Cancer Institute. It was my understanding that when the various institutes were originally formed, the scientific directors of each were asked if they wanted a pathology department. The Cancer Institute apparently was the only institute which said "yes." The heart institute's scientific director at the time was Robert Berliner, and he said the NHI did not need a pathology department. (Later, fortunately for me he changed his mind.)

The pathology department—officially called the Laboratory of Pathology of the National Cancer Institute—consisted of a staff of probably 15, about 9 of whom did exclusively cancer research on non-human animals, and 6 of whom did surgical and autopsy pathology involving Clinical Center patients. There were 6 residents, 2 in each year of the 3-year program. It was a fun group of people. I had never been around pathologists before, except briefly in medical school. I enjoyed it. I enjoyed the gross and histology morphology. There was no clinical pathology. There was another department for that. The pathology residents did only surgical and autopsy pathology. Each resident did surgicals for 3-months each year (9 months in the 3-year program) and autopsy rotation each month. I did 150 autopsies—exactly 150—during the 3 years, 50 a year. I never did any clinical pathology. The second most common autopsy involved patients with heart disease. The staff was all interested in cancer. (Few go into pathology because they are interested in heart disease—you can't make a living.) Because of my interest in heart disease, plus the fact that none of the other residents or staff were interested in heart disease, and the fact that none liked to present at NHI's mortality conference (partly because Glenn Morrow would give them a hard time), virtually from the beginning, I was "the cardiac pathologist" and, as a consequence, did nearly all of the autopsies on the heart cases and presented the finding at the monthly mortality conferences.

That was the period when patients with aortic valve stenosis were treated operatively with a tri-radiating dilator inserted into the apex of the left ventricle. Glenn Morrow, the cardiac surgeon, would insert that dilator and the stenotic aortic valve would crack at 3 sites. The consequence was that each of the first 5 or 6 patients died. Glenn Morrow mentioned to me that when he inserted that tri-radiating dilator into the stenotic aortic valve in patients who also had mitral stenosis, which he would treat similarly, that the patient survived and actually did well. He asked me "Why was that? Double valve stenotic patients did well but stenotic single aortic valve patients died?" The answer was that nearly all of the patients with isolated aortic valve stenosis (normal mitral valves) had bicuspid or unicuspid aortic valves and the tri-radiating dilator was made for 3-cuspid aortic valves, not for bicuspid or unicuspid valves. The patients with mitral stenosis had 3-cuspid aortic valves and the tri-radiating dilator was made for them. The tri-radiating dilator cracked the bicuspid and unicuspid valves in the leaflet itself, not at commissures between cusps.

At one of the early mortality conferences I presented a patient with a bicuspid aortic valve. Glenn Morrow came up to me and said "No way." I showed him the heart and the aortic valve. I said, "What do you call that?" He said, "I think you are right." That was my introduction to Glenn Morrow and to the NHI.

Charles: *When was that?*

William: August or September 1959.

Charles: *For 3 straight years, you presented monthly autopsy findings at the cardiovascular mortality conferences?*

William: I did.

Charles: *Who was the director of cardiology at that time?*

William: When I came to NIH in 1959, Eugene Braunwald had just returned to the NIH from The Johns Hopkins Hospital where he had done a year of medical residency. Before that he was in the physiology laboratory of the NHI for 2 years. He needed another year of medical residency to take his boards in internal medicine. Glen Morrow had hired Gene Braunwald to head the Cardiology Section of the Surgery Branch (always called "Clinic of Surgery" by Glenn Morrow). When Braunwald joined the Surgery Branch, he saw all the patients before a cardiac operation and also 6 months after operation when they returned for repeat cardiac catheterization. Within 2 or 3 years, Gene Braunwald convinced Robert Berliner that cardiology deserved to be a separate branch and as a consequence the Cardiology Branch was created on equal footing with the Surgery Branch. (Glenn also hired me later, and I was in the Surgery Branch for my first 5 years in the NHI.)

Charles: *Your first publication was June 1961, and it concerned mitral valve disease. That means you were in the Cancer Institute for nearly 2 years before your first publication came out.*

William: Correct, but the interval from manuscript acceptance to publication at that time was usually 9 to 12 months or even more. It's not like that today. That was the time when abstracts were published in 4 to 6 months and that short lag time made abstracts popular. Today, a manuscript can be published as quickly or sometimes more quickly than an abstract. When Braunwald started the Cardiology Branch, all heart patients were referred to the Cardiology Branch initially and if they needed an operation, then referred to the Surgery Branch. A number of patients at the time had congenital heart disease. A particular common defect was variously called *atrioventricular canal, endocardial cushion defect,* and now *atrioventricular septal defect.* This condition is a syndrome typically consisting of a defect in the lowermost portion of the atrial septum, a cleft in the anterior mitral leaflet, partial absence of a portion of septal tricuspid leaflet, anomalous insertion of chordae tendineae from the anterior mitral leaflet to the crest of the ventricular septum, and "ventricular septal defect" (actually an absence of a portion of ventricular septum in its most posterobasal portion). In 1960, a 14-year-old boy with wide open mitral regurgitation was admitted. Rather than having mitral regurgitation secondary to rheumatic heart disease, at operation he was found to have a large cleft in the anterior mitral leaflet and a very small defect in the lowermost portion of the atrial septum, so small that a shunt was not detected preoperatively. This youngster thus had an unusual form of mitral regurgitation, and unfortunately, the operation was not successful. I was asked to present the morphologic features of this case at a symposium Gene Braunwald initiated. I presented the 5 previously mentioned features of this condition and also those of 11 other patients with atrioventricular septal defect who had been studied at autopsy at NIH. I studied each of the hearts (the organs were saved at NIH) and presented the findings in those 11 patients along with the findings in the 14-year-old boy.

Charles: *Was anybody in the department of surgery an expert in cardiovascular morphology at that time?*

William: No. Furthermore, none of the staff pathologists in the National Cancer Institute were interested in cardiovascular disease. I think the pathology department was pleased that there was now someone to take care of the interests of the cardiologists and cardiac surgeons, and I was happy to be that person. It sort of made me feel like a staff person—I was wanted.

Charles: *How did you go about acquiring morphologic cardiac knowledge?*

William: I started reading the writings of Jesse Edwards, whose name had been mentioned to me by Glenn Morrow, and additionally, Jesse Edwards had been a member of the *Laboratory of Pathology* before World War II. On the heart autopsies, I figured out quickly that I had to be able to show pictures of the heart that attendees at the mortality conference could understand. When I came to NIH, the hearts were always opened according to flow of blood. An incision was made in the right lateral border of the right atrium, right ventricle, and then from the right ventricular apex into the pulmonary trunk. The left side of the heart was opened similarly on its lateral border and then from the left ventricular apex into the ascending aorta. The consequence was that this hollow 3-dimensional organ became a flattened organ. (It is like incising a rubber tire perpendicular to its circumference and then stepping on both ends, such that it becomes a straight line.) I learned quickly not to open the heart when it was "fresh," but to let it fix in a separate container of formaldehyde.

I spent a lot of time, often 6 hours a week, with Kensie Edwards, who had come to NIH initially as a grass cutter. He took lessons in photography at the YWCA. He became the best photographer at NIH as far as I was concerned. To get good photos of the heart not only is a good photographer needed, but also an expert who knows how to open the heart to illustrate the lesions properly. I studied Jesse Edwards' articles and learned much through his photos and writings. Jesse is good with his hands, a requirement for opening the heart properly, and, if that is not done well, good photographs are impossible, irrespective of the expertise of the photographer. Jesse Edwards was my mentor through his writings. Jesse wrote the section—about 275 pages—on congenital cardiovascular anomalies in *Gould's Pathology of the Heart,* a 900-page book. Every time, for example, we had a tetralogy of Fallot case I'd read that chapter by Edwards again. I probably read that chapter 20 or 30 times.

I got comfortable with cases such as corrected transposition of the great arteries, an entity which Edwards greatly simplified in the early 1960s. He emphasized that it was crucial to decide initially whether the patient had situs solitus or situs inversus. In the former, the left ventricle switches over to the right side and the right ventricle to the left side; the great arteries switch so that physiologically it's a normal connection. With situs inversus, normally the left ventricle is on the right and the right ventricle on the left, so with corrected transposition superimposed on situs inversus, the left ventricle is where it should be, namely on the left and the right ventricle is on the right. The atria do not switch. Corrected transposition inverts the atrioventricular valves, the ventricles, the conduction system, the great arteries, and the coronary arteries. Jesse Edwards made corrected transposition simple by requiring the designation of the situs initially. When I went to Hopkins as an assistant resident in medicine, a patient presented with pure mitral regurgitation and was found to have corrected transposition. I gave a talk on this entity at one of the cardiology conferences and not long thereafter got an offer to stay at Hopkins with appointments in both cardiology and pathology. If one knows the definition of corrected transposition, the entity is a piece of cake! Jesse Edwards uncomplicated that complex entity. Jesse also made classification of pulmonary hypertension simple. His simplifying complex entities impressed me.

Charles: *This period in your training was also the time in which you wrote your first manuscript for publication. Did you derive satisfaction from that?*

William: Tremendous satisfaction. I attended the weekly Friday afternoon NHI's cardiac catheterization conferences, presented monthly at the NHI mortality and morbidity conferences, spent 3 months annually on surgical pathology, and constantly on autopsy call, and at the same time tried to write some papers, and bathe 2 babies in the evenings. I was busy. But I was learning an enormous amount and loved it. I came to NIH looking like a blank sheet of paper, and every day I poured lines of new information (for me) on it. It was thrilling.

Charles: *Towards the end of the second year, you had to decide what to do again.*

William: Yes. By then I would have fulfilled my military obligation, so I had to decide whether to stay another year or leave, and if I left what would I do? I decided to stay 1 more year because then I would be board eligible in anatomic pathology. Additionally, I had a lot of research projects going and they would not be completed if I left. I completed a lot of studies that third year.

The big decision for me came during that third year. I applied to Duke's surgery residency program. I was told that they could probably give me a job, but I'd have to start as an intern because I had not interned in surgery. I told them that I couldn't do that. I had 3 kids, by then, 3 years of anatomic pathology training, and 1 year of internal medicine training. Surely, that experience would be useful to me. We went back and forth and finally, Dr. Bill Anlyan, the chairman of surgery at the time, said, "Ok, you can start as a first year resident." In the interim, Glenn Morrow offered me a job to stay at NIH and start a pathology section in his surgery branch. I said, "Thank you, but I don't know what I want to do eventually yet. I'll do it if you give me a year away so that I can take a year of internal medicine and then a year of cardiology when I come back." (Only 1 year of cardiology was required in the early 1960s for cardiology board eligibility.) Glenn said he would have to talk to Robert Berliner, the NIH Scientific Director, about that. The Duke surgical residency was for several years, and I had no money and they paid little. Soon, Glenn called me and told me that Berliner approved my request. That meant I could go elsewhere for a year of medical residency on a full Public Health Service salary, and could come back to the NIH for a year in cardiology also on a full Public Heath salary. The choice was easy. By then I had 2 kids, another on the way, and no money. The additional training would make me board eligible in both internal medicine and cardiology.

Charles: *So you went to Hopkins, Osler Medical Service, for 1 year. Tell about that year.*

William: It was wonderful. I loved it. Johns Hopkins is a great institution. Actually, I had applied to Grady Hospital and Willis Hurst's residency program, but I didn't hear anything from him for 2 months. Because Gene Braunwald had gone to Hopkins for a year, I decided to apply there. By that time, I had quite a few publications. I sent the application in on a Wednesday as I recall. Dr. A. McGehee Harvey, the chairman of medicine at Hopkins, in the interim called Braunwald and asked about me. Braunwald apparently gave me a great review. While visiting Carey's parents in Cincinnati, I received a call from Dr. Harvey, who asked if I wanted the job. I said "Yes, sir!" That was it. A week or so later, Willis called me. I told him I already had a job.

Charles: *So, on June 30, 1962, you went to Baltimore?*

William: Yes. I was trying to finish up several projects at NIH, and on the day we left Bethesda for Baltimore I got home about 6:00 A.M. Carey and I then left for Baltimore and Hopkins. About 2 miles down the road, I pulled to the side and told Carey that I couldn't stay awake and that she would have to drive. (I had not slept in 2 nights trying to finish papers at NIH.) We drove to the Hopkins compound. It was about 103° on June 30 when we moved in. Hopkins was 1 of the best years of my life. I loved it. I think Carey liked bonding with all the spouses. The kids played in the enclosed "compound" and learned to fend for themselves. The year was great in every way.

Charles: *The Glancy's were your neighbors?*

William: Yes. Carey and Eileen Glancy hit it off right away. Luke Glancy also was on the first ward I was assigned to.

Charles: *Tell us about Luke Glancy because he's been a lifelong friend of yours.*

William: Luke is a great guy. He's originally from Atlanta. After completing college at Emory, he went to the Johns Hopkins School of Medicine. Because I had been an anatomic pathology resident at NIH the previous 3 years, my fellow medical residents assumed that I knew little clinical medicine. About my third day on the ward, a 14-year-old African-American boy with sickle cell crisis was admitted. I heard a classic murmur of tricuspid regurgitation and so wrote that in the chart. The chief resident, Gottlieb Christian Freisinger ("Bud"), came around, read my workup and was doubtful of my diagnosis of tricuspid regurgitation. I took him to the patient and when the boy took a deep breath and the murmur increased considerably in intensity, Bud agreed. That simple episode established me a bit with the other medical house officers. All year I ate lunch, whenever I could, at the Welch Library, where the famous painting of Osler, Welch, Halsted, and Young was hung. The Welch Library served as the faculty club at the time. I went to the autopsy suite when I could to see what was going on, and met some of the pathology house officers also.

Assistant residents in medicine had to present patients on Saturday mornings at medical grand rounds. My first week there, I was asked to present a patient and I had never even been to a Hopkins grand rounds before. The patient was brought into the auditorium on a gurney or in a wheelchair and the house officer stood adjacent to the patient and presented the patients' story. The patient who I presented had tried to commit suicide. I described what had happened. One physician thought I should not have shared how many pills she took. Other physicians defended me. But, I broke in quickly there. Medical grand rounds on Saturday mornings were a huge deal. There were many very good discussions.

During that year I met Victor McKusick, who later became chairman of the department. Dick Ross, who was chief of cardiology, and Ivan Bennett, who was director of the department of pathology, offered me a faculty position in both departments. I told them that I couldn't do it because I was obligated to go back to NIH. But it was nice to be offered a faculty position. I probably would have had a much different career subsequently. Before I went to Hopkins, I had never met Dr. McGehee Harvey and before going I went through Index Medicus to find his publications, which numbered about 75. I got copies of many of them, and read them. I was prepared to meet the chief. The department chairman, Dr. Harvey, had an open house on July 2 for the house staff and that is when I met Dr. Harvey for the first time. I introduced myself to him and as we talked I was hopeful that some of the things he had written about would come up. It turned out that he loved baseball, so we talked about the Baltimore Orioles for about 45 minutes. I had read his publications without benefit.

Charles: *Did you write any papers during your year at Hopkins?*

William: Yes, Luke Glancy and I wrote a paper on pheochromocytoma occurring in a few patients with cyanotic congenital heart disease (WCR #25). The patient with corrected transposition, as I mentioned earlier, who had pure mitral regurgitation, also was reported (WCR #24).

Charles: *After your year in medicine at the Johns Hopkins you returned to the NIH as a clinical associate?*

William: Yes.

Charles: *How long were you a clinical associate?*

William: One year.

Charles: *Tell about that year.*

William: It was a great year. I spent 8 months on the cardiac surgery service and 4 months in the cardiac catheterization laboratory in that order. I hadn't been in an operating room since medical school, and the first day I assisted Mort Buckley in opening and closing the chest in a patient with coarctation of the aorta. I had a terrible cold that day. My mask was wet from the dripping nose.

Charles: *Mort Buckley was a surgical associate at that time? Who were the staff surgeons at the time and what was the time period?*

William: The staff surgeons were Andrew Glenn Morrow, Nina Braunwald (Gene Braunwald's wife), and Joseph Gilbert. I was a clinical (actually surgical) associate from July 1, 1963, to June 30, 1964. It was an absolutely fantastic year.

Charles: *Did you operate with all 3 of them? Were you first assistant or second assistant?*

William: I was the first assistant for opening and closing and the second assistant when the staff surgeon was there. There were never more than 3 operators at the table. (Glenn Morrow didn't believe in a large operating group.) Joe Gilbert and I hit it off, and Joe did the adrenalectomy operations for Fred Bartter's patients with hyperaldosteronism, and I assisted him during several of those procedures.

Charles: *Did he operate above and below the diaphragm?*

William: No. He did a V-shaped incision in the abdomen beginning in the midline and below the 12th rib on each side. I enjoyed it. I was flattered by Joe Gilberts' asking me to help him on those procedures. I enjoyed it immensely.

Charles: *During those 8 months in cardiac surgery, what operations were being done?*

William: Valve replacement was #1. Various congenital anomalies: ventricular septal defect with and without right ventricular outflow obstruction, atrial septal defect, atrioventricular septal defect, patent ductus arteriosus (in adults), hypertrophic cardiomyopathy. There was no coronary artery bypass grafting at that time.

Charles: *The first successful valve replacement was what year?*

William: 1960. Valve replacement at NIH started in 1962.

Charles: *How many operations were being done a week?*

William: None were done on Mondays. That was the day that Glenn Morrow made rounds with the entire staff. There was either 1 or 2 on each of the other 4 days. There were never more than 2 a day. A big week would be 7 or 8 operations. On average, 5 or 6 operations a week. But they were big cases: atrioventricular septal defect, tetralogy of Fallot, hypertrophic cardiomyopathy, double valve replacement.

Charles: *The 30-day mortality was fairly high in those days?*

William: As I recall, the mortality rate of the first 85 mitral valve replacements done was astronomically small, then from case 86 to 100, it was astronomically high. Bob Reis came as a cardiac surgeon when Joe Gilbert left the following year. Maybe Bob Reis said this to flatter me, but he liked the idea of using smaller sized protheses, particularly in the mitral position. He told me that he hadn't done a single valve replacement until he came to NIH and the first 85 he did without a death. He put a sized 2M Starr-Edwards prothesis into virtually every patient irrespective of the patient's size. Whether that had anything to do with his low mortality or not, I don't know. I liked to think that it did.

Charles: *Did you carry on the pathological morphologic studies at the same time you were involved clinically?*

William: I tried to, but my time was not my own. I opened a lab, and got it started. It was hard because I couldn't do the autopsies. I catered to the pathology residents. I got the heart put in a container with formaldehyde, and I would open the heart later. It was a very busy year.

Charles: *Your goal was to have a full-functioning laboratory when the clinical year was over?*

William: Correct. That was my goal.

Charles: *Did you gain anything from those 8 months in cardiac surgery?*

William: Yes, much. It was wonderful. It was the most enjoyable professional year I ever had. I gained an appreciation of surgery. It's physical work. It requires focus. It is not a casual endeavor. It takes time dealing with patients. I got a good appreciation of the discipline. You have to stay in physical shape for surgery. I felt that I could talk to surgeons well after that year. I wish all cardiologists were so lucky to have that experience. Heart disease is relatively straightforward. There is a narrowing or obstruction or a leak or a hole or a wrong connection. If it is a hole, it must be closed. A stenotic area, be it a valve or coronary artery, must be opened or bypassed. A leakage must be stopped. I liked the straightforwardness of it all. I think when one brings in "remodeling" and "endothelial dysfunction" relatively simple things are made unnecessarily complex.

Charles: *Did you take call during your clinical year at the Clinical Center? Did you take calls from home?*

William: Yes. As a surgical associate I was on call for my patients each week night. I alternated on Friday and Saturday nights with the other first year surgical associate. On Sunday, all the new patients were admitted and each of the 2 first year surgical associates worked them up. So Sundays were always busy. There were no admissions on days other than Sundays.

Charles: *What about the experience in the cardiology branch during those 4 months?*

William: It was great. Two cardiologists were in charge of the 2 cardiac catheterization laboratories. By the time Bob Brawley and I were assigned to this rotation, the 3 cardiologists were a bit weary from 8 straight months in the lab. As a consequence, Brawley and I essentially alternated cases. Although I was in the cath lab only 4 months and that was a precoronary angiography period, the patients had complex valve disease or shunts or hypertrophic cardiomyopathy, and we did extensive studies on them. In the complicated congenital heart diseases, I wasn't doing the thinking. It was John Ross or Dean Mason standing there telling me what to do next, because the purple people have all kinds of different shunts and obstructions. I was busy learning the technical aspects. It was not just getting a catheter into a coronary artery and injecting contrast material. These patients were very complex, and a great deal of data was being collected for research purposes. Every patient with hypertrophic cardiomyopathy inhaled amyl nitrate, and we watched the left ventricular pressure tracings jump off the paper. Those were great times. Gene Braunwald ran the show. There was never a doubt as to who was in charge.

Charles: *Was your catheter access the arm or the leg? I don't suppose there were any percutaneous interventions?*

William: It was the arm. In patients with aortic stenosis, we did direct left ventricular punctures from the precordium with an arterial needle in an artery in the arm.

Charles: *Braunwald was the head of the cardiology branch at that time?*

William: Yes. He was clearly the boss. Every Friday afternoon the cardiac catheterization data for the week was presented at the 2 to 4 P.M. joint cardiology–cardiac surgery conference. After one Friday conference, Braunwald called several of us into his office because he thought that the conference that afternoon had been a bit casual, i.e., sloppy. It was never sloppy again. He ran a disciplined ship. He is the best I have encountered, bar none.

Charles: *By July 1964, you had completed your post graduate training, so effectively you had 4 years of college at SMU, 4 years of medical school at Emory, and had completed multispecialty training in a 6-year period. What boards were you eligible for at that time?*

William: I was eligible for anatomic pathology, internal medicine, and cardiology.

When I finished June 30, 1964, I took the anatomic pathology boards that September and passed them. I never took the other 2. It would have been nice if I had, but I tell you, (1) it would have required a good bit of study for both of them; (2) I had a lot of projects rolling; (3) I wanted to get them out and not spend any more time just studying. I have never regretted that decision, although taking and passing the other 2 would have looked good on my CV.

Charles: *In July 1964, you were in your first so-called "real job" in the sense of having completed your training.*

William: Right. By then, however, I had been in the Public Health Service for 5 years.

Charles: *You were in charge of the pathology section within the surgery branch ("Clinic of Surgery")?*

William: Correct. The first 5 years in the NHI, I was chief of the pathology section in the surgery branch. My publications dealt mainly with complications of cardiac operations, and I was in the surgery branch! That is a difficult scenario. Every manuscript I had went through Glenn, of course, and he was co-author. Obviously, one has to have a lot of confidence to write about one's own complications. My manuscripts, which involved mainly surgical complications, complicated the relationship between Glenn and me and understandably so. Glenn would hold up my manuscripts, and I couldn't get them out. I eventually went to Robert Berliner and told him that I wasn't here to make money—that I was here to publish my findings. My studies weren't being done elsewhere. Berliner talked to Glenn, who was obviously annoyed by my going to Berliner, but our relationship was quite smooth from then on. Glenn was a very smart man and a very good writer. What happened after that episode was that Glenn trusted me too much. No matter what I did thereafter, he sort of approved it, which disappointed me because I wanted his input. Then I was moved to the section of pathology under the scientific director, by then Donald Fredrickson, which meant nothing, because I was doing the same thing. Then about 1976, Jack Orloff, who had taken Fredrickson's place as the scientific director, set up a pulmonary branch in the NHI. Ronald Crystal was appointed as head. I checked Crystal's publications and found that I had 5-times more publications than Crystal had at that time. I wrote Jack Orloff saying "This is my record and this is Ron Crystal's record. You made him a branch chief; I believe that I should be a branch chief also." I got back on the memo I had sent to him, "Okay." So I became chief of the pathology branch, but essentially my duties were the same from 1964 until I left in 1993. Jack Orloff was great. I never bothered him, and he never bothered me. If I had not been productive, however, I am sure I would have heard from him fairly regularly.

Charles: *Was there any similar laboratory in the country or elsewhere focusing exclusively on cardiovascular disease to your knowledge?*

William: Yes. In St. Paul and Minneapolis (Jesse E. Edwards); Rochester (Jack L. Titus); in Chicago (Maurice Lev); Boston (Richard Van Pragh); Washington, DC (William Manning); London (Reginald E.B. Hudson and M.J. Davies); Amsterdam (Anton E. Becker); Toronto (Malcolm D. Silver); Milan (Giorgio Baroldi), among others. Jesse Edwards, by that time, had moved to St. Paul, Minnesota, from the Mayo Clinic. When Jesse moved to St. Paul, he immediately started a relation with the University of Minnesota, where he obtained numerous heart specimens and bought them back to his "cardiac registry" in St. Paul. Jesse did general pathology and surgical pathology at his hospital as well as run his "cardiac registry." At NIH, I realized quickly that I wasn't going to make much progress if I was totally dependent on NIH for specimens. NIH had only about 25 heart autopsies a year. I couldn't do much with that.

Charles: *How did you go about expanding your database?*

William: Dr. Proctor Harvey, head of cardiology at Georgetown Hospital in Washington, DC, who had already invited me to give a couple of talks there, invited me to do a cardiac pathology conference at his hospital. Abner Golden, chairman of Georgetown's department of pathology and a former professor at Emory who I had known in medical school, was agreeable to Proc's proposal. I started going to Georgetown every week. Initially, the conference was in the autopsy room, which is not a very pleasant place to have conferences. After a while, Proc arranged for it to be held in one of the clinical conference rooms. Then, Gordon Ewy and Frank Marcus, former Proc Harvey fellows, invited me to the District of Columbia General Hospital to give a monthly cardiac pathology conference. Joe Lindsey, an Emory classmate of mine, who was head of cardiology at the Washington Hospital Center, invited me there for a monthly conference. Then, I was invited to George Washington University Hospital, to the National Naval Medical Center, to the National Children's Hospital to do a monthly conference at each. Richard Ross, chief of cardiology at The Johns Hopkins Hospital, invited me there to do a bimonthly cardiac pathology conference. Then, the chief of pathology at Howard University Hospital set up a monthly conference there for me, and the cardiologists were jointly involved. About the same time, I was invited to put on the same type conference at the District of Columbia Medical Examiner's Office. That was a bonanza. I could get as many as 20 cases in a month from that institution. Then, Suburban Hospital, across Georgetown Road from the NIH campus, began saving all of their hearts for me. The pathologist there and I became friends. He did a lot of autopsies and would save the hearts for me. I sent him notes on each one with a description of the heart. All of these hospitals let me take the hearts back to NIH, and then we (my fellows and I) would send them reports and photographs of the hearts. Hopefully, that arrangement was good for them and good for me. I went from 25 cases at NIH to 500 to 600 a year, all of which had some type of cardiac disease. Eventually, I went to 11 or 12 hospitals, all monthly, except Hopkins bimonthly, and Georgetown, weekly.

Charles: *You would go to the hospital, give a conference, and then take the hearts back to NIH?*

William: Correct. Each hospital would usually have 3 or 4 heart cases. I would examine them as unknowns, try to predict the clinical history, and hemodynamics. The conferences were well attended.

Charles: *Based on the morphologic examination, you tried to predict the clinical scenario?*

William: Correct. I would try to predict the patients' age and sex and the various signs and symptoms. One time I came into a conference (this sounds a bit arrogant), and put my gloved hand into the heart container, and without looking at the heart stated, "This is amyloid heart disease." This specimen felt like a handball. My diagnosis was correct. That impressed those in attendance.

Charles: *You asked a lot of questions. What happened over those 28 years to all those hearts?*

William: I kept them.

Charles: *When you went to Dallas in 1993, what happened to all the hearts?*

William: I took them to Dallas.

Charles: *And roughly, how many are we talking about?*

William: Several hundred a year for about 25 years.

Charles: *Where are they stored?*

William: Presently, they are stored in an air conditioned room in the parking lot but they are soon to be moved.

Charles: *Has any faculty or family member ever inquired about these hearts?*

William: No. Now I use them mainly for teaching purposes. If I had more money and personnel, more studies would be done on them.

Charles: *What appeals to you about studying hearts on a table?*

William: I just fell into it. That wasn't my intent initially. I found studying the heart itself to be very interesting. Studying the whole heart provides the whole picture. Function is easy to predict with the heart in one's hand.

Charles: *You made drawings, and photographs, and described the specimen.*

William: I have always tried to quantify things. If it's coronary disease, how bad was it? The entire lengths of the 4 major coronary arteries were divided into 5-mm long segments and each was examined histologically.

Charles: *Every necropsy case got a chart.*

William: Yes.

Charles: *You wrote on the chart's cover and the data gathered (cath, ECG, etc.) was placed in the chart.*

William: Yes. Visiting so many hospitals allowed the opportunity to build a huge quantity of morphological data. Of the multiple reasons I left NIH in 1993, one included simply getting weary of traveling to so many different hospitals or institutions to acquire the heart specimens. I spent probably in total nearly 2 days a week visiting the other hospitals. About 2 years before I left NIH, the scientific director asked me why I went to all these other hospitals. I asked him how he thought I got 200 cases of rupture of the heart to study because none came from NIH. Where did he think they came from? If one is to be a real "cardiac pathologist," no single hospital can supply enough "material" to make one an expert. One needs a whole city. What happened fairly frequently is this scenario: I would get a case let's say from the Medical Examiner's office and the patient's physician was a cardiologist at Georgetown University Medical Center. I would call the cardiologist and inform him/her that I was bringing the patient's heart to his/her hospital on such and such a day. Thus, he/she would get the morphologic follow-up on his/her patient.

I also received many hearts of patients who had been studied at NIH but died at home or elsewhere. Glenn Morrow, whenever he discharged a patient at NIH, would tell him/her: "If anything happens to you, good or bad, I want you to let me know right away." As a consequence of that simple request, Glenn would be notified immediately if a patient had died. He would then call me, send me the patient's record, and I would try to arrange for an autopsy, and then the heart would be sent to me. We obtained invaluable follow-up information by this means. As a consequence, we were able to study many cases late after valve replacement or myotomy/myectomy.

Charles: *You also received many cases by mail from a variety of hospitals around the country?*

William: Yes, many. I would always send the submitter a full report and photographs of the heart.

Charles: *The submitter wanted another opinion?*

William: Yes.

Charles: *Many sudden death cases?*

William: Yes, a lot. In the late 1970s, when you and your siblings were about ready to go to college, I started getting calls from lawyers to give expert opinions, depositions, and I enjoyed that for a bit. Many were sudden death cases. I was virtually always on the defense team. That experience altered my approach to research and to teaching. "Can you prove it in court?" It helped me identify "yes" or "no" questions. I found the medico-legal work a very useful exercise for both teaching and research. The last 10 years I was at NIH, I did little medico-legal work and the last 3 years at NIH employees were not allowed to do so. I found analyzing cases a very helpful exercise for a period.

Charles: *How many hearts do you think you have thoroughly examined at necropsy?*

William: Probably about 15,000 with cardiovascular disease, and also a lot of normal or near normal ones. When at NIH, there was an autopsy conference at the Clinical Center the day following an autopsy, at 8:30 A.M. If I was in town I tried to go to those sessions, because I thought it was important to see the normal as well as the abnormal. I wrote quite a few papers on cancer of the heart. All organs in autopsies at the Clinical Center were saved. Luke Glancy, my first fellow, and I, for example, examined and reported on 70 cases of melanoma studied at necropsy. We reported on 196 cases of lymphoma. We also compared electrocardiograms in a large number of lymphoma cases studied at autopsy and found a similar percentage of electrocardiographic abnormalities in those with versus without lymphoma in the heart. Saving organs is important. They do that at the Mayo Clinic and at the Johns Hopkins. Autopsies, of course, are less often done now than in the past, so some of the necropsy studies I was involved in are more important now than ever before.

All but 2 of those visits to hospitals in the Washington, DC, area were set up by cardiologists. The 2 exceptions were Howard University and the District of Columbia Medical Examiner's Office, which were set up by the pathologists at those institutions. "Chiefs of the Autopsy Service" can be roadblocks to specialists. Heads of autopsy services have been problems for me periodically in my career.

Charles: *Do you believe that your experience during those 28 years as laboratory director was unique.*

William: Absolutely.

Charles: *In what respect?*

William: My position can't be replicated today. If you take a heart from one hospital to another today you might get reprimanded, "Oh, I didn't know we had given permission for that!" If you are going to have an autopsy and you have heart disease, do you want the general pathologist to look at your heart or do you want a student of heart disease to do the examination? The general pathologist does not read *Circulation* or *The American Journal of Cardiology* or *The Journal of the American College of Cardiology*, or the *Journal of Thoracic and Cardiovascular Surgery*, or *Annals of Thoracic Surgery*, and few cardiovascular articles appear in pathology journals. Apparently, many physicians think that answers just jump from the autopsy table. It's not that way. As Hurst and others have said: "We see what we know and we find only what we look for." Physicians do not go into pathology because they are interested in heart disease. You can't make a living in pathology as a "heart expert." I was lucky and in the right place at the right time.

Charles: *Has it been your purpose to bridge the gap between the bedside and the necropsy table? In other words, bring your knowledge gained from the laboratory to the bedside?*

William: Yes, absolutely. Autopsies are not to serve pathologists, but to serve clinicians. The information is useful only if it's related back to the people who are caring for patients. Autopsies are vehicles for learning. They provide checks on clinical judgments and on clinical "instruments of precision."

Charles: *When you conduct a conference seated at a table with trainees or guests and a heart is presented, what goes through your mind on how to examine the specimen?*

William: I wrote a paper one time on how to examine the heart and had a hard time getting it published. It was declined by several journals before it was finally accepted. When it was published, however, I received several hundred reprint requests despite the fact that I had had a hard time getting it published! How I open a heart is determined by what I think is there. How you examine a patient is determined by what you think the problem is. If it's valvular heart disease, then I approach it differently than if its coronary or congenital heart disease. Unfortunately, around the country, most hearts are opened according to flow of blood, which is not ideal. I try to maintain the heart as close as possible to how it was in life. Thus, I never open a heart as most pathologists do "according to flow of blood." I try never to open a heart before it is fixed in formaldehyde. I put it in a container of formaldehyde with a string through the atrial veins so the specimen can dangle in the formalin in the container. We die in peak ventricular systole. (It takes less energy to contract than it does to relax the ventricles), so if no materials are placed in the ventricular cavities and the specimen is allowed to float freely in a container during fixation a true characterization of the size of those chambers during life can be visualized after life. Photographs are far better when the heart is opened after it has been fixed. Good gross photographs and radiographs of the heart specimen are essential for good teaching and publishing.

Charles: *Would you typically draw right on the chart?*

William: Yes.

Charles: *How did you prepare illustrations for publications?*

William: I would draw them out myself. Then, I was blessed for many years at NIH by having the opportunity to work with Mr. Leon Schlossberg, a wonderful human being and the best medical illustrator since Max Brodel. I worked with him for 20 years.

Charles: *How often did he come over to NHI from Hopkins?*

William: At least once a month. Every 2 weeks on occasion.

Charles: *How many illustrations do you think he made for you ended up published?*

William: I don't know how many were published, but he drew at least 500 for me. I would spend a lot of time with him on those illustrations. As good an illustrator as he was, I knew the heart better than he did. I was pretty picky and critical. It was Glenn Morrow who introduced me to Schlossberg. Schlossberg would come to NIH and make operative drawings for a number of Glenn's cases. After awhile, Glenn would call me to his office when Schlossberg came over with his illustrations and get my opinion regarding accuracy. That always pleased me. The original illustration of hypertrophic cardiomyopathy at operation shows a big bump right under the aortic valve. That drawing has led many in the cardiovascular community to believe that the greatest thickness of the ventricular septum is immediately below the aortic valve. It's not that way. Illustrations are very important, but they must be accurate.

Charles: *Did you retain all those originals done by Leon Schlossberg?*

William: Yes. They are in my home.

Charles: *What about Kinsey Edwards? He was your photographer for years?*

William: I am truly indebted to Kinsey Edwards. When I opened up the heart pathology laboratory in the NIH, Dr. Louis B. Thomas, who headed the pathology department in the National Cancer Institute, allowed me to utilize the services of Kinsey Edwards. For many years from 9:00 A.M. to 12:00 noon on Tuesdays and Thursdays I spent most of that time with him. After awhile, I would leave the surgical valves with him because he knew the way I liked the valves to be photographed. He was a splendid photographer. It was wonderful working with him because if he didn't finish photographing all the valves, for example, he would always call me and tell me what he hadn't finished. That's a wonderful relationship. I always knew whether something was done or not done. There were no surprises. Kinsey Edwards, an African-American, was a wonderful man. He played the piano. He came over to my house. His wife was an elegant woman who was a secretary for Lyndon Johnson's wife. These were classy people who didn't have the good fortune of getting a good education, but were very smart, and honorable, and worked hard.

Charles: *Any other co-workers in your laboratory that remained with you for many years at NIH?*

William: Yes, Filipina Giacometti ran the histology lab. Her first daughter, Andrea, was born on the Andrea Doria ship during their passage from Italy to the USA. She has 2 daughters: 1 is a physician and the other, a lawyer. Fili headed my histology lab for 25 years. She is a dear friend, a wonderful human being, and a dedicated worker. We still talk on the phone occasionally.

Charles: *How do patients with coronary atherosclerosis present and how do they die?*

William: The most common presentation is angina pectoris, probably about 50%; another 25% present with acute myocardial infarction, and the other 25% present with cardiac arrest, obviously the worst way to present. Sudden death in them is their first and usually their last manifestation of coronary heart disease. With angina pectoris, the left ventricular myocardium is usually normal or nearly so and the ventricular cavities are usually of normal size. With myocardial infarction, of course, a portion of the heart muscle is destroyed. Of all the options, angina pectoris is the best one to present with and the one most responsive to therapy because the myocardium in general is in good shape. There is a rare patient whose first manifestation of coronary disease is dyspnea alone or a nonfatal arrhythmia.

Charles: *How have your morphological studies helped you come to an understanding of atherosclerosis?*

William: Some studies in my lab beginning in the late 1970s had not been done before, namely those quantitating degrees of luminal narrowing and those quantitating the composition of the atherosclerotic plaques in the 5-mm segments of each of the 4 major epicardial coronary arteries. These studies showed that irrespective of the type of fatal coronary event that every 5-mm coronary segment contained atherosclerotic plaque and about 35% of the segments are narrowed >75% in cross-sectional area by plaque alone; another 30% or so would be narrowed 51% to 75% in cross-sectional area by plaque alone and then the remaining ones would be narrowed ≤50% in cross-sectional area. Those studies established the fact that atherosclerosis was a very diffuse disease in patients with fatal coronary disease. A 2007 study of endarterectomy specimens of the right coronary artery in live patients having coronary bypass disclosed just as much narrowing in these specimens as in the right coronary artery of patients with fatal coronary disease. The patients whose first manifestation of coronary disease was cardiac arrest had the same amount of coronary narrowing as did patients who had had previous coronary events. In other words, there is very little difference in the quantity of atherosclerotic plaque in patients with fatal coronary disease and in those with nonfatal coronary events. The greatest quantity of plaque is built up before the first event, not between the first event and the last event.

Charles: *When were these morphological studies done in your laboratory?*

William: They were started in the late 1970s and throughout most of the 1980s. They compared degrees of narrowing and composition of plaques among patients with different coronary events, various complications of myocardial infarction, various systemic diseases (the Hurler Syndrome, systemic lupus erythematosus), older versus younger patients, etc.

Charles: *To your knowledge, had anyone previously removed the coronary tree and sectioned it systematically and examined cross sections in this fashion?*

William: No. The right coronary artery, in general, in adults is about 10 cm in length and, therefore, if one divides it into 5-mm segments, that results in 20 segments in that artery. The left main in general is about 1 cm in length and therefore that produces two 5-mm segments. The left anterior descending is also about 10 cm in length and therefore that produces as a rule about twenty 5-mm segments. The left circumflex, of course, is quite variable but may average 6 cm if one includes those in whom that artery is dominate with those in whom it is not dominate. In general, one has about 54 five-mm segments to examine per patient. It is essential that these segments be stained with an elastic tissue stain to show the internal elastic membrane, because if that's not clearly visible one cannot estimate properly the degree of luminal narrowing. Via a computer, we could calculate accurately the area of the plaque and the area of the lumen.

Charles: *How does your analyses of distribution of coronary atherosclerosis compare with angiographic findings?*

William: The angiogram, of course, is the best "instrument of precision" during life to determine the presence of and the degree of coronary narrowing. That dimension is a diameter reduction, not a cross-sectional area narrowing. An angiogram is a luminogram, so the wall of the artery is not visualized. The area of greatest narrowing is simply compared to an adjacent area, which is not normal but only less narrowed. Intravascular ultrasonic imaging, of course, uses the unit of cross-sectional area narrowing and those studies compare very favorably with the necropsy studies.

Charles: *Is it correct to say that coronary atherosclerosis is diffuse and not focal in patients with symptomatic coronary artery disease?*

William: Absolutely. Every 5-mm segment contains plaque and about 35% of the segments are narrowed >75% in cross-sectional areas. Also, the total quantity of plaque in the right, left anterior descending, and left circumflex coronary arteries is similar at necropsy irrespective of the type of coronary event. If a patient presents with an anterior wall acute myocardial infarct, that indicates that the thrombus is present in the left anterior descending coronary artery. It does not indicate that that artery is more narrowed by plaque than is the right or the left circumflex coronary arteries. The same cholesterol level flows down all 3 major arteries, so in general the quantity of plaque in each is similar. There may be larger mountains in focal areas in 1 artery than in another, but if you add up the total quantity of plaque present in these 3 arteries, it's about the same. Since 1 mountain may be bigger in 1 artery than in another, the angiogram may show only 1 artery to be severely narrowed or just 2 of the 3 arteries to be quite narrowed. But if one could look at each 5-mm segment in those cases, the quantity of plaque is similar in all 3 arteries.

Charles: *When does atherosclerosis begin to appear in human beings in the Western World?*

William: By age 20 years in all societies in the world, irrespective of cholesterol levels, intimal thickening is approximately equal to medial thickening. That is a 360° circumferential thickening. That thickening, which is fibrous tissue plus smooth muscle cells, appears to be simply a reaction to the intra-arterial pressure. The same thing occurs when you put a saphenous vein into an arterial system. The intima quickly becomes as thick as the media. In societies whose total cholesterol is >150 mg/dl or so, the plaque build up continues, whereas in societies with very low total cholesterol levels, lets say 120, 110 or 130 mg/dl, the process does not develop further than the intima's being about the same thickness as the media. The rapidity of development of plaque is determined by the cholesterol level in my view. The higher that level, the more rapid plaques develop. Patients with homozygous familial hypercholesterolemia, individuals whose total cholesterol levels are >800 mg/dl from birth, generally die about age 10, and they have a huge quantity of plaque in the coronary arteries by that time as a rule. The arteries in patients with heterozygous familial hypercholesterolemia, whose total cholesterol levels average about 300 mg/dl, generally also develop large quantities of plaque, and they usually die before age 50. The rest of us, in my opinion, have non-familial hypercholesterolemia, which is dietary induced, and the age of death and the quantity of plaque develops much slower and death is much later.

Charles: *In light of the obesity epidemic, do you predict more or less atherosclerosis in the future?*

William: I predict more. People get obese because of eating too many calories and not using them up. The most concentrated calories come in the form of fat, which is stored, and the result is obesity. As a rule, overweight people have higher cholesterol levels than those of similar age and sex whose weight is ideal (body mass index ≤25 kg/m^2). I predict that coronary disease is going to get even worse in the near future in younger people. Diabetes mellitus, type 2, is appearing now in teenagers. Statin drugs, however, are having a major effect on frequency of atherosclerotic events, but that's mainly in the older population. These young obese people are not going to be on protective drugs, with certain exceptions, until after events occur. Yes, I think we are going to see more plaques with time and earlier events. Diabetes mellitus is already present in >20 million Americans, and the number affected increases yearly.

Charles: *What is the composition of an atherosclerotic plaque in a cross-section of a coronary artery in patients with fatal coronary disease?*

William: The dominate component of atherosclerotic plaques in patients with fatal coronary disease and in the endartectomy specimens of right coronary artery among patients having coronary bypass is fibrous tissue, which makes up about 70% of most plaques. Another 10% or so is calcium, about 10% lipids, and about 10%, miscellaneous materials.

Charles: *How do statins affect the atherosclerotic plaque in your view?*

William: Intravascular ultrasonic imaging has shown that plaque quantity can be reduced by lipid lowering therapy, mainly statin therapy. Coronary angiography is not a good method to determine reversibility, although several studies using so-called quantitative coronary angiography did show a slight reduction in degrees of luminal narrowing among patients treated with stains compared to control groups.

Charles: *What happens in an acute coronary event in an atherosclerotic plaque?*

William: I think the cardiology community is convinced that plaque rupture is responsible for sudden coronary death, for unstable angina pectoris, for conversion from stable to unstable angina, and for acute myocardial infarction. In my experience, plaque rupture has only been seen essentially on a natural history basis only in patients with acute myocardial infarction and that's in about 70% of them, so 30% do not have plaque rupture. Virtually all patients with acute myocardial infarction have a thrombus superimposed on a plaque. The plaque underneath may or may not have ruptured. From studies in my own laboratory at NIH, plaque rupture is not responsible for sudden coronary death, or for unstable angina pectoris. (It's very difficult to get patients to study at necropsy whose only coronary event was unstable angina because most of them either have coronary angioplasty or coronary bypass or they go on to develop acute myocardial infarction.) In my view, the most common cause of plaque rupture today is coronary angioplasty, which works by cracking the plaque, and yet few of those patients form thrombi over the ruptured plaque in the post procedure state. I'm aware that those individuals are getting heparin and some clopidogrel after the procedure but, nevertheless, plaque rupture is the reason angioplasty is effective. Likewise, every patient who has coronary bypass has an incision into the wall of the coronary artery and plaque is always on the intimal surface at the site of the incision. Whether it is an arterial conduit like a mammary artery or a venous conduit like a saphenous vein, the incision in the wall of the native coronary artery at the anastomosis site ruptures plaque at that site and thrombus formation at the site of the ruptured plaque thereafter is rare. In my view, the issue really comes down to whether one believes that quantity of plaque is the more important item or plaque rupture the more important item. I come down firmly on the side of quantity of plaque ("plaque burden"), not on the side of plaque rupture as the cause of most coronary artery events. The great majority of all plaques consist of fibrous tissue, not pultaceous debris (lipid material)!

Charles: *Do you believe that atherosclerosis is a systemic disease?*

William: Absolutely. If there is a lot of plaque in the coronary arteries, then there is a lot of plaque in the aorta and in the peripheral arteries, which include the carotid arteries. The same cholesterol level is flowing through all of our arteries, and if that level is high enough to cause plaque in one place, then it is high enough to cause plaque in another. Clinically, of course, as you know, patients tend to present with involvement clinically of only 1 arterial system. One patient might present with a transit ischemic attack due to large quantities of plaque in an internal carotid artery; another might present with peripheral arterial insufficiency and claudication; another, abdominal aortic aneurysm, and, most commonly, of course, with myocardial ischemia or infarction. The coronary arteries are different from other arteries in that they are perfused by a diastolic pressure, whereas all of the other arteries are perfused by a systolic pressure. The coronary arteries are unique also in that they are the only arteries arising from the aorta at obtuse angles; all of the others come off at acute angles. Blood stays in the coronary arteries longer and flows more slowly because it perfuses them only during ventricular diastole and that fact may play some role in the fact that the coronary system produces more clinical events than do the other arterial systems.

Charles: *What is the role of infection or inflammation in atherosclerosis?*

William: If one thinks of inflammatory cells as the defining feature of inflammation, inflammatory cells are uncommon in atherosclerotic plaques. Occasionally, a lipid accumulation contains a lot of cholesterol clefts and even giant cells, and there is a minor inflammatory reaction to that, but most plaques contain essentially no inflammatory cells. When physicians state that atherosclerosis is "an inflammatory disease" that generally means I think that the C-reactive protein and/or certain cytokines are elevated in the serum. Russell Ross, who first said that "atherosclerosis is an inflammatory disease," studied atherosclerotic plaques experimentally produced in non-human animals. I believe that opine has led the cardiovascular community astray. In my view, atherosclerosis is a consequence of a cholesterol problem, not an inflammatory problem. Societies where infectious disease is rampant, namely, some of the undeveloped countries where malaria is devastating and some parasitic diseases are common, generally have little atherosclerosis. In other words, the higher the infection frequency, the lower the atherosclerotic frequency.

Charles: *What is your view of primary and secondary prevention of atherosclerosis?*

William: I don't think atherosclerosis is a multi-factorial disease. The Framingham studies, which began in 1948, have emphasized that the greater the number of atherosclerotic risk factors present, the greater the chance of an atherosclerotic event, and that study has emphasized that cigarette smoking, diabetes mellitus, systemic hypertension, and elevated serum total and low-density lipoprotein (LDL) cholesterol levels are equivalent risk factors. But what was their definition of "elevated cholesterol"? For years, it was a serum total cholesterol level >250 mg/dl. If a level that high is used for "elevated cholesterol," that factor does not shake out as essential for atherosclerosis to occur. If one asks of each of the various atherosclerotic risk factors whether or not it has to be present for atherosclerosis to occur, then, in my view, the only one that shakes out as essential is an elevated total cholesterol (>150 mg/dl) or LDL cholesterol (>70 mg/dl) level.

Charles: *What is the best way to prevent atherosclerosis?*

William: The best way is to be a vegetarian–fruit eater, a non-flesh eater and a non-saturated fat eater. Animal eating, of course, is not the only way to take in saturated fat. Palm kernel oil, for example, is 90% saturated fat. Very few people are willing to be vegetarian–fruit eaters, and therefore, these cholesterol-lowering drugs are needed. They represent true life insurance. Life insurance as we generally know it is death insurance. The person who buys "life insurance" dies and then somebody else gets the money.

The statin drugs and other lipid-lowering drugs are true life insurance policies. People who take them live longer than those who do not take them. Pure vegetarians over decades infrequently get symptom-producing atherosclerosis, high blood pressure, gallbladder disease, gallstones, kidney stones, diverticulitis, appendicitis, hemorrhoids, certain cancers (colon, breast, and prostate gland), osteoporosis and osteoarthritis. We could all improve our health and diminish our health care bills if we would decrease our flesh-eating meals from too often 21 per week to no more than 5 a week. And the cows would jump for joy and our planet's health would also improve enormously.

Atherosclerosis is infrequently genetic in origin. Studies by Brown and Goldstein indicate that it's a genetic problem in 1 of 500 people. That means that the rest of us, namely 499 of 500, have atherosclerosis because of what we put in our mouths 21 times a week when we pull out chairs up to the table. Family members eat the same food and family members tend to get the same diseases. There are not many tables where 1 family member eats a 16 oz steak while sitting next to a vegetarian–fruit eater.

Charles: *Are you a vegetarian?*

William: No. I was a vegetarian for 18 months nearly 2 decades ago. I eat fish.

Charles: *When did you alter your eating habits? Was there any specific motivation or influential book?*

William: Yes. I read John Robbins' book called *A Diet For A New America*. John Robbins is the son of the Robbins of Baskin-Robbins fame, the ice cream producer. In his book he showed what damage to planet earth is being done by our constant demand for the flesh of cows, pigs, chickens, etc. Up to that point I had not thought about it. He convinced me that if we were all vegetarian–fruit eaters not only would we be better off, but the planet would be far better off. He also provided the list of diseases that are uncommon in non-flesh eating people. Subsequently, I've read a number of pieces about that to convince me that that is the situation.

Charles: *What is your view of body weight?*

William: The most important thing for our health that any of us can do in my view is to have an ideal body weight. If one gains weight, the levels of serum total cholesterol, blood pressure, blood glucose, and blood insulin levels increase, and if we are overweight and lose weight, the levels of serum total cholesterol, blood pressure, blood glucose, and insulin fall. Over 60% of American adults are overweight and half of them are obese, meaning body mass index >30 kg/m^2. About 100 of the 180 million adults in the USA are overweight and about 50 million are obese. Our health care will not be changed by nuclear cardiology. It will be changed by each of us doing our share to stay healthy so that our health care bills will not be astronomical. Health care in the USA presently uses 16% of our gross national product, higher than any country in the world, and yet the US population is far from the healthiest population on the planet.

Charles: *What is your view of percutaneous coronary intervention and of coronary artery bypass grafting?*

William: I think both are useful procedures. If I had an *acute* coronary syndrome, I would want to be taken to the cardiac catherization laboratory and have coronary angiography. If I had a severe narrowing in 1 or more of my major coronary arteries, I would want strong consideration for revascularization. Very few interventional cardiologists have ever looked at a coronary artery after they have blown up a balloon in it or after having inserted a metallic stent. It's really a miracle to me that this procedure works as well as it does, but it works because plaques are cracked and that cracking allows the lumen to open up more. It does not work because plaques are pushed more peripherally than they had previously been. It's a miracle to me that more complications do not occur. Often when cracking a plaque, the media is also torn. Angioplasty is successful because the external elastic membrane is an extremely strong structure, maybe the strongest structure in our body.

Coronary artery bypass, of course, has been around for 40 years (since 1967). It must provide more nourishment to ischemic myocardium than does any percutaneous intervention procedure. The down side, of course, is that operative incisions are necessary and that means damage to some human tissues in order to provide benefit to other human tissues. Nobody wants a median sternotomy unless you have to, but that procedure in 40 years has proved itself to be a very good one. A patient with a first coronary event usually (>80%) dies from a repeat coronary event. Patients who have coronary bypass and survive for a year after the operation only have a 50% chance of having a fatal coronary event later. That observation supports the view that the coronary bypass operation prolongs life by letting patients survive long enough to die from a non-coronary event, most commonly cancer. There is no data on whether percutaneous coronary intervention prolongs life. Both percutaneous coronary intervention and coronary bypass are highly useful procedures and both will be around for as long as we continue our present lifestyle habits, which keep our serum cholesterol levels out of bounds.

Charles: *What is your view of heart failure?*

William: It's important to divide heart failure etiologically. Heart failure due to valve disease needs operative or percutaneous intervention depending on the valve type. Heart failure due to systemic hypertension is generally diastolic left ventricular failure, and in that circumstance the left ventricular cavity does not dilate. Heart failure due to hypertrophic cardiomyopathy or to amyloid heart disease or sarcoid heart disease requires different therapies. If we talk about the most common cause of heart failure, namely, myocardial infarction, which heals, according to Framingham about 90% of those patients had pre-existing systemic hypertension. Patients with healed myocardial infarcts who have heart failure always have dilated left ventricular cavities and the cardiac mass, i.e., heart weight, is virtually always increased. (The normal heart weight in adult women is <350 grams and in adult men, <400 grams.) In patients with heart failure secondary to myocardial infarction which healed, the heart weight is virtually always increased, and I think that increase is more reasonably attributable to previous systemic hypertension than anything else. Of course, if one has bad heart failure from a large myocardial infarct which healed, the blood pressure elevation may be entirely eliminated. Large myocardial infarction usually lowers elevated blood pressure to normal or subnormal levels. Because coronary disease is the most common cause of heart failure, the prevention of heart failure from coronary disease requires early therapy of serum lipids and blood pressure. We have presently 6 statin drugs, 2 fibrates, 1 small intestinal blocker of cholesterol absorption, and 70 anti-hypertensive drugs. Heart failure therapy needs to start long before heart failure appears, and the major prevention is anti-lipid therapy and anti-hypertension therapy.

Charles: *What is your view of aortic dissection?*

William: Acute aortic dissection is nearly always a consequence of systemic hypertension. The reported clinical frequency of systemic hypertension in patients presenting with acute aortic dissection is about 70%, but a number of those patients are in shock by that time and had not sought medical care previously. The heart weight in patients with aortic dissection, whether the tear is in the ascending, transverse, or descending thoracic aorta, is virtually always increased, and I attribute that increased mass to previous systemic hypertension. The way to prevent aortic dissection is to prevent the occurrence of systemic hypertension. Today only, about 35% of the 65 million adults in the USA with systemic hypertension are having their blood pressure "controlled", i.e., <140/90 mm Hg. (In 1972, that control figure was 15%), so we could do much better.

Charles: *Your father wrote an article on systemic hypertension and you have views on systemic hypertension. Do they differ?*

William: When my father died in 1941, there were no anti-hypertensive drugs available, with the exception of sublingual nitroglycerin and some sedatives such as phenobarbital. My father wrote a paper in 1936, providing advice to patients whose blood pressure was elevated and that advice centered around a more quiet and peaceful life (See *AJC* From-The-Editor column #181). Today, we have plenty of splendid antihypertensive drugs, but they are inadequately utilized. I believe that all adults should know their blood pressure, and that it should be taken regularly at home and recorded. If it is elevated, it should be quickly treated.

Charles: *What's the cause of a fusiform abdominal aortic aneurysm?*

William: In my opinion, abdominal aortic aneurysm is a combination of atherosclerosis and systemic hypertension. If you have hypertension and a total cholesterol <150 mg/dl, it's very unlikely that abdominal aortic aneurysm will occur. On the other hand, if the serum cholesterol level is high and the blood pressure is <120/80 mm Hg, it is also very unlikely that abdominal aortic aneurysm will occur. In my experience, people with abdominal aortic aneurysm who have come to autopsy essentially always have hearts of increased weight, a finding I attribute to systemic hypertension. There is a view that genetics play a big role in abdominal aortic aneurysm and that it is often familial. My research assistant, Jamie Ko, recently looked at the medical records of 31 patients who had had operative resection of abdominal aortic aneurysm and found that 2 patients (6%) had another family member who also had had an abdominal aortic aneurysm.

Charles: *Have you studied carotid arterial plaques in necropsy or in surgical specimens?*

William: Yes, in operative specimens. My impression is that the quantities of lipid in the internal carotid arteries, which are narrow enough to warrant operative intervention, i.e., endarterectomy, contain more lipid than do the coronary plaques. Quantitating the composition of plaques in operatively excised internal carotid artery specimens has not been done, and it is a bit trickier to do than in coronary specimens. I'm a bit fearful of percutaneous intervention therapy for significant narrowing of internal carotid arteries associated with cerebral ischemia. Carotid endarterectomy is a very straightforward, relatively safe, predictable operation, and a huge amount of data on its effectiveness and safety is available. Furthermore, the operative incisions are relatively small, no bone is incised, and the hospital stay is short. The amount of data available on effectiveness and safety of percutaneous carotid intervention is small. Because a good bit of the carotid plaque is lipid, I worry about the effectiveness and safety of percutaneous intervention in the carotid arterial system.

Charles: *Is it fair to say in your roughly 3 decades as a laboratory chief that you studied atherosclerosis in the second 2 decades but not really in the first decade?*

William: That's correct. At NIH, relatively few coronary patients were studied clinically. I didn't start studying coronary disease until I started getting heart specimens from non-NIH hospitals and institutions and that started in the late 1960s. My first article on coronary disease was in 1972, and I had come to NIH in July 1959.

Charles: *How long did it take for these ideas on atherosclerosis to marinate in your mind to the point that you began to focus on prevention and give presentations on prevention?*

William: In the 1960s, the few talks I gave usually concerned valvular heart disease, complications of valve replacements, and occasionally cardiomyopathies. When my first publication on coronary artery disease (with Max Buja) appeared in 1972, my invitations to give talks absolutely skyrocketed. I think actually I was always cholesterol oriented. I'm not sure why but it always appealed to me, and the idea that you could produce plaques by giving cholesterol, mainly egg yolks or saturated fat, namely animal fat, hit home to me quite early. The fact that plaque could not be produced by making herbivores hypertensive or by blowing cigarette smoke in their faces for a lifetime also intrigued me. In 1969, I had a trip to Israel to present at a meeting there, and I asked the scientific director, namely Robert Berliner, if it would be possible for me to travel through central Africa, particularly Kampala, Uganda, on the way to Israel because I had heard that they did a lot of autopsies at MaKerere College Medical School and Mulago Hospital and saved the hearts. I had done some work on carcinoid heart disease and wanted to make sure that endomyocardial fibrosis, which was common there, was not similar to carcinoid heart disease. Dr. Berliner agreed. In the rear of the Mulago Hospital was a separate building where autopsies were performed. Families would wait outside for their loved ones' bodies while the procedures were being done. The pathologists retained the hearts. They must have had 500 hearts, and I looked at many of them. Many of the hearts were very heavy. Hypertension was a major problem there, but the coronary arteries were clean as a whistle. I asked about serum total cholesterol levels and was told they usually were 90 to 130 mg/dl, twice as low as they were in the

USA. That struck me that although hypertension was crucial in stroke and aortic dissection, it by itself seemed not to produce atherosclerotic plaques.

Then in 1976, your mother and I went to New Zealand. I was the "New Zealand Heart Foundation Lecturer" for that year. Their annual lecturer traveled the country for 2 weeks while they raised money for their heart foundation. (The visiting lecturer had to speak English.) While traveling around that country during that period, I was interviewed by numerous radio and television stations, and I realized quickly what people wanted to talk about were risk factors for heart disease. I had to come to grips with the cardiovascular risk factors, what causes coronary heart disease, and how could it be prevented. In 1976, there were no good cholesterol-lowering medicines. Bile acid resins and niacin were available, but few people took them at the time. That trip allowed me to focus on prevention earlier than I probably would have otherwise.

Charles: *Let's talk about your Williamsburg, Virginia, conference on heart disease. When did it begin and how long has it gone on?*

William: It began in 1973 and has been continued every year since, except for 2005 when the Williamsburg Conference Center was renovated. The sponsor of the conference for the first 32 years was The American College of Cardiology and now it is Imedex, a splendid private continuing medical education organization. The conference starts the first Sunday afternoon in December and continues to Wednesday at noon. Enrollees receive 18.5 hours of continuous medical education credit for their attendance. Each speaker, usually 13 per conference, gets 90 minutes and more than 1 topic can be discussed by each speaker. We have averaged about 200 enrollees per conference.

Charles: *Why Williamsburg?*

William: About 1972, the College asked if I would direct 1 of their extracurricular courses, and I was given a choice of where to have it. I selected Williamsburg, which is about 150 miles from the Washington, DC, area where I lived at the time.

Charles: *You have invited a number of different speakers during those 3+ decades. What did you learn from that activity?*

William: That's an interesting question. I learned a lot of different things about people who attended the meeting and about the faculty who presented at the meeting. Most enrollees have been repeaters, which mean that they had been to 1 or more previous meetings. One physician has come to 29 of the 33 meetings. I became friends with quite a few physicians who came to the meeting regularly, and that has been a source of pleasure. (Once I had been invited to give a talk in California when living in Bethesda, Maryland, flew the distance of the country, and gave a 10-minute talk. I thought that that was foolish and a waste of time. That program in California went on for 2-1/2 days, the same amount of time that the Williamsburg program goes on and yet they had something like 35 faculty members.) At Williamsburg, I thought the speakers should talk long enough so that the enrollees could have time to evaluate them, and also there would be time for questions and answers and audience comments. The faculty members were given 90-minutes for their presentations, and they could talk about more than 1 topic. I invite presenters based on their contributions to our fund of knowledge and on their ability to communicate with an audience. I let the presenters select their own topics. I try never to invite a speaker unless I have previously heard him/her present to an audience. Giving each speaker 90 minutes limits the number of faculty. There is a faculty dinner on Sunday and Monday evenings. Speakers who get good marks from the enrollees are invited back. Those who do not get good marks are not invited back. The enrollee evaluations at the end of the meeting are carefully considered for future meetings. I learned that the only way to know if a faculty member would attend the faculty dinners was to know his/her flight schedule. I was never obligated, as are some chairs of cardiology or chairs of departments of medicine, to invite their own faculty members to pay them back for this or that favor. I always could select whomever I thought was the best at the time.

Charles: *What makes a good speaker and what makes a bad speaker?*

William: That is an interesting question. Some people communicate well and others don't. Arrogant people rarely make good speakers. People who strive to inform others, not to show how smart they are or what interesting work they have done recently, generally are pretty good. Just because one has been a good investigator or has a splendid reputation is no guarantee that that person is a good speaker (communicator). It's interesting that there are not many absolutely wonderful speakers in the medical arena. There are a lot of wonderful political speakers or lawyers or motivational speakers, but the number in medicine is relatively limited. Humility, data, desire to inform, and enthusiasm are key ingredients.

Charles: *Let's talk about your own speaking engagements. You have spoken in >2,000 cities. In the first 6 months of 2006, there were 42 presentations, 17 in Texas and 25 outside of Texas, and those outside of Texas were in 8 states and in 1 foreign country. Have you always maintained this high frequency of speaking engagements?*

William: Since 1972 the answer is "yes." I have overdone presentations. They are not something that I'm that particularly proud of. I put the list of presentations in my CV simply so I can remember them and the places I have visited. At NIH, we had certain limitations. There, I got 30 days of vacation a year. If I gave a talk when I was at NIH for those 32 years and received an honorarium for it, I had to be on vacation, unless it was a weekend or a local evening presentation. As a consequence, I used my vacation time almost entirely when at NIH for presentations. I needed the income, because at NIH I was either a civil servant or a public health servant and had 4 offspring with many expenses. I enjoy meeting new people, and these trips have allowed me to do that. I also get a good bit of work done on airplanes and in hotel rooms. At NIH, I was in the laboratory and didn't see patients, and because I enjoy talking to people, the trips filled a void for me. I have always felt it a privilege and an honor to be invited various places. Also, I thought I had a message. During the last 3 years at NIH, governmental employees were not allowed to take an honorarium no matter if the talk was on a Saturday or Sunday or at night. My speaking dropped enormously, not that I did the speaking exclusively to have additional income, but speaking does take energy if one does it well. One period at NIH, I didn't accept any speaking invitations for 6 months, and during that period I found that I missed it. Then, when I started speaking again invitations were relatively slow in coming initially. William F. Buckley, for example, who has given numerous talks through the years, about 3 or 4 years ago, cut it off entirely. I actually give relatively few talks proportional to the invitations I get, and I do not mean to say that in an arrogant way. I can look at my computer screen nearly every day, and there is an invitation. I found that if I'm going out of town on a Friday or Thursday night, then I'm more productive the previous 4 days than when I'm not going on a 1-night trip. The speaking breaks stimulate me in a way. Ideas have occurred to me on trips. But trips wear me down a bit more now than 30 years ago.

Charles: *How many foreign countries have you visited?*

William: I think 65. Some I have visited several times.

Charles: *Were there any spectacular trips during your career?*

William: Absolutely. I was unsophisticated from a travel standpoint growing up. I hadn't even been to Alabama when I went off to college. I'd been to very few places in Georgia before I went to college. So having traveled very little in the first 20 years of life, for doors opening to see many different places was thrilling. Have I had spectacular trips? I've had many fantastic trips; very exciting, educational, and broadening.

Charles: *I noticed that you went to South Africa early in your career and to the USSR?*

William: John Barlow of mitral valve prolapse fame invited me along with 3 other Americans in 1974. Barlow and I became friends after that. That was one of my earliest international trips and my ex-wife accompanied me on it. It was a major eye-opening trip. I was on a delegation to study sudden death in the Soviet Union in 1973 and thought at the time there was probably no better place to go if that was the topic. That trip allowed me to learn a little about the communist empire. The traveling group was headed by Bernard Lown, who had invented the defibrillator. I found him to be very impressive. I've now been to most continents on the planet, and to some multiple times. I'm a blessed and lucky human being.

Charles: *If you were required to live in a country other than the US, which country would you choose?*

William: Canada or the United Kingdom.

Charles: *I gather that most of your talks deal with atherosclerosis and its prevention?*

William: That's the case now. Early on I talked a lot about valvular heart disease, prosthetic valve complications, cardiomyopathies, congenital heart disease, and infective endocarditis—multiple topics. Since 1990, most of my talks have been on preventive cardiology. I never was invited to give a talk sponsored by a pharmaceutical company until 1986. Prior to that time, it was always an invitation from a hospital or medical school. Medical education has changed enormously in the past 20 years. Pharmaceutical companies sponsor a lot of my talks, and I have not been hesitant in speaking under the sponsorship of a pharmaceutical company. Five pharmaceutical companies have sponsored presentations I have given recently. I give the same presentation irrespective of the sponsor. Some meetings have large audiences. I enjoy it.

Charles: *How would you characterize your relation with pharmaceutical companies?*

William: I have no stocks in any pharmaceutical company or in any medical device company. My relation is almost entirely speaker-related. I've been on an advisory board for Johnson & Johnson/Merck for 7 years, trying to get lovastatin over-the-counter, something I believe in but the Federal Drug Administration up to now has not believed in. The United Kingdom, in contrast, put simvastatin over the counter in about a year.

Charles: *Has your presentation technique changed over the years?*

William: Yes. When I moved to Dallas in March 1993, I had several talks scheduled during those first couple of months. I told Baylor's President, Boone Powell, Jr., that I probably should delay my coming for a couple of months because I would be gone several times during the first 2 months. He said, "Come on." When I drove from the Washington, DC, area to Dallas, I threw the slides I used most often for talks in a bag, which I placed in the trunk of my car. When I arrived in Dallas, I had forgotten that I had put slides in a bag, which felt empty to me from the outside, and I threw it in my closet, thinking it was empty. When I was preparing for my first trip, I couldn't find my slides. Since I did not have time to prepare new slides, I went to the first few talks without slides and simply spoke from the podium. After 1 such talk, a listener at the Lahey Clinic came up to me and said, "Don't ever show another slide." That was all I needed at the time, and then a couple of talks later there was a flipchart on the stage, and I used it. I have used a flipchart ever since. Then, about 3 months later after coming to Dallas, my son John visited me. As he was leaving, he asked if I had a bag that he could have. I went into the closet and low and behold there found my slides in the loose cloth bag. Nevertheless, I have never used the slides again.

Charles: *Do you plan to learn PowerPoint?*

William: I more or less know how to do it, but I have not taken the time to prepare slides or convert slides.

Charles: *Let's talk about writing. I am deeply aware that you have a keen interest in the English language. How do you suppose you acquired that interest?*

William: I majored in English in college but those courses were more in history than in English. The college gave me English credit for some history courses. When arriving at NIH, I quickly sensed that the ability to write medical papers was the great separator. I loved the challenge. I learned quickly that good writing meant clear thinking. I remember an English teacher in college told me, "Outline, outline outline." I never did it in college. Then, when I came to NIH and realized my career was essentially dependent on my pen, I started outlining. At least for discussion portions of manuscripts, I always outline what I am going to say before I write anything. I do not start writing a manuscript until all the data are in, the tables are finalized, the figures are finalized, and the message is clear. Writing is the last thing I do on any particular project. Selling an idea and convincing others of its correctness requires clear thinking and precise writing. I enjoy all of it.

Charles: *What books on writing have influenced you?*

William: I have probably 50 books on writing, words, composition, editing. The one which has probably helped me the most is "*On Writing Well*" by William Zinsser. His chapter on "clutter" is magnificent. Of course, "*The Elements of Style*" by William Strunk, Jr, and E.B. White is masterful. My mother gave me a copy of that book in 1959. One paragraph in that book is the key to writing:

> "Vigorous writing is concise. A sentence should contain no unnecessary words, a paragraph no unnecessary sentences, for the same reason that a drawing should have no unnecessary lines and a machine no unnecessary parts. This requires not that the writer make all his sentences short, or that he avoid all detail and treat his subjects only in outline, but that every word tell."

And "*The Writer's Art*" by James J. Kilpatrick provides a finely crafted, witty guide to writing well. And all of the books by Theodore M. Bernstein are useful: "*The Careful Writer, Miss Thistlebottom's Hobgoblins; Dos, Don'ts & Maybes of English Usage.* And H.W. Fowler's "*A Dictionary of Modern English Usage*" is a must. And there are many more. I have mentioned only a few. If one's career is dependent on his/her pen, clear thinking and clear writing are mandatory. Abraham Lincoln was great because he could think clearly and write clearly. I strongly recommend *Lincoln's Sword. The Presidency and the Power of Words* by Douglas L. Wilson. Lincoln's sword was his pen!

Charles: *You said 2 or 3 times that your career was dependent on your pen. Do you write with one?*

William: No, I write with a pencil.

Charles: *Do you use a computer when you prepare a manuscript?*

William: No. I use a yellow pad as a rule.

Charles: *How has writing a manuscript changed over the years?*

William: Manuscripts to get published have to be much better now and more crisp than when I started 47 years ago. Most are shorter, more concise; illustrations, figures, and tables are better; and statistics, which were nearly nonexistent when I started, are now needed in all manuscripts with data.

When I went to NIH in July 1959, there were no xerographic machines or computers. Copies of originals were made on carbon paper. Because I was last in line to get things typed when I first went to NIH, I would write the manuscript in pencil and then re-work it on my initial draft until I thought it was fine and then I would hand it in to be typed. I would revise that typed version, of course, but the number of changes would be *relatively* minor. The next typing would be the final one sent to the journal. Now, with computers, I still write my manuscripts out on paper, but now they may go through 10 drafts before being sent to an editor. To make changes in a manuscript now is a piece of cake. Forty years ago, every change was a big deal. Standards improve with time, so manuscripts today must be much better than in the past. The demand for editorial pages is greater than ever in history and to get published manuscripts must be good.

Charles: *Do you particularly admire any writer, medical or non-medical?*

William: Yes. Of those I have read William Osler is the best. Eugene Braunwald, Michael E. DeBakey, Denton Cooley, Dean Mason, Eric Topol, and Rob Califf are superb writers among others. Abe Lincoln, Ulysses S. Grant, William T. Sherman, Benjamin Franklin, Theodore Roosevelt, and Winston Churchill were all superb writers. James J. Kilpatrick, William F. Buckley, George Will, David McCullough, Erik Larson, Simon Winchester, to name just a few, are some of my favorites.

Charles: *In 1982, you became editor in chief of The American Journal of Cardiology (AJC). Tell about that period. You were 50 years of age. How did you acquire that position?*

William: In 1975, Dean Mason was elected president of the American College of Cardiology and the chairman of the publications committee had just fulfilled his term. Dean appointed me chairman of the publications committee of the College and that committee oversaw the AJC. We had a meeting once a year at the time of the American College of Cardiology's Annual Scientific Sessions. I prepared for that meeting by studying the AJC, which was edited then by Dr. Simon Dack, its first editor. At each of the annual meetings I invited the publisher of the AJC, who had never been invited previously, and he came. At the meeting I would raise issues which I thought might improve the quality of the journal. Members of that committee were appointed for 3-year terms with an option to serve another 3 years. I was renewed after 3 years and actually held that position for 6 years. During the sixth year, the American College of Cardiology wanted the publisher of the AJC, which at the time was the official journal of the American College of Cardiology, to share its financial statements with them. The college had no idea how much money the publisher was making on the AJC. The publisher of the journal, however, refused to do that. (The AJC journal title was owned by the publisher, not by the college.) The College wanted to have its own journal, i.e., to own its own journal's title, and the College ceased its relation with the AJC and started the *Journal of the American College of Cardiology (JACC)*. When the college decided to publish JACC, Simon Dack, who was editor of the AJC, was asked to become the editor of JACC and that opened up the editorship of the AJC. The publisher of the AJC had known me for 6 years, having attended the annual publications committee's meetings each year. He saw how I operated, and he heard the ideas I had to improve the journal. The publisher asked me if I would like to be editor in chief of the AJC. I accepted after some brief negotiations. I had to get permission from the director of the NHI. I was advised not to take the position, because it would interfere too much with my NIH work. I asked if there was a law against my accepting the editorship. I was told "no. " Thus, in June 1982, I became the second editor of the AJC. I took to the AJC editorship with great enthusiasm, and the ideas I had presented at the publications committee annually for 6 years, none of which were ever acted on, were instituted when I became editor within 3 months—something which shows the weakness of a publications committee and the strength of an editorship. Simon

Dack had been editor of the AJC from it's inception in 1958. We both have had prolonged tenures.

Charles: *How much time do you give to this responsibility weekly and has that changed over the years?*

William: The year I became editor, 1982, the journal received 1,100 manuscripts. By 1985, we were up to 1,600, and fairly quickly we rose to 2,100 to 2,200 per year, and stayed at that number for many years. In 2005, the number of manuscripts submitted increased by 500 to 2,650. In 2006, it increased another 500 to nearly 3,200. Thus, during my 25-year tenure, the number of manuscripts submitted has increased by two-thirds (from 1,100 to nearly 3,200). Although the number of manuscripts submitted has increased by nearly 2,000, the number of editorial pages available for publication has not changed one iota. We still publish nearly 700 articles in the AJC each year, but they are much shorter now than in the past. The acceptance rate has dropped (to 21% in 2006).

Charles: *Do you have difficulty making a decision about a manuscript?*

William: Usually not. Manuscripts which I think should be strongly considered for acceptance I print out and take them home to examine and edit. When I have a problem making a decision, I put the manuscript aside. The next day the decision usually is much easier. Occasionally, I ask an associate editor (Paul Grayburn, Clyde Yancy) for their opinion. In April 2005, the journal went on-line, that is, all manuscripts are submitted online, sent out for review online, returned to authors online, and all revised manuscripts are returned online.

Charles: *What's the most common revision you require of manuscripts before publication?*

William: Shortening the manuscript, particularly the discussion, and improving the tables.

Charles: *What do you look for in a reviewer?*

William: I want to know if the information in the manuscript is new or if not, does it confirm a previous observation or does it present data, even though not new, in an interesting or unique way. Being newsworthy for the readership also helps. The AJC is an independent journal. Readers do not receive it because they are members of this or that society. Subscribers have to pay for it directly. If its contents are not useful to the readers, subscriptions fall. I like manuscripts that are helpful to physicians and ideally would be useful when they see their next patient. I think the AJC is the most clinical of the U.S. cardiology journals. We do not publish studies on non-human animals. I discontinued publishing them about 1984. They take up the most space and are the least read. The journals that come as part of the medical society's dues can afford that luxury.

Charles: *Can you summarize your philosophy on each section of a manuscript: title, abstract, introduction, discussion, etc?*

William: Nobody has ever asked me that question before. The title should be descriptive of the contents of the manuscript. I try to avoid subtitles, abbreviations in titles, and the message of the manuscript in the manuscript's title. Subtitles are often more descriptive of the contents of a manuscript than is the primary title, and subtitles are often neglected in references. Thus, I avoid subtitles except in maybe editorials. I alter 95% of the titles and try to make them descriptive of the contents. I don't like structured abstracts. Structured abstracts take up more space than nonstructured ones. An abstract should be a single paragraph of no more than a single double-spaced manuscript page. The last statement in the abstract is the conclusion ("In conclusion, ..."). The *Introduction* should be no more than a single paragraph—1/2-page in length. The *Methods* and *Results* sections are the most important portions of manuscripts. (Some journals place those 2 sections in smaller type than that used for the rest of the manuscript. I think that is a mistake.) The methods and results sections should be in exquisite detail. If you don't know how a study was done, you can't evaluate the results. The first paragraph of the discussion should briefly summarize the major findings of the study. Previous studies on the topic should be discussed next, including how the present manuscript differs from those previously published on the topic. The discussion I view as a tree trunk. If you make the whole discussion the trunk of the tree, each paragraph might best represent 1 limb of the tree. The limbs selected to be discussed should be fully discussed, from the trunk to the end of the limb. If the tree trunk has 15 limbs on it, select only 3 or 4 and discuss them fully, don't cut them short. A conclusion at the end of a discussion is unnecessary. I usually eliminate them. References can usually be limited to no more than 30. The word *reference* is not needed to headline this section. By not using the word *references* we save 3 editorial pages a year! References should include the names of all authors, not just the first 3, and full inclusive pages should be used to separate articles from abstracts. I look for good figures and good tables. Good tables and figures are the things that make a manuscript, not the words in it, as a rule. I spend a good bit of time on tables and titles in my own manuscripts and in those submitted to my editorship.

Charles: *How has the AJC changed structurally under your editorship over these 25 years?*

William: It has changed considerably. If you look at the journal in June 1982 and then again in October or November 1982, the changes were fairly radical. And these changes were made without any outside consultant. The managing editor in New York and I did them without expense to the publisher. The journal previously had highlighted a few articles on the cover. I thought that was risky because sometimes the worth of a manuscript is not apparent until 5 years or so later. The manuscripts were subdivided into those having to do with coronary artery disease, arrhythmias and conduction disturbances, heart failure, valvular heart disease, cardiomyopathy, miscellaneous topics, historical topics, and editorials. They were divided by type of disease, not by "instruments of precision" (echo, etc). We had a section called *brief reports*—very short manuscripts—for years, but in the last 2 years all manuscripts are subdivided by topic, not by manuscript length. The latest alteration was prompted by the publisher, but it was actually something I wanted also. The brief reports were published back to back, so there was no wasted space at the end of the article. We have lost that advantage by starting all manuscripts on a separate page. Both authors and readers I believe like each manuscript to start on a separate page. That change means that we can't publish quite as many manuscripts as previously. We now put the table of contents on the cover, at least as much as we can get there, and readers like that. The reason the number of manuscripts submitted has increased so much in the last 2 years is not entirely clear, but at least 2 factors seem important: (1) going online has allowed authors to send in manuscripts without a lot of effort or expense, and (2) featuring brief reports in the same way as long reports. Short reports now have the same subheadings as long reports as a rule. The length of a manuscript does not determine its quality! James Watson and Francis Crick won a Nobel Prize for a 1-page article!

Charles: *What is your view of so-called "case reports"?*

William: We publish case reports in the AJC, about 10 a year. I like case reports as long as they are crisp and short. There are some topics that only lend themselves to the case report format. Few cardiology journals publish case reports now. We are the exception. I like them and wish that we could publish more, but we do not have the space. Doctoring is one patient at a time.

Charles: *What's your philosophy about abbreviations in a manuscript?*

William: Abbreviations save space, but I like to limit them mainly to phrases in the manuscript's title and to no more than 5 per manuscript. If a manuscript, let's say, concerns the frequency of atrial fibrillation in mitral stenosis, you know that both "atrial fibrillation" and "mitral stenosis" are going to be used a lot in that manuscript. So the 2 obvious abbreviations are AF and MS. I spend too much time on abbreviations. One manuscript—the champ during my editorship—had 26 abbreviations. I've counted 24 or 25 on several occasions. "Histories" and "physicals" written by house officers often contain (I have counted) as many as 75 abbreviations. Manuscripts are much different and require a different discipline than writing "histories and physicals."

Charles: *What red flags in a manuscript suggest to you that the manuscript is probably not worthy of publication?*

William: That's a good question. If the abstract is structured, I suspect that the manuscript had earlier been sent to another journal which declined it, and that the authors probably made little effort to respond to the previous reviewers' suggestions before submitting the manuscript to the AJC. If references are not in the style of the AJC that suggests that the authors are not in the upper ranks of research sophistication. Sloppy writing, poor tables, and cluttered figures are signs of non-excellence.

Charles: *Do you pay any attention to where a manuscript originates?*

William: I do. Since being online, I initially see the manuscripts without the authors' names on them or their locations. In general, manuscripts coming from the USA or UK or Western Europe or Israel or Japan or Hong Kong are better than those coming from other countries, but some excellent manuscripts come from other non-mentioned countries also.

Charles: *Do you write "From the Editor" columns?*

William: Yes. When I became editor in June 1982, we had 15 issues a year beginning in 1983. I wrote 15 columns a year for 5 years and never missed one. Now I'm down to 4 or 5 a year in the AJC. It's a funny thing; I've never had one of these *From the Editor* columns declined. I am also editor in chief of the *Baylor University Medical Center Proceedings*, a quarterly, and have been since 1994. I have a column entitled "Facts and Ideas From Anywhere" in every issue. These are relatively long columns, and 2 books have been published incorporating these columns (1994 to 2000) (2000 to 2005).

Charles: *Do you publish your own scientific articles in the AJC?*

William: Yes, absolutely. Probably too much. Early on, I sent almost all of my own manuscripts to the AJC. I keep all the reviews of my own articles. They get 2 reviews like most other manuscripts. The associate editor, Paul Grayburn, handles manuscripts with my name on them.

Charles: *You became editor of the AJC in 1982. Up to that point nearly all of your first nearly 500 publications were scientific. After 1982, there were many editorials. Discuss that.*

William: I wrote a few editorials before becoming editor of the AJC. When becoming editor I thought it important to put my stamp on the journal and started the From the Editor column. I thought it was important for readers of the journal to know some of the editors' views. I've known editors who've been editors for 5 to 25 years, and I never knew what they thought about anything. So right or wrongly, I think it's a useful endeavor. Subsequently, the editors of *JACC* and *Clinical Cardiology* have written monthly or at least frequent From the Editor columns in their journals.

Charles: *Which is more difficult for you, editing or writing?*

William: Writing. Much more difficult.

Charles: *Which activity brings more satisfaction— editing or writing?*

William: Writing. That I had written a lot before I became editor helped me enormously. The annual book, *Cardiology* 1982, *Cardiology* 1983, etc, required a lot of writing and a lot of editing, and that also improved by editorship. I have learned more about editing from my own manuscripts going through the peer-review process than from any other endeavor. I believe it useful that editors continue to publish scientific articles, i.e., other than editorials, to maintain understanding and humility.

Charles: *Let's talk about the move from NIH to Baylor University Medical Center (BUMC) in Dallas in 1993. Let me ask first, did you seriously consider any other job offers during your years as a laboratory director at NIH?*

William: I was offered the chairmanship of the department of pathology at Baylor College of Medicine (Houston) in 1972 by Dr. Michael DeBakey, and I regrettably accepted that position for a 4-month period but never moved to Houston. Finally, I realized that I really wanted to stay in cardiovascular disease, and I was not certain I could do that as a pathology department chairman. It was a job that involved 4 hospitals, a lot of administrative work, and I was very happy at NIH. I enjoyed the projects that I was doing and decided why leave a situation where I was professionally very happy. The other side of that issue was that I had 4 offspring, all of whom would eventually go to college and probably also to graduate school. I felt selfish from a family standpoint in staying at NIH, but hoped that things would work out and they did. Shortly after declining the Baylor College of Medicine position, I was offered the chairmanship of the department of pathology at Vanderbilt Univer-

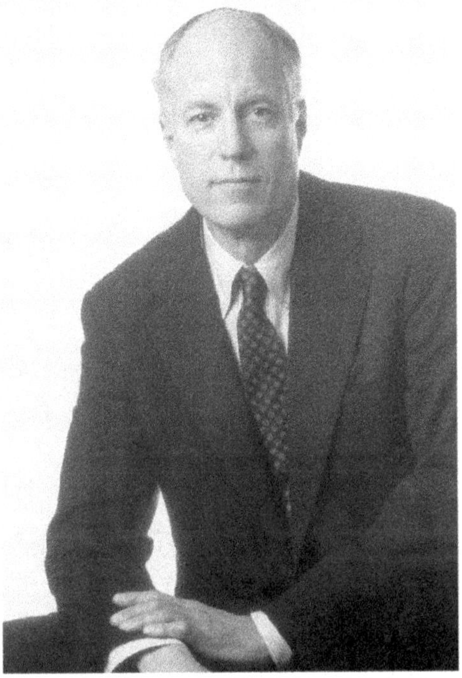

Figure 12. WCR when he came to Baylor University Medical Center, Dallas, in 1993 when he was 60 years of age.

sity, and I declined that position for the same reason, although I liked Vanderbilt and Nashville a great deal. Then, I was asked to interview for the chiefship of the department of pathology at the Massachusetts General Hospital (Boston), but I was not offered the position. Thereafter, I didn't look at any other offer until about 1990, and then I was asked to look at the chairmanship of pathology at the Medical College of Virginia in Richmond, Virginia. Although I liked Richmond, I still was not anxious to be a pathology department chairman. At the same time, however, NIH was changing. The surgery branch in the National Heart, Lung, and Blood Institute (NHLBI) had been eliminated and that decision bothered me greatly. I sensed a future demise of the cardiology branch at the NHLBI. Then in 1991, my marriage split up. NIH was putting major emphasis on molecular biology. Suddenly, recruiting good fellows became difficult. (Medical schools wanted to retain their best.) The honoraria were eliminated for speaking and then there was discussion that NIH was going to put a 500-hour limit on any non-NIH activities of the scientists. I was spending >500 hours a year at that time on the AJC. I was never allowed to do editorial work on the AJC from 8:30 am to 5:00 pm on non-holidays, Monday through Friday, and I honored that requirement. But that 500-hour annual requirement, if put in place, bothered me because my time on the AJC at nights and weekends would add up to considerably more than 500 hours annually. (Fortunately, it was never put into effect.)

The scientific director, to my surprise, became aware that I was going to a lot of hospitals in the Washington, DC, area during weekdays. (The scientific director was a non-MD, a PhD who worked on amoebas.) I didn't think that the clinical operation was getting a fair shake and was worried that it would change even more. Additionally, in 1992, I reached retirement (30 years) in the Public Health Service, and NIH favored eliminating retirees. I was fortunate to be renewed for 3 more years (to 1996), but I didn't like the idea of having to be renewed every 3 years.

Charles: *Tell how the Baylor Dallas offer came about. Who offered you the job? What position did you take?*

William: In early 1992, Dr. Jack Hyland, who was chief of the cardiology division of the department of internal medicine at Baylor University Medical Center (BUMC) in Dallas, invited me to speak at medical grand rounds there in August 1992. I accepted and went to Dallas, gave medical grand rounds, and about a week later, I was called by 1 of the administrators (Tim Parris) at BUMC to inquire if I might be interested in coming to Dallas and becoming a part of their medical center. I told him that I would like to pursue it, because I had been to SMU and I knew Dallas a bit. I knew very little about BUMC. He said he would come to Washington, DC, and talk to me. He visited me at NIH, looked at my lab and office. I was impressed that somebody interested in me wanted to see my present operation. Nobody had done that before or even inquired. Tim Parris and I had dinner, and we hit it off quite well, I became intrigued, and Tim invited me to Dallas to visit BUMC more thoroughly, which I did. About 2 weeks after that visit, Boone Powell, Jr., who was President of the Baylor Health Care System (BHCS) (BUMC owns 8 other hospitals in the Dallas Ft. Worth community and many free-standing clinics) came to Washington, and we had dinner together at the Cosmos Club. He offered me the position of executive director of the Baylor Cardiovascular Institute, which was going to be the research and educational arm of the Baylor Heart and Vascular Hospital, which they intended to build. They had not started it yet, but hoped to get it underway in the relatively near future. He presented me with a nice proposal and told me that Baylor would move a good bit of my laboratory to Dallas, give me a lab, nice office setting, etc. I decided that this was the thing to do. I liked the people I had met at BUMC. I liked their philosophy, and decided that it was for me. I started on March 1, 1993 (Figure 12), and I've been here ever since, and I have been happy the entire time. This is only my second job. I've been well supported.

Charles: *Compare Dallas and Washington, DC, having lived in Washington for over 3 decades.*

William: Washington is a wonderful city but we lived in Potomac, Maryland, which at the time was 45 minutes from the White House. (Now, it's probably 75 minutes from the White House because of the increased traffic.) And although Washington had an incredible variety of activities, (Smithsonian, etc.) working in Bethesda and living in Potomac did not allow those advantages to be fully utilized. By the 1990s, all my kids had left home, all had finished college and postgraduate schools, and all were working. I found a home in Dallas in late 1992 in a very nice community (Highland Park), 3.5 miles from BUMC and 4 miles from downtown Dallas. I thought it was an ideal work and home situation, and it has proven to be so.

Charles: *What is your position at BUMC at the moment?*

William: My title is Executive Director, Baylor Heart and Vascular Institute. I am also Dean, A Webb Roberts Center for Continuing Medical Education, and also editor in chief of the *Baylor University Medical Center Proceedings*.

Charles: *What responsibilities did you assume at BUMC?*

William: I hadn't been at Baylor long when it became apparent that the Heart and Vascular Hospital wasn't going to be built in the very near future. There were disagreements, which eventually were resolved, and the hospital was finished in 2002. In the interim, Baylor had a journal called the *Baylor University Medical Center Proceedings* and the founding editor wanted to retire. He asked me if I would be interested in being editor of the journal, and I said, "Of course I would." In January 1994, after I had been there about 10 months, I was appointed editor of that journal. I've enjoyed immensely that opportunity. It gave me an opportunity to participate in the broad Baylor community, which included all of the departments.

I started interviewing some of the BUMC staff and subsequently have done over 60 interviews of them. When I became editor, I tried to decide how I could put my stamp on this journal and decided to start a column, which was initially called *Facts and Ideas from Elsewhere* (later changed that to *Facts and Ideas from Anywhere*). That became a fun column for me and involves a variety of topics. It is published every 3 months. That 90-day interval comes around quickly! I keep a basket at home and throw interesting items I've read in it and then every 3 months I summarize them. Initially, I wrote those columns by hand, but because they are relatively long I found that method too tedious. The first 5 and second 5 years of these columns were each compiled into books. It has been heartwarming for me to see how successful this adventure has been. The journal has expanded from a circulation of 1,000 to a circulation of nearly 7,000. We are now on PubMed, the journal is published on acid-free paper, and the number of articles published in each issue has increased >5 times the number published in 1992. That journal has been a fun activity for me.

Not long after I had been at BUMC, I was also appointed Dean of the A. Webb Roberts Center for Continuing Medical Education. Obviously, I had had a long experience with the Williamsburg meeting, so it seemed reasonable for me to head that activity.

I have done the cardiovascular surgical pathology since I've been at Baylor. These specimens include operatively-excised valves, tumors, and aortas that are resected by vascular and cardiac surgeons. Until the last 3 years I examined all the autopsy hearts and actually opened them and spent time with the cardiology fellows and pathology residents on those particular cases. I have a 90-minute conference once a week with the cardiology fellows. We have 5 other cardiology conferences each week: a journal club, a vascular conference with the vascular surgeons, an echocardiography conference, a coronary angiographic conference, and a general cardiology lecture. In addition, I attend the medical grand rounds lecture series and have invited a number of speakers to present at that department's grand rounds.

Charles: *You have been editor of the* Baylor University Medical Center Proceedings *since 1994 and I noticed that in each of the 4 issues per year you have a column which has variously been called "Facts and Ideas from Everywhere" and "Fact and Ideas from Anywhere". Two of your books are collections of these articles published in the BUMC Proceedings. Where do you get these facts and ideas from?*

William: I take several general medical journals such as the *New England Journal of Medicine*, *Annals of Internal Medicine*, *JAMA*, *Lancet*, *British Medical Journal*, as well as the cardiology journals, and each week or so I go through the most recently received journals and tear out the articles that I think might be of interest to a general audience. Then, for several days before the quarterly manuscript is due, I sit down with a recording device and go through these medical articles I have ripped out and dictate a few comments on the ones that I think are newsworthy. Additionally, any articles I read in newspapers or magazines, I also tear out and put them in the basket and each 3 months go through them and dictate summaries of those articles I think are potentially interesting to the readers. Often, I summarize a book I have encountered. Although this journal is quarterly, the *Facts and Ideas from Anywhere* column has gotten to be relatively long, namely about 10 editorial pages, which amounts to about 40 manuscript pages.

Charles: *From your vantage point of 50 years in medicine, where are we now in cardiology, cardiovascular surgery, and in cardiovascular pathology?*

William: Probably no subspecialty of medicine has made more progress in the last nearly 45 years than has cardiovascular disease. When President John Kennedy was killed in 1963, β blockers had just become available. There were no calcium channels blockers, no angiotensin-converting enzyme inhibitors, no α-receptor blockers, no statins, no intestinal cholesterol blockers, no coronary angioplasty, and no coronary bypass. Aspirin was not recognized to be cardioprotective. Clopidogrel was not available. Coronary angiography was being performed probably in only 3 hospitals in the USA. Cardiac valve replacement, which started in 1960, was just getting underway in many hospitals. Coronary care units were not in existence yet. Multicenter placebo controlled double blind studies in cardiovascular disease were not being performed. The developments in cardiovascular radiology in the past 45 years have been phenomenal. It would have been difficult to have predicted so many of these developments in 1963, and to predict today what the developments will occur in this area in the next 50 years would be impossible. Certainly, genetics will come to the forefront and therapy will be more individualized based on genetic makeup than ever before. I believe we will have good drugs to lose weight, better drugs to lower blood glucose, blood cholesterol, and blood pressure levels. In actuality, in 50 years from now, atherosclerotic plaques except in patients with homozygous familial hypercholesterolemia and possibly in patients with heterozygous familial hypercholesterolemia should be nonexistent. Of course, if that happens, so many of the technological developments

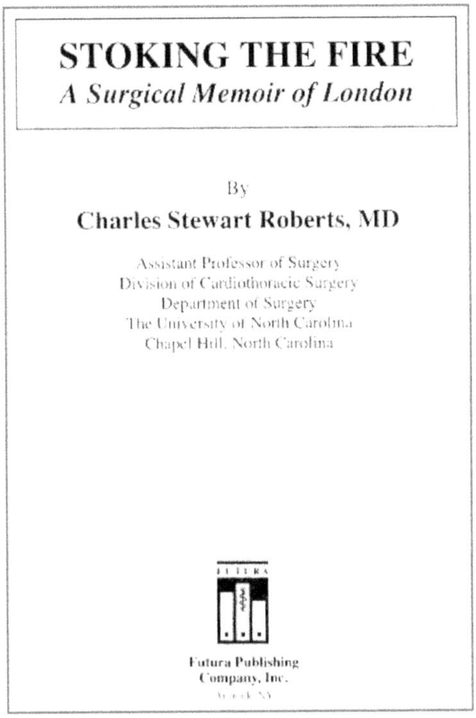
STOKING THE FIRE
A Surgical Memoir of London

By
Charles Stewart Roberts, MD

Assistant Professor of Surgery
Division of Cardiothoracic Surgery
Department of Surgery
The University of North Carolina
Chapel Hill, North Carolina

Futura Publishing
Company, Inc.

Figure 13. Title page of a book written by the interviewee, Charles Stewart Roberts, MD, after spending 1 year in London training under Mr. Christopher Lincoln in pediatric and adult cardiac surgery. Reprinted with permission of Blackwell Publishing.

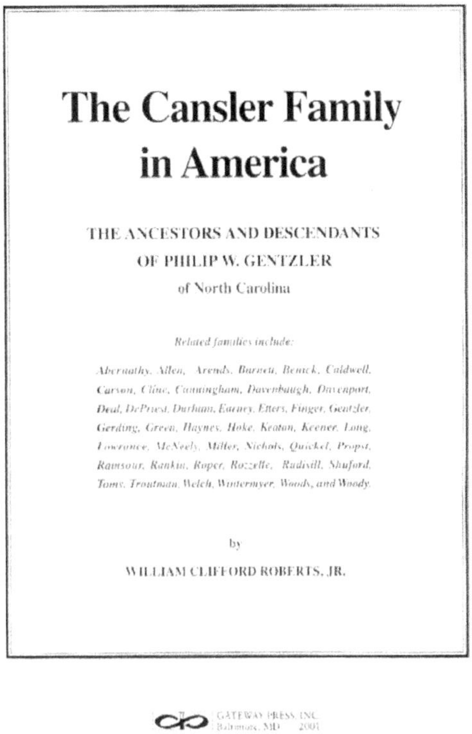
The Cansler Family in America

THE ANCESTORS AND DESCENDANTS
OF PHILIP W. GENTZLER
of North Carolina

Related families include:

Abernathy, Allen, Arends, Barnett, Benick, Caldwell, Carson, Cline, Cunningham, Davenbaugh, Davenport, Deal, DePriest, Durham, Earney, Etters, Finger, Gentzler, Gerding, Green, Haynes, Hoke, Keaton, Keener, Long, Lowrance, McNeely, Miller, Nichols, Quickel, Propst, Ramsour, Rankin, Roper, Rozzelle, Rudisill, Shuford, Toms, Troutman, Welch, Wintermyer, Woods, and Woody.

by

WILLIAM CLIFFORD ROBERTS, JR.

GATEWAY PRESS, INC.
Baltimore, MD 2001

Figure 14. Title page of a large book written by WCR's oldest son, William Clifford Roberts, Jr, and published by the Gateway Press of Baltimore, Maryland in 2001. The book is about the family of his mother—Carey Cansler Roberts'. Reprinted with permission.

in heart disease, namely, angioplasty with or without stents and bypass, will be unnecessary. There will be more pressure on Americans to eat properly, quit smoking, etc. Hanging a pig up in the backyard to barbecue will be taboo in 25 years. Killing 100,000 eleven-hundred pound cows everyday in the USA will be reduced in my view in the next 30 or so years, and those developments, of course, will be greatly beneficial to our health. Cardiovascular surgery will always have a place: I can't envision changes to prevent congenital cardiovascular anomalies, which include hypertrophic cardiomyopathy and congenitally bicuspid aortic valve and mitral valve prolapse, in the next several decades. Trauma to lungs, heart, and blood vessels will always need operative therapy. Cardiovascular pathology will for the most part be limited to cardiac transplantation, operatively excised cardiac valves, and tumors, because autopsies will continue to decrease in frequency. I think that is unfortunate, because despite enormous developments of our "instruments of precision," there are still new findings at necropsy by specialists in cardiovascular disease.

Charles: *Do you have an interest in medical history?*

William: Yes.

Charles: *Have you published any articles in medical history?*

William: Yes, 15, but most of them have been short. The most fully developed ones concern Tomlinson Fort (WCR #72), Simon Dack (WCR #317), Norman Jefferies Holter (WCR #556), George Edward Burch (WCR #693), Benjamin Franklin (WCR #926), and small vignettes on Sir William Osler, Stewart Ralph Roberts, Ruby Holbrook Roberts, J. Willis Hurst, Jeffrey Isner, and James Watson.

Charles: *What physician or physicians of the past would you have liked to have known?*

William: That is an interesting question, and one that I have not been asked previously. Sir William Osler would lead the list, but I would also include Sir Thomas Clifford Allbutt, Daniel Drake, James B. Herrick, Silas Weir Mitchell, Thomas Sydenham, and Sir James MacKenzie among others. Of surgeons, I would have loved to have known John Hunter and his brother William Hunter, James Marion Sims, Sir James Paget, Thomas Beville Peacock, William and Charles Mayo, and Harvey Cushing among others. Among pathologists, I would be intrigued by Carl von Rokitansky, Friedrich von Recklinghausen, Rudolph Virchow, and Giovanni Battista Morgagni. Also, I would add Oliver Wendall Holmes and Arthur Conan Doyle, Marie Curie, and Florence Nightingale.

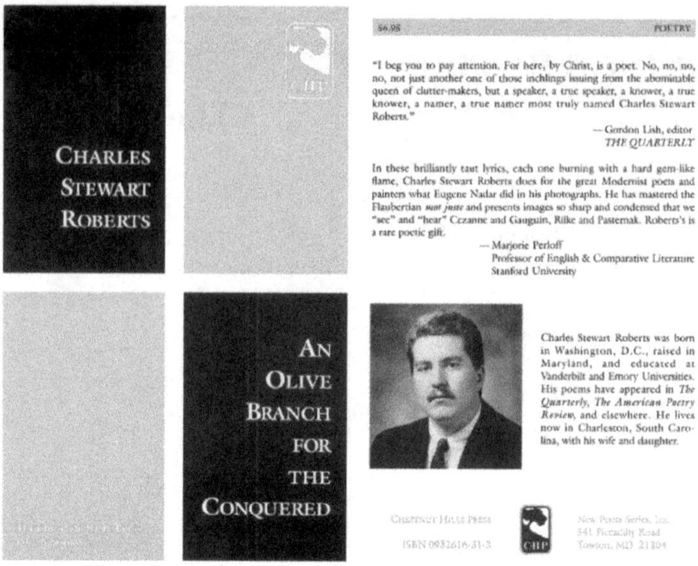

Figure 15. Cover of a book of poetry entitled *An Olive Branch for the Conquered* written by the interviewee, Charles Stewart Roberts and published by the Chestnut Hills Press in 1990 when CSR was 29 years of age. The page on the right is the back cover which shows some comments from the editor of the quarterly and Dr. Marjorie Perloff of Stanford University. Reprinted with permission of Brick House Books, Inc./Chestnut Hills Press.

Charles: *Tell about the American Osler Society?*

William: The American Osler Society is a group comprised predominately of physicians interested in Sir William Osler in particular but in medical history in general. The society meets once a year and papers are presented during the 2-day meeting. About half of the papers have something to do with William Osler. It's an organization into which the members are elected and membership essentially requires a presentation by the new members. Dr. Marvin Stone at BUMC invited me initially and provided the path for my successful election. It is a wonderful organization and I have, since being made a member, never missed a meeting. I enjoy it immensely. I have presented 3 papers at that meeting: 1 on Dr. Tomlinson Fort of Milledgeville, Georgia; 1 on the commonalities of the interviewees I have interviewed and published in *The American Journal of Cardiology*, and 1 on the late Dr. George Burch of New Orleans.

Charles: *What are your most treasured medical books?*

William: My 3 most treasured books are the collected reprints of my father, which are bound into 2 volumes; the book by Charles Stewart Roberts (you!) entitled *Life and Writings of Stewart R. Roberts, M.D., Georgia's First Heart Specialist* (Figure 8); the book by Charles Stewart Roberts (you!) entitled *Stoking the Fire, a Surgical Memoir of London* (Figure 13). It's not often that a son writes a biography about his father's father, and you did!) Next in line of my favorites would be my father's book, Stewart Ralph Roberts, MD, entitled *Pellagra. History, Distribution, Diagnosis, Prognosis, Treatment, Etiology* published by C.D. Mosby in 1914 (Figure 9). The book by William Clifford Roberts, Jr., my oldest, entitled *The Cansler Family in America. The Ancestors and Descendants of Philip W. Gentzler of North Carolina* is a prized possession (Figure 14) as is a book written by Charles Stewart Roberts entitled *An Olive Branch for the Conquered* published by The Chestnut Hills Press in 1990 (Figure 15).

Next would be my William Osler books. I have his first edition (1892) of *The Principles and Practice of Medicine Designed for the Use of Practitioners and Students of Medicine*, and every word of the 1,079 pages was written by Osler. Another book, I am delighted to have is the Sir William Osler Memorial Number, *Appreciations and Reminisces* edited by Maude E. Abbott, MD, and published in 1926. My father, Stewart R. Roberts, had a chapter in that book entitled *William Osler, Clinician-Teacher (*pages 431 to 434). A classified and annotated bibliography occupying 156 pages is included in this splendid book. I am enormously fond of the *Sir William Osler, Bart. Brief Tributes to his Personality, Influence and Public Service* written by his Friends, Associates, and Former Pupils, In Honor of his Seventieth Birthday and First Published in the *Bulletin of the Johns Hopkins Hospital* for July 1919. My favorite is the chapter entitled "OSLER THE TEACHER" by W.S. Thayer. A *Year with Osler 1896 to 1896, Notes Taken at His Class in The John Hopkins Hospital* by Joseph H. Pratt (1949) is a front-row seat book on Osler which I have.

The 2 major biographies of Sir William Osler I am pleased to have: The Pulitzer-Prize winning 2-volume book entitled *The Life of Sir William Osler* by Harvey Cushing, appearing in 1925, and the 1999 *William Osler. A Life in Medicine* by Michael Bliss. Other Osler books I am most proud to have are: *An Alabama Student* and *Other Biographical Essays* by William Osler published in 1908; Shigeaki Hiohara and Hisae Mike's book entitled *Osler's "A Way of Life" and Other Addresses with Commentary and Annotations* published in 2001. William Osler's collected papers on the cardiovascular system edited and introduced by W. Bruce Fye and published in 1985 is perfect for those interested in both Osler and cardiovascular disease. One of my very favorite books on Osler is entitled *OSLER Inspirations from a Great Physician* by Charles S. Bryan. I keep it on my bedside table. This book appeared in 1997 and truly brings Osler back to life.

W. Bruce Fye's American Cardiology. *The History of a Specialty and Its College* published in 1996 is a must for all in cardiovascular disease. Tomlinson Fort's *A Dissertation on the Practice of Medicine, Containing an Account of the Causes, Symptoms, and Treatment of Disease and Adaptive to the Use of Physicians and Families* published in Milledgeville, Georgia, in 1849 is a prize possession. Three reference books have been very useful to me: *An Introduction to the History of Medicine with Medical Chronology, Suggestions for Study and Bibliographic Data* by Fielding S. Garrison and published in 1913; a *Biographical History of Medicine X. Excerpts and Essays on the Men and their Work* by John H. Talbott published in 1970; and *Classic Descriptions of Disease with Biographical Sketches of the Authors* by Ralph H. Major, published in 1932, are highly useful for any student of the history of medicine. Since I have always been intrigued by Harvey Cushing, the book *Harvey Cushing A Biography* by John F. Fulton published in 1946 and *Meningiomas. Their Classification, Regional Behavior, Life History and Surgical End Results* by Harvey Cushing with collaboration of Louise Eisenhardt are prized possessions.

The book *Anomalies and Curiosities of Medicine* by George M. Gould and Walter L. Pyle published in 1900 is a classic. I also have the *"Final Report of the Commission on Medical Education,"* because this book was signed by my father, December 20, 1932. Sir James MacKenzie has always been a hero of mine, and I am fortunate to have his *Diseases of the Heart* published initially in 1908 and his book entitled *Angina Pectoris* published in 1923. The biography entitled *The Beloved Physician— Sir James MacKenzie* by R. MacNair Wilson and published in 1926 is an inspiring book. The book entitled *On Malformations, & C., of the Human Heart with Original Cases* by Thomas B. Peacock published in 1858 is a classic which I am pleased to have. (It was a gift from Dr. Bruce Waller.) A book I have always admired is *Facts on the Heart* by Richard C. Cabot appearing in 1926. My father had William Withering's book *An Account of the Foxglove and Some of its Medical Uses: With Practical Remarks on Dropsey, and Other Diseases* published in 1785. It was saved during the fire which burned our house. Obviously, I am elated to have the copy. Otto Juettner's *Daniel Drake and his Followers. Historical and Biographical Sketches* is a prized possession. This book appeared in 1909 and was purchased by my father and again saved in the fire. A wonderful book in more recent times is *Exploring the Heart. Discoveries in Heart Disease and High Blood Pressure* by Julius H. Comroe and published in 1983.

Charles: *Do you collect books?*

William: Yes. Some of them are described above. Now I collect medical books almost entirely on cardiovascular disease and William Osler.

Charles: *Do you read in subjects outside of medicine? And if so, how much do you read, I presume, mainly at night?*

William: I try to read as Osler suggested about 30 minutes before turning my light out at night. In contrast to Osler, who spent the last half hour of the day in communion with "the Saints of humanity," I tend to pick up a book, most often a biography, of Lincoln or other famous personalities. I love Abe Lincoln, who is our best American in my view. For some reason in recent times, I have collected some books on natural disasters and some even unnatural ones, such as *Krakatoa* by Simon Winchester; *Rising Tide* by John M. Barry; *When the Mississippi Ran Backwards* by J. Feldman; *Triangle* by David von Drehle; *San Francisco is Burning* by Dennis Smith; *The Great Deluge* by Douglas Brinkley; *Lusitania* by Dianna Preston; *Sudden Sea; The Great Hurricane of 1938* by R.A. Scotti, among others.

Some wonderful books on medicine are now being written by non-medical people and some are superb: *Doctors from Hell* by Vivian Spitz; *The Barbary Plague* by Marilyn Chase; *Rats* by Robert Sullivan; *Leonard Wood* by John McCallum; *The Mold and Dr. Florey's Coat* by Eric Lax; *The Miraculous Fever Tree* by Fiammetta Rocco; *The Speckled Monster* by Jennifer Lee Carrell; *The Great Influenza* by John M. Barry; *The Great Mortality* by John Kelly; *Pox* by Debra Hayden; *Splendid Solution* by Jeffrey Kluger; *The Colony* by John Tayman; *Goldberger's War* by Alan M. Kraut; *The Knife Man* by Wendy Moore; *The Great Starvation Experiment* by Todd Tucker, among many others.

I also have collected a number of biographies of prominent US businessmen, mainly those in the 19th century, but including Josiah Wedgwood, Robert Fulton, Thomas Edison, Andrew Carnegie, Henry Clay Frick, John P. Morgan, Henry Ford, William Randolph Hurst, Andrew Mellon, John D. Rockefeller, Sr., Milton S. Hershey, Alexander Graham Bell, Charles Goodyear, Henry Morrison Flagler, Bertrand Russell, among others. I have a set of short biographies on the US Presidents, and I like them very much. The general editor of the series is Arthur M. Schlesinger, Jr.

Charles: *What are a few books that would be on your "desert Island" list?*

William: I think most readers would answer that by saying the Holy Bible, the complete works of William Shakespeare, and *Don Quixote* by Miguel de Cervantes. I think these 3 would be good choices. I would prefer to have an annotated Bible. My edition of *Don Quixote* is 940 pages in length, and one can open that book on virtually any page and read an interesting conversation. E.H. Gombrich's book entitled *The Story of Art* would be nice to have along. I would definitely take Howard Zinn's *A People's History of the United States 1492–Present.* I would also take Charles S. Bryan's *OSLER Inspiration from a Great Physician,* because I never get tired of looking at those pages. If there was space, I would take Walter Isaacson's book on some of Franklin's major writings entitled *A Benjamin Franklin*

Reader and also the Library of America's *Speeches, Letters, Miscellaneous Writings, the Lincoln—Douglas Debates, Presidential Messages and Proclamations of Abraham Lincoln.*

Charles: *What non-medical persons in history would you like to have dinner with, if that could be arranged?*

William: If I had my choice, I believe I would pick Sir Isaac Newton, Benjamin Franklin, Abraham Lincoln, Charles Darwin, Theodore Roosevelt, and David McCullough.

Charles: *What Americans outside of family and media do you admire?*

William: Certainly Benjamin Franklin, Abraham Lincoln, Theodore Roosevelt, David McCullough, David Herbert Donald, Doris Kearns Goodwin, and many others.

Charles: *Describe your home in Highland Park, Dallas, Texas.*

William: I live on Harvard Avenue, which is near the southernmost end of Highland Park. It is located 3.5 miles from BUMC and about 4 miles from downtown Dallas. The house is approximately 4,100 square feet, 2-story, and is situated on a quiet street. I have a small study downstairs, which is enclosed in wood, and that is where I pay bills, etc., and where my desktop computer is located. The living room, dining room, and kitchen areas are spacious and warm. There is 1 small bedroom downstairs adjacent to the enclosed garage. There are 4 bedrooms upstairs. One of the larger ones I have converted into my medical study. It is surrounded on 3 sides by book cases and the 4th is windows. It contains 2 desks back-to-back. On 1 desk I do editing, and on the other I do my own writing. One bedroom is used for storage of medical journals and for 3 pieces of exercise equipment (Nordic track, stationary bicycle, and rowing machine) and the other is the guest bedroom. The last is the master bedroom, which is relatively large. The hallway upstairs and my own bedroom each contain 3 large bookcases, mainly for non-medical books. There are 2 large bookcases in the living room, which contain non-medical books and some bookcases in the small study downstairs. The yard is small. I am very comfortable in this house which is close to downtown and yet is quiet.

Charles: *How is your house furnished?*

William: Mainly with Stickley furniture, which is produced in upstate New York and comes in cherry or oak. Mine is oak and painted with a dark mahogany type color. The floors are covered with Persian rugs and the walls are filled with Carrita Smith paintings, which are very realistic and mainly outdoor scenes from various parts of the USA.

Charles: *Do you spend much time at home?*

William: Yes I do. When I was at NIH for those 32 years, virtually every Saturday I worked all day long at NIH as you might remember. In Dallas, in contrast, I infrequently go into my Baylor office on Saturdays or Sundays, but I still work almost all of Saturday and for varying hours on Sunday. If I can keep up with the editorial work during the week, I can do non-journal things on the weekend, but if I don't then I do mainly editing on the weekends. I am very happy at home. Most of the work I do is pleasurable. I feel quite fortunate to have so many rewarding activities.

Charles: *Do you have domestic help?*

William: Yes I do. I am a bit spoiled. A dear lady comes

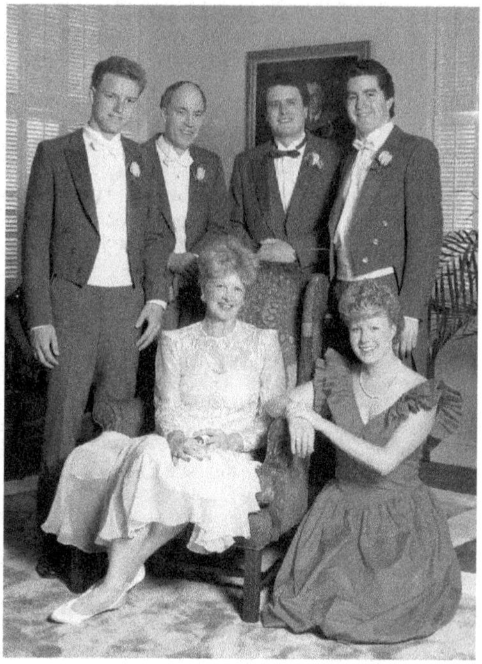

Figure 16. A photograph of WCR's clan at the time of WCR Jr's wedding. Carey Cansler Roberts is seated and Francis Carey Roberts is beside her. The boys (left to right) are John David, WCR, William Clifford Jr, and Charles Stewart.

a half day twice a week. Also, a yard man comes once a week or bi-weekly depending on the season of the year.

Charles: *What sports have you played and what sports do you currently play?*

William: As a kid I played football, basketball, baseball, tennis, and golf, but I was not good enough to make any of the high school teams. I gave up golf decades ago. As you know, I play tennis twice a year when we go on our family vacations.

Charles: *Do you follow sports? Do you have any sports heroes?*

William: Yes, I have had my sports heroes through the years. Gary Player (golf), Rick Barry (basketball), Jimmy Connors (tennis), Jerry West (basketball), Bill Bradley (basketball), Roger Staubach (football). The sports section is the first thing I read in the newspaper each day still. I do not attend the sporting events because that takes too much time.

Charles: *What newspapers or periodicals outside of medicine do you take?*

William: I take *The Dallas Morning News*, USA Today, *The Wall Street Journal*, *Barron's* (Saturday only), *The New York Times* (Sunday only). I also take *National Geographic*, *US News and World Report*, and *Forbes*. I used to take *Newsweek* or *Time* magazine, *The Atlantic*, *Scientific American*, and some others but I found that I wasn't spending

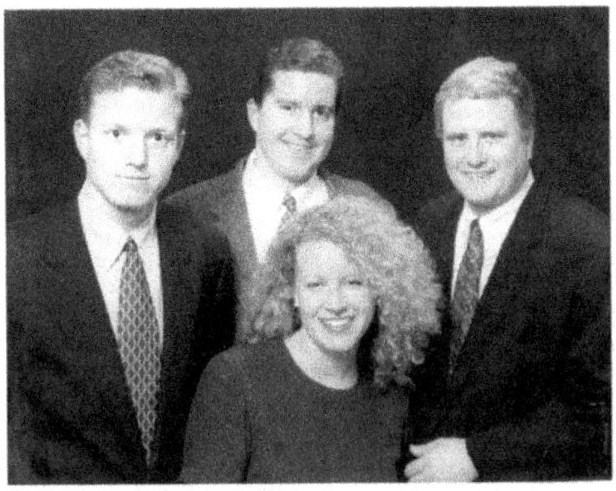

Figure 17. WCR's offspring about year 2000. Daughter, Francis Carey, with John, Charles, and Cliff Behind going *left to right*.

enough time reading them to make it worthwhile so I eliminated those subscriptions.

Charles: *Do you watch television–which shows?*

William: I turn the television set on when dressing or undressing or when I am eating a meal. On weekends, I watch when I can Book TV on C-Span. I try to watch *The McLaughlin Group* on PBS on Sunday mornings. That's my favorite news program. That's about it.

Charles: *What private clubs do you belong to?*

William: In Dallas, I belong to the Crescent Club and to the Montaigne Club. I have retained my membership in the Cosmos Club in Washington, DC, and try to stay there when I am in that area.

Charles: *Do you exercise regularly?*

William: I used to, but dropped off for nearly a year, but now I am back. As mentioned earlier, I have a Nordic track, a stationary bike, and a rowing machine in 1 of the converted bedrooms. I use those machines now about 5 days a week. For years I wore a pedometer and would keep a record of the number of miles I walked each day during regular activities at the hospital. I still try to use the stairs. My weight for decades was never over 165 pounds, but in the last year or so that number has moved to 175. I like it better at 165 and certainly no more than 170. My goal now is to get those 5 or 10 pounds off. I'm 72 inches tall, so fortunately it doesn't show too much.

Charles: *Your father apparently did not drink alcoholic beverages, do you?*

William: Yes I do. I did not have my first drink of alcohol until I was 27, and until I was 50 I would drink alcohol only on weekends. Now, I generally have 2 glasses of wine each night. Occasionally, I have a cocktail at a social occasion. I enjoy it.

Charles: *On a personal level, describe your marriage and children.*

William: Frances Carey Cansler and I married on August 20, 1955, when she was 20 and I was 22. It was too young for both of us. She had finished 2 years of college and I, 1 year of medical school. She did not finish college at that time, but worked to support our union in a physician's office at Emory University. Our first child, *William Clifford Roberts, Jr.*, was born on December 10, 1958, when I was interning in Boston. Our second, *Charles Stewart Roberts*, was born June 23, 1960; our third, *Frances Carey Roberts* on February 12, 1962, and our fourth, *John David Roberts* on November 24, 1966. Carey and I were married for 36 years. We separated in 1991 and were divorced not long thereafter. We both have always had busy lives. Carey was the major raiser of the offspring. I tried to do my share when the youngsters were small with bathing, etc. Carey taught Evelyn Wood Speed Reading for a brief period in Bethesda, Maryland, and also at the Williamsburg Heart Conference for 3 years. She was the Director of the Montgomery County Bi-centennial Commission for 2 years, marketing director of the Bethesda Bank for 2 years, and then public relations director at Suburban Hospital in Bethesda for 2 years. As mentioned earlier, she was the author of 3 books, one a historic novel and 2 were murder mysteries. She supported my work quite well in that I was never limited on how much I could work or travel and every Saturday I spent the entire day at the NIH. My time with the family was about 3 week nights and all day Sundays.

The 4 offspring have turned out quite well (Figures 16 and 17). Cliff and Charles went to Vanderbilt; then Cliff got an MBA at Emory and was in the trucking business for quite a few years, eventually forming his own oil-moving company. He sold that and then became a teacher in public school and loves it, and that is where he is now. Charles also went to Vanderbilt and then to Emory University School of Medicine. His internship and first year residency in surgery was at Barnes Hospital in St. Louis; followed by 2 years in the Surgery Branch in the National Heart, Lung, and Blood Institute at NIH in Bethesda; then 3 years at the University of South Carolina in Charleston in general surgery, and then a fellow in cardiovascular surgery at the University of North Carolina–Chapel Hill. He then spent 1 year in pediatric cardiac surgery with Mr. Christopher Lincoln at the Brompton Hospital in London, UK, then returned to Chapel Hill and was on the faculty there for 4 years, and then in 2001 moved to Winchester, Virginia, where he is head of the section of cardiovascular and thoracic surgery. He is very happy and very busy.

Frances Carey graduated from the engineering school of SMU in Dallas, Texas, and for a number of years was a programmer with several companies. Then she worked with Oracle and became a quite successful salesperson. At age 37, she met her future husband, Brian Willard, also an engineer, and when she was 38 and he 40 they married. The next year they had a daughter, and 2 years later a son, and 2 years after that another son. All seem to be healthy and doing quite well. Frances now is a stay-at-home mother as was her mother most of the time. She reads extensively and stays up well with world affairs.

John, the fourth child, has dyslexia and school was a bit difficult for him. He graduated from Virginia Commonwealth University, and there became extremely interested in computers and software. After working with IBM for nearly 2 years, he moved to San Jose, California, and Silicon Valley, his goal. In 2004, he formed his own company SugarCMR, and he is its CEO. He now has received well over $30 million from venture capitalists. In February 2007, he was featured in an interview in the *San Francisco Chron-*

San Francisco Chronicle

BUSINESS

SECTION C

Tuesday, January 30, 2007

"SugarCRM will do for the software industry what Southwest Airlines did for the airline industry."

JOSH STEIN, *venture capitalist*

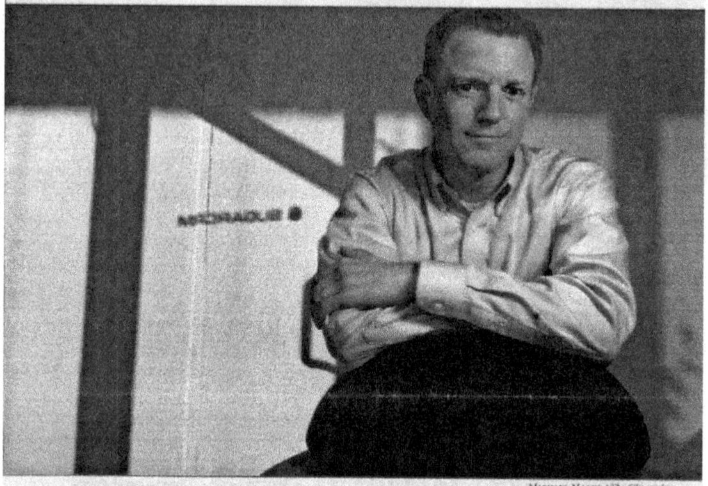

MICHAEL MACOR / The Chronicle

John Roberts, who battled dyslexia, is the founder of SugarCRM, a Cupertino software company.

OPEN-SOURCE SUCCESS IS SWEET

Company founder, forced to look at problems from different angles, comes up with new approach

By Benjamin Pimentel
CHRONICLE STAFF WRITER

Growing up with dyslexia was tough for John Roberts.

He had a hard time spelling, struggled with poor grades and became the only one in his family not to get into a top university.

But he said the learning disability, which makes it hard for him to read and write, forced him to constantly find new, even odd, angles from which to view a problem.

Roberts used that unique vision three years ago when he quit his job to start a company based on an untested concept: making business software applications and essentially giving them away.

SugarCRM is now seen as a pioneer in what some analysts describe as an emerging market: commercial open-source software applications that businesses use for such tasks as managing sales and keeping track of customers.

The Cupertino company is viewed by some industry observers as a potential threat to the rising star of the software industry, Salesforce.com.

SugarCRM has snatched away a few of the on-demand software company's customers, prompting Marc Benioff, Salesforce.com's high-profile founder and chief executive officer, to personally step in to win his old clients back.

Roberts, 40, and his team still face skepticism in the technology world, where some analysts doubt the company's long-term prospects.

But Josh Stein, a venture capitalist with Draper Fisher Jurvetson and a SugarCRM board member, said the firm is blazing a trail.

"SugarCRM will do for the software industry what Southwest Airlines did for the airline industry," he said. "It's cheaper. It might be slightly less comfortable, but it's a much more efficient system."

Roberts grew up in the Washington area where his dad worked as a physician at the National Institutes of Health and his mother wrote fiction. Encouraged by their parents to aim high in education, his three siblings got into well-known universities.

But dyslexia and his poor grades forced Roberts to settle for a public university in Virginia. "I couldn't remember how to spell simple words, and standardized tests would just crush me," he said.

"It was certainly frustrating," he added. "Your parents aren't wealthy, but they believe in academics so much that they'll pay

▸ ROBERTS: *Page C3*

Figure 18. A copy of the first page of the business section of the San Francisco Chronicle, January 30, 2007 featuring John David Roberts, the fourth offspring of WCR. John started his own company, SugarCRM, about 2 years earlier. The third page of the business section is also half filled about John and his company.

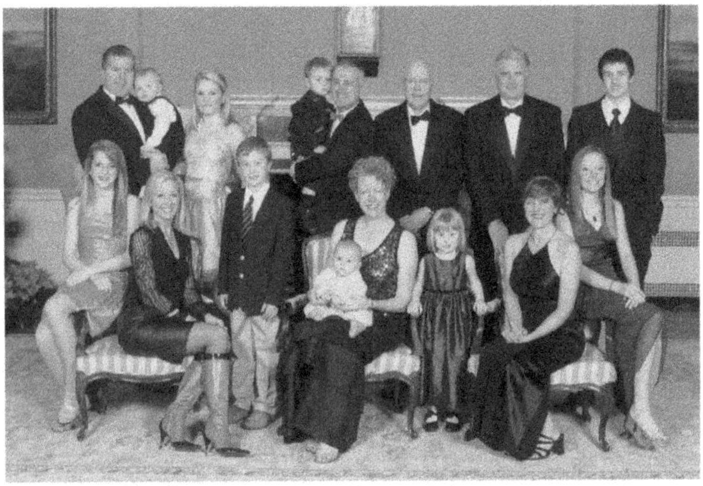

Figure 19. WCR's clan showing 3 of the WCR offspring and their children which now total 11 grandchildren. John, and his family are not in the picture but are shown in Figure 20.

icle (Figure 18). He now has lectured at Stanford University, the University of California at Berkley, and spoken at numerous business meetings. His company looks as if it will be a winner. The number of employees is over 100. They have opened another office in Dublin, Ireland, and have representatives in several other cities.

Cliff, the oldest, has a boy and a girl; Charles has 2 girls and 2 boys; Frances has 1 girl and 2 boys; and John has a boy and a girl. I am the lucky grandfather of 11 and I am very proud and happy about that.

Charles: *Did you sit down as a family every night for dinner?*

William: Yes, if I was home. After the first 3 left home, I'm afraid that sitting down for dinner vanished, but I do believe it is a good idea.

Charles: *Did you go to church while living in Bethesda and Potomac, Maryland?*

William: Yes. We virtually always went to Sunday School and then to church as a family. Then we would come home for lunch and then we would go on "an adventure." The adventures included going downtown to the Smithsonian Museum, or to the C&O Canal, or to a local historic site. When the kids were young, they would also accompany us to Williamsburg, Virginia, during the first week of December at the Williamsburg Heart meeting, which I directed. The Sundays were generally a family day where we all did something together.

Charles: *What was your view of the education of your 4 children?*

William: I think the 4 offspring understood how important education was to both their mother and me. The first 3 were always interested in books. The fourth found reading difficult, but as he has gotten older he has read extensively. He gets probably most of his information on the computer. I think all 4 offspring are pushing education appropriately in their children.

Charles: *How often do you see your children and their families during the year?*

William: That's variable. When I became a single grandparent in the early 1990s, I worried about being a reasonable grandfather as a single person. About 1995, I invited all of the grandchildren and their parents to explore New York City for a week. We all got together there, and it turned out to be a very educational and enjoyable visit. That started the yearly city adventure, and subsequently we have spent about a week in Chicago, Boston, Philadelphia, Montreal, San Francisco, and another visit to New York City. A couple of years ago there was some desire to have purely a "vacation" rather than a city visit, and therefore the last couple of years we have spent a week, usually in July, at The Homestead in southwest Virginia. Also, during the past 10 years, many of us have met at either Christmas time or New Year's for 4 or 5 days at the Greenbrier in White Sulpher Springs, West Virginia (Figures 19, 20). Both are beautiful resorts. Both my offspring and their children look forward to these trips, and there is a good bit of bonding during that concentrated period. During most years, my own kids visit with me in Dallas bringing 1 or more of their kids at the same time. Whenever I can get a trip to Atlanta, or northern Virginia, or the San Francisco area, I try to go so I can visit my children. The oldest now lives in Atlanta, Georgia; Charles lives in Winchester, Virginia; Fran lives in Leesburg, Virginia; and John lives in Los Gatos (close to San Jose), California. We also often talk on the telephone on Sundays or at least try to.

Charles: *What are your expectations for your 11 grandchildren?*

William: Of course, I wish them all successes that life can bring. I realize that that requires a great deal of work, and I hope and pray that they are willing to put in the time and effort to be smart enough to make their society and their environs better than what it was when they first appeared on planet Earth. I talk to some of the grandchildren periodically

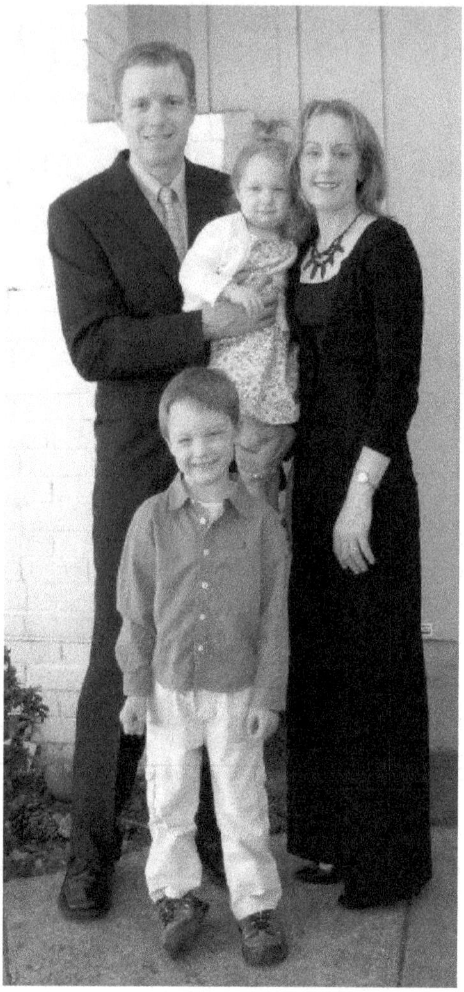

Figure 20. John and Kathy Roberts and their 2 children taken in 2007.

about "delayed gratification." By that I mean hard work during these first 2 decades pays huge dividends during the decades that follow. It's like saving money; the earlier one can save money, the more dividends and interest comes (Einstein said that compound interest was our greatest invention). I hope, of course, that the grandchildren will be informed, wise, and humble. The earlier we can stuff our brain full, the better off we are. I hope the 11 grandchildren will have healthy habits, keep an ideal body weight, and be examples to their offspring, associates, and colleagues.

Charles: *When asked to give advice to the young, Ezra Pound said, "Curiosity." What is your advice?*

William: I think that is good. Curiosity, desire to learn, making learning fun rather than a chore, is the key to success. I have been so lucky in that what I do to earn a living for me is fun. Developing a specific interest as early as possible in life I think is also helpful. So many successful people knew what they wanted to do early on. My son, John, as soon as he first encountered a computer knew that he wanted to be in the technology arena, and he made it. The others essentially have done the same thing.

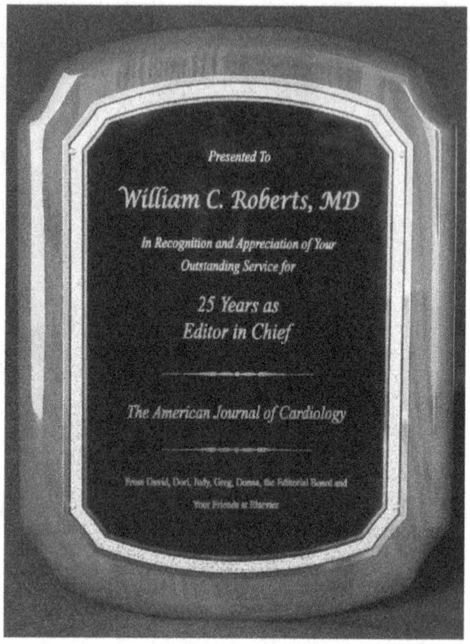
Presented To
William C. Roberts, MD
In Recognition and Appreciation of Your
Outstanding Service for
25 Years as
Editor in Chief
The American Journal of Cardiology

Figure 21. A copy of the plaque presented to WCR by David Dionne, the publisher of *The American Journal of Cardiology*, at the editorial board meeting in March 2007 commemorating 25 years of the WCR editorship.

Charles: *What are the biggest problems on planet Earth right now?*

William: I would say the number 1 problem is what to do with atomic power. We can destroy the planet now with the push of a button. The number of hydrogen bombs available on the planet is astronomical, and with more than 6 billion people on the planet, somebody is going to push that button purposefully or inadvertently. Problem number 2 in my view is the pollution of and warming of the planet. (Apparently Albert Einstein was asked what would happen if planet Earth was destroyed? Einstein answered, "Well, it's one of the minor planets anyway.") Global warming appears to be a real thing. We must slow down our consuming in the USA. No country in the world consumes like we do. No wonder the rest of the world dislikes us. We use about 25% of the natural resources of the planet, and yet we constitute only 5% of the world's population. We must cut down on our consumption. We can become more energy efficient, and that must be done on a rapid basis. The planet's population is a problem. The population of the USA at the time of the revolution was 4 million people; at the

Table 1
Types of articles published by WCR June 1961 to December 2006.

1. Studies involving multiple patients	524
2. Studies involving single patients	208
3. Editorials	288
From-the-editor columns in *The American Journal of Cardiology* - 187	
From-the-editor columns in *Baylor University Medical Center Proceedings* - 49	
Others - 58	
4. Chapters in books	131
5. Interviews	122
American Journal of Cardiology - 63	
Baylor University Medical Center Proceedings - 62	
6. Non-human animal studies	31
7. Miscellaneous	83
Total	**1,387**

Table 2
Topics of articles published by WCR June 1961 to December 2006

1. Coronary artery disease	220
2. Valvular heart disease	206
3. Congenital heart disease	102
4. Cardiomyopathy	93
5. Heart in systemic disease (amyloid, lupus, sarcoid, etc.)	83
6. Neoplasms involving the heart including consequences of irradiation and/or chemotherapy	43
7. Sudden cardiac death	26
8. Non-human animal studies	31
9. Pulmonary disease ± pulmonary hypertension	24
10. Aorta and/or its branches (excluding coronary)	21
11. Techniques or methods	34
12. Systemic hypertension	11
13. Pericardial heart disease	9
14. Non-cardiac, non-vascular disease patient studies	7
15. Biography	15
16. Miscellaneous cardiac conditions	34
17. Interviews	122
In *The American Journal of Cardiology* - 65	
In the *Baylor University Medical Center Proceedings* - 57	
18. Facts and Ideas from Anywhere	48
19. Preventive cardiology	54
20. Editing, writing, reviewing manuscripts, medical journals	43
21. Non-cardiovascular disease editorials	44
22. AJC 25 Years Ago columns	48
23. Summaries of annual AJC board meetings	22
24. Annual columns on Good Books in Cardiovascular Disease	21
25. International cardiology	10
26. Book reviews	8
27. Forewords in books	4
28. Editor's Roundtable	1
29. Summaries of Williamsburg heart meetings	3
Totals	**1,387**

time of the Civil War (1861 to 1865), 31 million; 1915, 100 million: by 1967, 200 million; and by 2006, 300 million. Both China and India are well over 1 billion people now. The majority of the 6 billion are poor, and the difference between the rich and the poor continues to widen.

Charles: *What is your view of Darwin's Theory of Evolution?*

William: I am a Darwinian through and through. Darwin knew he was going to cause a revolution, and that's a major reason he waited nearly 30 years to publish his first book.

Charles: *What is your view of war?*

William: There are always wars going on somewhere on planet Earth. Germany and Japan were major enemies of ours in World War II. Now some of our best friends are the Japanese and the Germans. We lost the Vietnam War, and yet the Vietnamese apparently now look very favorably toward Americans. The USA has the largest controlling stick on the planet but that doesn't mean that it has to be used. The Iraqi War is a disaster in both lives lost (>3,000) and seriously (≥20,000) injured, and cost (>$400 billion). Power does not mean that it has to be used. Wars now are too costly in human destruction and money waste. We simply cannot afford the destruction, when there are so many people on the planet starving to death! A cultural clash is occurring between the Christian-Judaic religion and Islamism. Both claim monopoly for their God. The rest of the religions around the world do not. We have heated up the clash by our army's entering the Middle East.

Charles: *What is your philosophy on personal finance?*

William: I believe in saving money, and the earlier one can save in life, the better. The earlier one can save a dollar, the more that dollar can compound. We all spend too much money. I try to be generous with my family and friends, but I don't like to waste money. I do my own stock picking. I mainly buy the large companies. I am diversified. I get the most useful information from *Barron's* and *Forbes*. *MorningStar* is also helpful. Fortunately, I have done quite well in the stock market, and I am very grateful for that.

Charles: *What medical accomplishments are you most proud of?*

William: Certainly one is that you have become a physician and a very successful one. And, of course, I am pleased that you are in cardiovascular disease, a cardiovascular surgeon. I am pleased that I have been able to come up with a number of ideas which hopefully have added to our body of cardiovascular knowledge, and that I have been able to do that over nearly 5 decades. When I first started, I thought I might have ideas for 1 or 2 years, and then I realized that I had ideas for 10 years, then 20 years, then 40 years. It has never been a problem finding new projects to work on. I'm particularly pleased with my accomplishments in coronary heart disease and in valvular heart disease. I was fortunate in the Washington, DC, area to have access to so much "material." That took a lot of effort and teaching time, but it certainly paid big dividends. I'm also pleased that I was also able to influence a few very bright people who were fellows with me through the years.

Charles: *What award are you most proud of?*

William: I'm most pleased with being made a member of Alpha Omega Alpha about 25 years after I graduated from medical school. I missed being AOA in medical school by 1 or 2 slots. Getting the award 25 years after graduation was more heart-warming in a way than receiving it in medical school. It might be good, in actuality, to give the AOA award 25 years after completion of medical school than during the junior and senior years in medical school. I have also received the SMU Alumni Association Award and the Emory Medical School Alumni Award and am pleased to have received them. Both SMU and Emory were very good to me. I have been the fortunate recipient of a number of awards and 1 honorary doctorate degree.

Charles: *What advice would you have for a young person interested in pursuing a career in medicine?*

William: I have not been in any career, of course, other than medicine, but medicine is a wonderful vocation. To be able to help others is a beautiful thing in life. There are so many options in medicine. One can be a practicing surgeon or practicing clinician or purely a laboratory person or purely an administrative type person. I would advise the young person to choose carefully which area of medicine he/she selects. If one loves surgery, then go into surgery. If one loves internal medicine, then go into internal medicine. If one loves pediatrics, then go into pediatrics. But first learn what those specialists do day in and day out before making that choice. Talk to physicians who have been out there awhile. Don't be timid when young. Ask questions. My confidence developed when I began to ask questions. That's when I really started learning. I never asked questions hardly until I had finished medical school. Questions are the key to life. They are the key to conversation. If one asks questions to others, they start talking and they think that you are such a good conversationalist because you brought this or that out of them. Questions have been the key to learning for me.

Charles: *How long would you like to work at BUMC?*

William: I would like to work as long as I am healthy. I enjoy going to work every day. There is nothing more exciting than trying to come up with a new idea every day and then gathering the data to prove it right or wrong, and then putting a nice ribbon around it so that it might be published. We have a lot of data at Baylor, and I intend to milk it as much as possible as long as I'm here. I also enjoy being the editor of *The American Journal of Cardiology* (Tables 1 and 2) and also the *Baylor Proceedings*. I hope to retain both of those positions for some time. Both have brought out things in me that I did not know were there.

Charles: *What are your present goals?*

William: I would be disappointed in myself if I do not produce a book summarizing most of the studies that I have been involved in through the years. That's my goal now.

Charles: *What do you wish to be written on your headstone? And where do you want that headstone to be?*

William: When my time is up, I want to be cremated. I'm not against having a small headstone at the Roberts's graveyard in Oxford, Georgia. I would want put on it: "William Clifford Roberts, 1932 to . . . He was a medicine man, he loved it, and he recommends it to others." I'll have to think about this a bit.

Charles: *You have interviewed a number of successful people in medicine. What characteristics were common in them?*

William: That's a good question. I gave a talk on that to the American Osler Society a few years back on that topic. The most common finding was enormous emphasis by their parents on the importance of education. Study, study, study. . .. learn. It was emphasized to most of them that medicine was a very special area in that you had to have an expertise that was not available to anyone else in the population, except those who had trained in medicine. That medicine degree can never be taken away. So many of the parents of physicians and surgeons whom I interviewed had not been to college but knew the importance of education. They knew that education was the route out of the slums and the road to success. Of 63 interviewees in the AJC, only a couple of the parents had divorced. The parents of the successful offspring appeared to be fairly close. Many had extended families, and there were often family gatherings frequently during the year. Often they worked in their father's business when teenagers. Education was the dominant emphasis, no doubt about that.

Charles: *Homo sapiens as a species have been on planet Earth roughly 100,000 years. You have been a Homo sapien on planet Earth for roughly 3 quarters of a century. How do you like it so far?*

William: I love it. I'm a happy man. I feel incredibly fortunate. I have a wonderful family, 4 offspring, 11 grandchildren, all of whom are healthy and are striving toward success. I'm healthy. I have a wonderful professional position.

I have opportunities galore professionally. I am provided support to do certain research projects and honored to be the editor of 2 medical journals; 1 for 25 years and the other for just over 13 years (Figure 21). Editorship provides great opportunities not only for the editor, but for the editor to provide opportunities for others. It's rewarding to be a vehicle for others. I have been honored multiple times by my professional colleagues and, of course, that is rewarding. Unfortunately, I have not been as good a friend as I should have been. Friendship takes a great deal of time, and I must say I have not used my time well enough to be nearly as good a friend as I think I could be. I do hope I am around for awhile, because there are still a lot of things I want to do. I want to see what is going to happen to these offspring and their offspring. It's a joy to have the opportunity to observe and watch.

Charles: *Thank you for this insight into your life and may your next quarter century be fruitful.*

William: Chuck, I am honored to be your interviewee, and I appreciate your examining my life as you have and developing so many questions which have made me think a good bit about where I have been and where I hope to be. Thank you.

1. Charles S. Roberts, MD. Life and Writings of Stewart R. Roberts, MD. Georgia's First Heart Specialist. Spartanburg, SC: The Reprint Company Publishers, 1993:138.
2. Wilder Penfield and Lamar Roberts. Speech and Brain Mechanisms. Princeton, New Jersey: Princeton University Press, 1959:286.
3. Stewart R. Roberts, SM, MD. Pellegra, History, Distribution, Diagnosis, Prognosis, Treatment, Etiology. St. Louis: C.Y. Mosby, 1914:272.
4. John Laszlo, M.D. and Francis A. Neelon, MD. The Doctors' Doctor. A Biography of Eugene A. Stead Jr., MD. Durham, NC: Carolina Academic Press, 2006:346.
5. Roberts SR. Hypertension. *Journal of the Medical Association of Georgia* 1936; 25:413–417.
6. Roberts SR. Emory after twenty-five years. Emory Alumnus 1927; 3:7–10.
7. Roberts SR. Emory's Creed. Emory Alumnus 1928; 4:1.
8. Roberts SR. A medical center. Retiring address of the President of the Fulton County Medical Society, Atlanta, Georgia, 1915 (pamphlet).
9. Roberts WC. Dr. Stewart R. Roberts' "An Ideal of Modern Medicine." *Annals of Internal Medicine* 1969; 70:1016–1017.

Best Publications of WCR as Selected by WCR*

*The numbers correspond to their listing in his curriculum vitae. The number of articles listed may seem excessive, but most concern morphologic studies involving hearts—all collected and examined by WCR. Many of the studies will never be repeated again because the frequency of autopsies performed in hospitals continues to diminish and large collections of such specimens by one person will be unlikely in the future. In other words, these studies will not go out of date and possibly will become more valuable with time.

6. Andriole VT, Kravetz HM, *Roberts WC*, Utz JP. Candida endocarditis. Clinical and pathology studies. *American Journal of Medicine* 1962;32:251–285.
9. *Roberts WC*, Morrow AG, Braunwald E. Complete interruption of the aortic arch. *Circulation* 1962;26:39–59.
19. *Roberts WC*. The histologic structure of the pulmonary trunk in patients with "primary" pulmonary hypertension. *American Heart Journal* 1963;65:230–236.
22. *Roberts WC*, Sjoerdsma A. The cardiac disease associated with the carcinoid syndrome (carcinoid heart disease). *American Journal of Medicine* 1964;36:5–34.
23. Berry WB, *Roberts WC*, Morrow AG, Braunwald E. Corrected transposition of the aorta and pulmonary trunk. Clinical, hemodynamic and pathologic findings. *American Journal of Medicine* 1964;36:35–53.
28. *Roberts WC*, Morrow AG. Congenital aortic stenosis produced by a unicommissural valve. *British Heart Journal* 1965;27:505–510.
33. *Roberts WC*, Braunwald E, Morrow AG. Acute severe mitral regurgitation secondary to ruptured chordae tendineae. Clinical, hemodynamic, and pathologic considerations. *Circulation* 1966; 33:58–70.
60. *Roberts WC*, Morrow AG. Anatomic studies of hearts containing caged-ball prosthetic valves. *Johns Hopkins Medical Journal* 1967;121:271–295.
67. *Roberts WC*, Bodey GP, Wertlake PT. The heart in acute leukemia. A study of 420 autopsy cases. *American Journal of Cardiology* 1968;21:388–412.
71. Glancy DL, *Roberts WC*. The heart in malignant melanoma. A study of 70 autopsy cases. *American Journal of Cardiology* 1968; 21:555–571.
75. *Roberts WC*, Glancy DL, DeVita VT Jr. Heart in malignant lymphoma (Hodgkin's disease, lymphosarcoma, reticulum cell sarcoma and mycosis fungoides). A study of 196 autopsy cases. *American Journal of Cardiology* 1968;22:85–107.
82. Morrow AG, *Roberts WC*, Ross J Jr, Fisher Rd, Behrendt DM, Mason DT, Braunwald E. Obstruction to left ventricular outflow. Current concepts of management and operative treatment. *Annals of Internal Medicine* 1968;69:1255–1286.
86. *Roberts WC*, Liegler DG, Carbone PP. Endomyocardial disease and eosinophilia. A clinical and pathologic spectrum. *American Journal of Medicine* 1969;46:28–42.
98. *Roberts WC*, Friesinger GC, Cohen LS, Mason DT, Ross RS. Acquired pulmonic atresia. Total obstruction to right ventricular outflow after systemic to pulmonary arterial anastomoses for cyanotic congenital cardiac disease. *American Journal of Cardiology* 1969;24:335–345.
111. *Roberts WC*. The structure of the aortic valve in clinically-isolated aortic stenosis. An autopsy study of 162 patients over 15 years of age. *Circulation* 1970;42:91–97.
112. *Roberts WC*. The congenitally bicuspid aortic valve. A study of 85 autopsy cases. *American Journal of Cardiology* 1970;26:72–83.
113. *Roberts WC*. Anatomically isolated aortic valvular disease. The case against its being of rheumatic etiology. *American Journal of Medicine* 1970;49:151–159.
119. *Roberts WC*, Buja LM, Ferrans VJ. Loffler's fibroplastic parietal endocarditis, eosinophilic leukemia, and Davies' endomyocardial fibrosis: The same disease at different stages? *Pathology and Microbiology* 1970;35:90–96.
125. *Roberts WC*, Perloff JK, Costantino T. Severe valvular aortic stenosis in patients over 65 years of age. A clinicopathologic study. *American Journal of Cardiology* 1971;27:497–506.
130. Falcone MW, *Roberts WC*, Morrow AG, Perloff JK. Congenital aortic stenosis resulting from unicommissural valve. Clinical and anatomic features in twenty-one adult patients. *Circulation* 1971; 44:272–280.
131. Buja LM, *Roberts WC*. Iron in the heart. Etiology and clinical significance. *American Journal of Medicine* 1971;51:209–221.
142. *Roberts WC*, Buja LM. The frequency and significance of coronary arterial thrombi and other observations in fatal acute myocardial infarction. A study of 107 necropsy patients. *American Journal of Medicine* 1972;52:425–443.
143. Ferrans VJ, Morrow AG, *Roberts WC*. Myocardial ultrastructure in idiopathic hypertrophic subaortic stenosis. A study of operatively excised left ventricular outflow tract muscle in 14 patients. *Archives of Pathology* 1972;93:435–440.
146. *Roberts WC*, Buchbinder NA. Right-sided valvular infective endocarditis. A clinico-pathologic study of twelve necropsy patients. *American Journal of Medicine* 1972;53:7–19.
147. Buchbinder NA, *Roberts WC*. Left-sided valvular active infective endocarditis. A study of forty-five necropsy patients. *American Journal of Medicine* 1972;53:20–35.
149. *Roberts WC*, Cohen LS. Left ventricular papillary muscles. Description of the normal and a survey of conditions causing them to be abnormal. *Circulation* 1972;46:138–154.
154. *Roberts WC*, Perloff JK. Mitral valvular disease. A clinicopathologic survey of the conditions causing the mitral valve to function abnormally. *Annals of Internal Medicine* 1972;77:939–975.

161. *Roberts WC.* Valvular, subvalvular, and supravalvular aortic stenosis: morphologic features. *Cardiovascular Clinics* 1973;5:97–126.
162. *Roberts WC,* Ferrans VJ, Levy RI, Fredrickson DS. Cardiovascular pathology in hyperlipoproteinemia. Anatomic observations in 42 necropsy patients with normal or abnormal serum lipoprotein patterns. *American Journal of Cardiology* 1973;31:557–570.
165. *Roberts WC,* Bulkley BH, Morrow AG. Pathologic anatomy of cardiac valve replacement: A study of 224 necropsy patients. *Progress Cardiovascular Diseases* 1973;15:539–587, May/June.
170. *Roberts WC.* Operative treatment of hypertrophic obstructive cardiomyopathy. The case against mitral valve replacement. *American Journal of Cardiology* 1973;32:377–381.
173. Bulkley BH, *Roberts WC.* Ankylosing spondylitis and aortic regurgitation. Description of the characteristic cardiovascular lesion from study of eight necropsy patients. *Circulation* 1973;48:1014–1027.
175. *Roberts WC,* Dangel JC, Bulkley BH. Non-rheumatic valvular cardiac disease: A clinicopathologic survey of 27 different conditions causing valvular dysfunction. *Cardiovascular Clinic* 1973; 5:333–446.
206. Bulkley BH, *Roberts WC.* The heart in systemic lupus erythematosus and the changes induced in it by corticosteroid therapy. A study of 36 necropsy patients. *American Journal of Medicine* 1975;58:243–264.
210. *Roberts WC,* Fishbein MC, Golden A. Cardiac pathology after valve replacement by disc prosthesis. A study of 61 necropsy patients. *American Journal of Cardiology* 1975;35:740–760.
211. *Roberts WC,* Ferrans VJ. Pathologic anatomy of the cardiomyopathies. Idiopathic dilated and hypertrophic types, infiltrative types, and endomyocardial disease with and without eosinophilia. *Human Pathology* 1975;6:287–342.
219. Bulkley BH, *Roberts WC.* Dilatation of the mitral anulus. A rare cause of mitral regurgitation. *American Journal of Medicine* 1975; 59:457–463.
220. *Roberts WC.* The hypertensive diseases. Evidence that systemic hypertension is a greater risk factor to the development of other cardiovascular diseases than previously suspected. *American Journal of Medicine* 1975;59:523–532.
234. Arnett EN, *Roberts WC.* Acute myocardial infarction and angiographically normal coronary arteries. An unproven combination. *Circulation* 1976;53:395–400.
235. *Roberts WC,* Perry LW, Chandra RS, Myers GE, Shapiro SR, Scott LP. Aortic valve atresia: a new classification based on necropsy study of 73 cases. *American Journal of Cardiology* 1976;37:753–756.
236. Bulkley BH, *Roberts WC.* Atherosclerotic narrowing of the left main coronary artery. A necropsy analysis of 152 patients with fatal coronary heart disease and varying degrees of left main narrowing. *Circulation* 1976;53:823–828.
240. *Roberts WC,* Hammer WJ. Cardiac pathology after valve replacement with a tilting-disc prosthesis (Bjork-Shiley type). A study of 46 necropsy patients and 49 Bjork-Shiley protheses. *American Journal of Cardiology* 1976;37:1024–1032.
241. Arnett EN, *Roberts WC.* Valve ring abscess in active infective endocarditis. Frequency, location, and clues to clinical diagnosis from the study of 95 necropsy patients. *Circulation* 1976;54:140-145.
247. Maron BJ, Redwood Dr, *Roberts WC,* Henry WL, Morrow AG, Epstein SE. Tunnel subaortic stenosis. Left ventricular outflow tract obstruction produced by fibromuscular tubular narrowing. *Circulation* 1976: 54:406–416.
248. Arnett EA, *Roberts WC.* Prosthetic valve endocarditis. Clinicopathologic analysis of 22 necropsy patients with comparison of observations in 74 necropsy patients with active infective endocarditis involving natural left-sided cardiac valves. *American Journal of Cardiology* 1976;38:281–292.
252. Arnett EN, *Roberts WC.* Active infective endocarditis: a clinicopathology analysis of 137 necropsy patients. *Current Problems in Cardiology* 1976;1(#7):1–76, October.
254. *Roberts WC.* Choosing a substitute cardiac valve: type, size, surgeon. *American Journal of Cardiology* 1976;38:633–644.
266. Virmani R, *Roberts WC.* Aschoff bodies in operatively excised atrial appendages and in papillary muscles. Frequency and clinical significance. *Circulation* 1977;55:559–563.
270. *Roberts WC,* Spray TL. Pericardial heart disease. *Current Problems in Cardiology* 1977;2 (#3): –71.
273. *Roberts WC,* McAllister HA Jr, Ferrans VJ. Sarcoidosis of the Heart. A clinicopathologic study of 35 necropsy patients (Group I) and review of 78 previously described necropsy patients (Group II). *American Journal of Medicine* 1977;63:86–108.
276. Curry RC Jr, *Roberts WC.* Status of the coronary arteries in the nephrotic syndrome. Analysis of 20 necropsy patients aged 15 to 35 years to determine if coronary atherosclerosis is accelerated. *American Journal of Medicine* 1977;63:183–192.
291. *Roberts WC,* Buchbinger NA. Healed left-sided infective endocarditis: a clinico-pathologic study of 59 patients. *American Journal of Cardiology* 1977;40:876–888.
300. Crall FV Jr, *Roberts WC.* The extramural and intramural coronary arteries in juvenile diabetes mellitus. Analysis of nine necropsy patients aged 19 to 38 years with onset of diabetes before age 15 years. *American Journal of Medicine* 1978;64:221–230.
302. Hammer WJ, *Roberts WC,* deleon AC, Jr. "Mitral Stenosis" secondary to combined "massive" mitral anular calcific deposits and small, hypertrophied left ventricles. *American Journal of Medicine* 1978;64:371–376.
304. *Roberts WC,* Virmani R. Aschoff bodies at necropsy in valvular heart disease. Evidence from an analysis of 543 patients over 14 years of age that rheumatic heart disease at least anatomically, is a disease of the mitral valve. *Circulation* 1978;57:803–807.
305. Lachman AS, *Roberts WC.* Calcific deposits in stenotic mitral valves. Extent and relation to age, sex, degree of stenosis, cardiac rhythm, previous commissurotomy and left atrial body thrombus from study of 164 operatively-excised valves. *Circulation* 1978; 57:808–815.
316. *Roberts WC.* Coronary embolism: a review of causes, consequences, and diagnostic considerations. *Cardiovascular Medicine* 1978;3:699–710.
328. Isner JM, *Roberts WC.* Right ventricular infarction complicating left ventricular infarction secondary to coronary heart disease. Frequency, location, associated findings and significance from analysis of 236 necropsy patients with acute or healed myocardial infarction. *American Journal of Cardiology* 1978;42:885–894.
335. *Roberts WC.* Congenital cardiovascular abnormalities usually "silent" until adulthood: morphologic features of the floppy mitral valve, valvular aortic stenosis, hypertrophic cardiomyopathy, sinus of Valsalva aneurysm, and the Marfan syndrome. In Congenital Heart Disease in Adults, edited by Roberts WC, FA Davis Co., Philadelphia, pp. 407–453, May 1979. (*Cardiovascular Clinics* 1979;10(#1):1–574.)
339. Maron BJ, Epstein SE, *Roberts WC.* Hypertrophic cardiomyopathy and transmural myocardial infarction without significant atherosclerosis of the extramural coronary arteries. *American Journal of Cardiology* 1979;43:1086–1102.
341. *Roberts WC,* Brownlee WJ, Jones AA, Luke JL. Sucking action of the left ventricle. Demonstration of a physiologic principle by a gunshot wound penetrating only the right side of the heart. *American Journal of Cardiology* 1979;43:1234–1237.
343. *Roberts WC,* Jones AA. Quantitation of coronary arterial narrowing at necropsy in sudden coronary death. Analysis of 31 patients and comparison with 25 control subjects. *American Journal of Cardiology* 1979;44:39–45.
344. *Roberts WC,* Lachman AS. Mitral valve commissurotomy versus replacement. Considerations based on examination of operatively excised stenotic mitral valves. *American Heart Journal* 1979;98: 56–62.
347. Arnett EN, Isner JM, Redwood DR, Kent KM, Baker WP, Ackerstein H, *Roberts WC.* Coronary artery narrowing in coronary heart disease: comparison of cineangiographic and necropsy findings. *Annals of Internal Medicine* 1979;91:350–356.
348. *Roberts WC,* Giraldo AA. Bilateral oophorectomy in menstruating women and accelerated coronary atherosclerosis: an unproven connection. *American Journal of Medicine* 1979;67:363–365.
353. *Roberts WC,* Virmani R. Quantification of coronary arterial narrowing in clinically-isolated unstable angina pectoris. An analysis of 22 necropsy patients. *American Journal of Medicine* 1979;67: 792–799.
358. *Roberts WC.* The aorta: its acquired diseases and their consequences as viewed from a morphologic perspective. In The Aorta, edited by Lindsay J Jr, Hurst JW, Grune & Stratton, Inc., New York, 1979;51–117.

361. *Roberts WC*, Shemin RJ, Kent KM. Frequency and direction of interatrial shunting in valvular pulmonic stenosis with intact ventricular septum and without left ventricular inflow or outflow obstruction. An analysis of 127 patients treated by valvulotomy. *American Heart Journal* 1980;99:142–148.
366. *Roberts WC*, Jones AA. Quantification of coronary arterial narrowing at necropsy in acute transmural myocardial infarction: Analysis and comparison of findings in 27 patients and 22 controls. *Circulation* 1980;61:786–790.
375. Virmani R, *Roberts WC*. Quantification of coronary arterial narrowing and of left ventricular myocardial scarring in healed myocardial infarction with chronic eventually fatal, congestive cardiac failure. *American Journal of Medicine* 1980;68:83–838.
384. Maron BJ, *Roberts WC*, McAllister HA, Rosing DR, Epstein SE. Sudden death in young athletes. *Circulation* 1980;62:218–229.
395. Cabin HS, *Roberts WC*. True left ventricular aneurysm and healed myocardial infarction. Clinical and necropsy observations including quantification of degrees of coronary arterial narrowing. *American Journal of Cardiology* 1980;46:754–763.
397. Roberts CS, *Roberts WC*. Cross-sectional area of the maximal portions of the three major epicardial coronary arteries in 98 necropsy patients with different coronary events. Relationship to heart weight, age and sex. *Circulation* 1980;62:953–959.
399. Waller BF, *Roberts WC*. Amount of narrowing by atherosclerotic plaque in 44 nonbypassed and 52 bypassed major epicardial coronary arteries in 32 necropsy patients who died within 1 month of aortocoronary bypass grafting. *American Journal of Cardiology* 1980;46:956–962.
408. *Roberts WC*. Aortic dissection: anatomy, consequences, and causes. *American Heart Journal* 1981;101:195–214.
409. *Roberts WC*, Morrow AG, McIntosh CL, Jones M, Epstein SE. Congenitally bicuspid aortic valve causing severe, pure aortic regurgitation without superimposed infective endocarditis. Analysis of 13 patients requiring aortic valve replacement. *American Journal of Cardiology* 1981;47:206–209.
413. Brosius FC III, *Roberts WC*. Coronary artery disease in the Hurler syndrome. Qualitative and quantitative analysis of the extent of coronary narrowing at necropsy in six children. *American Journal of Cardiology* 1981;47:649–653.
415. Brosius FC III, Waller BF, *Roberts WC*. Radiation heart disease. Analysis of 16 young (aged 15 to 33 years) necropsy patients who received over 3,500 rads to the heart. *American Journal of Medicine* 1981;70:519–530.
416. Brosius FC III, *Roberts WC*. Significance of coronary arterial thrombus in transmural acute myocardial infarction. A study of 54 necropsy patients. *Circulation* 1981;63:810–816.
418. Haider YS, *Roberts WC*. Coronary arterial disease in systemic lupus erythematosus. Quantification of degrees of narrowing in 22 necropsy patients (21 women) aged 16 to 37 years. *American Journal of Medicine* 1981;70:775–781.
420. Virmani R, *Roberts WC*. Non-fatal healed transmural myocardial infarction and fatal non-cardiac disease. Qualification and quantification of coronary arterial narrowing and of left ventricular scarring in 18 necropsy patients. *British Heart Journal* 1981;45: 434–441.
422. Isner JM, Kishel J, Kent KM, Ronan JA Jr, Ross AM, *Roberts WC*. Accuracy of angiographic determination of left main coronary arterial narrowing. Angiographic-histologic correlative analysis in 28 patients. *Circulation* 1981;63:1056–1064.
432. Cabin HS, *Roberts WC*. Fatal cardiac arrest during cardiac catheterization for angina pectoris: analysis of 10 necropsy patients. *American Journal of Cardiology* 1981;48:1–8.
436. *Roberts WC*, Waller BF. Effect of chronic hypercalcemia on the heart. An analysis of 18 necropsy patients. *American Journal of Medicine* 1981;71:371–384.
441. Brosius FC III, *Roberts WC*. Comparison of degree and extent of coronary narrowing by atherosclerotic plaque in anterior and posterior transmural acute myocardial infarction. *Circulation* 1981; 64:715–722.
455. *Roberts WC*. Complications of cardiac valve replacement: characteristic abnormalities of prostheses pertaining to any or specific site. *American Heart Journal* 1982;103:113–122.
458. Siegel RJ, *Roberts WC*. Electrocardiographic observations in severe aortic valve stenosis: correlative necropsy study to clinical, hemodynamic, and ECG variables demonstrating relation of 12-lead QRS amplitude to peak systolic transaortic pressure gradient. *American Heart Journal* 1982;103:210–221.
466. *Roberts WC*, Siegel RJ, Zipes DP. Origin of the right coronary artery from the left sinus of Valsalva and its functional consequences: analysis of 10 necropsy patients. *American Journal of Cardiology* 1982;49:863–868.
474. *Roberts WC*. Reasons for cardiac catheterization before cardiac-valve replacement. *The New England Journal of Medicine* 1982; 306:1291–1293.
475. Maron BJ, *Roberts WC*, Epstein SE. Sudden death in hypertrophic cardiomyopathy: a profile of 78 patients. *Circulation* 1982;65: 1388–1394.
479. Cabin HS, *Roberts WC*. Comparison of amount and extent of coronary narrowing by atherosclerotic plaque and of myocardial scarring at necropsy in anterior and posterior healed transmural myocardial infarction. *Circulation* 1982;66:93–99.
480. *Roberts WC*, Honig HS. The spectrum of cardiovascular disease in the Marfan syndrome: a clinico-morphologic study of 18 necropsy patients and comparison to 151 previously reported necropsy patients. *American Heart Journal* 1982;104:115–135.
484. Fauci AS, Harley JB, *Roberts WC*, Ferrans VJ, Gralnick HR, Bjornson BH. The idiopathic hypereosinophilic syndrome. Clinical, pathological, and therapeutic considerations. *Annals of Internal Medicine* 1982;97:78–92.
486. *Roberts WC*, Curry RC Jr, Isner JM, Waller BF, McManus BM, Mariani-Constantini R, Ross AM. Sudden death in Prinzmetal's angina with coronary spasm documented by angiography. Analysis of three necropsy patients. *American Journal of Cardiology* 1982;50:203–210.
488. Waller BJ, Morrow AG, Maron BJ, Del Negro AA, Kent KM, McGrath FJ, Wallace RB, McIntosh CL, *Roberts WC*. Etiology of clinically isolated, severe, chronic, pure mitral regurgitation: analysis of 97 patients over 30 years of age having mitral valve replacement. *American Heart Journal* 1982;104:276–288.
489. *Roberts WC*, Dicicco BS, Waller BF, Kishel JC, McManus BM, Dawson SL, Hunsaker JC, Luke JL. Origin of the left main from the right coronary artery or from the right aortic sinus with intramyocardial tunneling to the left side of the heart via the ventricular septum: the case against clinical significance of myocardial bridge or coronary tunnel. *American Heart Journal* 1982;104: 303–305.
502. Cabin HS, *Roberts WC*. Quantitative comparison of extent of coronary narrowing and size of healed myocardial infarct in 33 necropsy patients with clinically recognized and in 28 with clinically unrecognized ("silent") previous acute myocardial infarction. *American Journal of Cardiology* 1982;50:677–681.
509. *Roberts WC*, Isner JM, Virmani R. Left ventricular incision midway between the mitral anulus and the stumps of the papillary muscles during mitral valve excision with or without rupture or aneurysmal formation: Analysis of 10 necropsy patients. *American Heart Journal* 1982;104:1278–1287.
512. Arnett EN, *Roberts WC*. Pathology of active infective endocarditis: a necropsy analysis of 192 patients. *Thoracic and Cardiovascular Surgeon* 1982;30:327–335.
516. Waller BF, *Roberts WC*. Cardiovascular disease in the very elderly. Analysis of 40 necropsy patients aged 90 years or older. *American Journal of Cardiology* 1983;51:403–421.
517. Glancy DL, Morrow AG, Simon AL, *Roberts WC*. Juxtaductal aortic coarctation. Analysis of 84 patients studied hemodynamically, angiographically and morphologically after age 1 year. *American Journal of Cardiology* 1983;51:537–551.
525. Warnes CA, Scott ML, Silver GM, Smith CW, Ferrans VJ, *Roberts WC*. Comparison of late degenerative changes in porcine bioprostheses in the mitral and aortic valve position in the same patient. *American Journal of Cardiology* 1983;51:965–968.
526. *Roberts WC*. Morphologic features of the normal and abnormal mitral valve. *American Journal of Cardiology* 1983;51:1005–1028.
529. Isner JM, Ferrans VJ, Cohen SR, Witkind BG, Virmani R, Gottdiener JS, Beck JR, *Roberts WC*. Clinical and morphologic cardiac findings after anthracycline chemotherapy. Analysis of 64 patients studied at necropsy. *American Journal of Cardiology* 1983;51: 1167–1174.

535. Virmani R, *Roberts WC*. Extravasated erythrocytes, iron, and fibrin in atherosclerotic plaques of coronary arteries in fatal coronary heart disease and their relation to luminal thrombus: frequency and significance in 57 necropsy patients and in 2958 five-mm segments of 224 major epicardial coronary arteries. *American Heart Journal* 1983;105:788–797.
540. *Roberts WC*, Waller BF. Cardiac amyloidosis causing cardiac dysfunction: analysis of 54 necropsy patients. *American Journal of Cardiology* 1983;52:137–146.
558. Byram MT, *Roberts WC*. Frequency and extent of calcific deposits in purely regurgitant mitral valves: analysis of 108 operatively excised valves. *American Journal of Cardiology* 1983;52:1059–1061.
563. *Roberts WC*. Cardiac valvular residua and sequelae after operation for congenital heart disease. *American Heart Journal* 1983;106: 1181–1187.
567. *Roberts WC*, Roberts JD. The floating heart or the heart too fat to sink: analysis of 55 necropsy patients. *American Journal of Cardiology* 1983;52:1286–1289.
571. Day PJ, *Roberts WC*. Relation of level of total serum cholesterol to amount of calcific deposits in operatively excised stenotic mitral valves: analysis of 155 cases. *American Journal of Cardiology* 1984;53:157–159.
572. Day PJ, McManus BM, *Roberts WC*. Amounts of coronary arterial narrowing by atherosclerotic plaque in clinically isolated, chronic, pure aortic regurgitation: analysis of 37 necropsy patients older than 30 years. *American Journal of Cardiology* 1984;53:173–177.
592. Sprecher DL, Schaefer EJ, Kent KM, Gregg RE, Zech LA, Hoeg JM, McManus B, *Roberts WC*, Brewer HB Jr. Cardiovascular features of homozygous familial hypercholesterolemia: analysis of 16 patients. *American Journal of Cardiology* 1984;54:20–30.
607. Warnes CA, *Roberts WC*. Comparison at necropsy by age group of amount and distribution of narrowing by atherosclerotic plaque in 2995 five-mm long segments of 240 major coronary arteries in 60 men aged 31 to 70 years with sudden coronary death. *American Heart Journal* 1984;108:431–435.
609. Warnes CA, *Roberts WC*. The heart in massive (more than 300 pounds or 136 kilograms) obesity: analysis of 12 patients studied at necropsy. *American Journal of Cardiology* 1984;54:1087–1091.
624. Waller BF, *Roberts WC*. Remnant saphenous veins after aortocoronary bypass grafting: analysis of 3,394 centimeters of unused vein from 402 patients. *American Journal of Cardiology* 1985;55: 65–71.
629. *Roberts WC*, Day PJ. Electrocardiographic observations in clinically isolated, pure, chronic, severe aortic regurgitation: analysis of 30 necropsy patients aged 19 to 65 years. *American Journal of Cardiology* 1985;55:432–438.
630. Silver MA, *Roberts WC*. Detailed anatomy of the normally functioning aortic valve in hearts of normal and increased weight. *American Journal of Cardiology* 1985;55:454–461.
631. *Roberts WC*, Podolak MJ. The king of hearts: analysis of 23 patients with hearts weighing 1000 grams or more. *American Journal of Cardiology* 1985;55:485–494.
656. Ross EM, *Roberts WC*. The carcinoid syndrome: comparison of 21 necropsy subjects with carcinoid heart disease to 15 necropsy subjects without carcinoid heart disease. *American Journal of Medicine* 1985;79:339–354.
667. Ross EM, *Roberts WC*. Severe atherosclerotic coronary artery disease, healed myocardial infarction and chronic congestive heart failure: analysis of 81 patients studied at necropsy. *American Journal of Cardiology* 1986;57:44–50.
668. Ross EM, *Roberts WC*. Severe atherosclerotic coronary arterial narrowing and chronic congestive heart failure without myocardial infarction: analysis of 18 patients studied at necropsy. *American Journal of Cardiology* 1986;57:51–56.
672. Maron BJ, Epstein SE, *Roberts WC*. Causes of sudden death in competitive athletes. *Journal of The American College of Cardiology* 1986;7:204–214.
685. *Roberts WC*. Major anomalies of coronary arterial origin seen in adulthood. *American Heart Journal* 1986;111:941–963.
686. Reis RN, *Roberts WC*. Amounts of coronary arterial narrowing by atherosclerotic plaques in clinically isolated mitral valve stenosis: analysis of 76 necropsy patients older than 30 years (From-the-editor column). *American Journal of Cardiology* 1986;57:1117–1123.
698. Maron BJ, Wolfson JK, Epstein SE, *Roberts WC*. Intramural ("small vessel") coronary artery disease in hypertrophic cardiomyopathy. *Journal of the American College of Cardiology* 1986; 8:545–557.
699. Barbour DJ, *Roberts WC*. Rupture of a left ventricular papillary muscle during acute myocardial infarction: analysis of 22 necropsy patients. *Journal of the American College of Cardiology* 1986;8:558–565.
700. Lester WM, *Roberts WC*. Diabetes mellitus for 25 years or more. Analysis of cardiovascular findings in seven patients studied at necropsy. *American Journal of Medicine* 1986;81:275–279.
704. *Roberts WC*. Congenital coronary arterial anomalies unassociated with major anomalies of the heart or great vessels. In Adult Congenital Heart Disease, edited by *Roberts WC*, FA Davis Company, Philadelphia, 1987:583–629.
705. *Roberts WC*. Congenital cardiovascular abnormalities usually silent until adulthood. In Adult Congenital Heart Disease, edited by Roberts WC, FA Davis Company, Philadelphia, 1987:631–691.
709. Sullivan MF, *Roberts WC*. Mitral valve stenosis and pure tricuspid valve regurgitation: comparison of necropsy patients having simultaneous mitral and tricuspid valve replacements with necropsy patients having simultaneous mitral valve replacement and tricuspid valve anuloplasty. *American Journal of Cardiology* 1986;58: 768–780.
710. Sullivan MJ, *Roberts WC*. Clinical and morphologic observations after simultaneous replacement of the tricuspid, mitral and aortic valves. *American Journal of Cardiology* 1986;58:781–789.
719. *Roberts WC*, Sullivan MF. Clinical and necropsy observations early after simultaneous replacement of the mitral and aortic valves. *American Journal of Cardiology* 1986;58:1067–1084.
735. *Roberts WC*, McIntosh CL, Wallace RB. Aortic valve perforation with calcific aortic valve stenosis and without infective endocarditis or significant aortic regurgitation. *American Journal of Cardiology* 1987;59:476–478.
746. *Roberts WC*, McIntosh CL, Wallace RB. Mechanisms of severe mitral regurgitation in mitral valve prolapse determined from analysis of operatively excised valves. *American Heart Journal* 1987;113:1316–1323.
751. *Roberts WC*, Kaufman RJ. Calcification of healed myocardial infarcts. *American Journal of Cardiology* 1987;60:28–32.
752. Kalan JM, *Roberts WC*. Comparison of morphologic changes and luminal sizes of saphenous vein and internal mammary artery after simultaneous implantation for coronary arterial bypass grafting. *American Journal of Cardiology* 1987;60:193–196.
760. Mann JM, *Roberts WC*. Fatal rupture of both left ventricular free wall and ventricular septum (double rupture) during acute myocardial infarction: analysis of seven patients studied at necropsy. *American Journal of Cardiology* 1987;60:722–724.
763. Motamed HE, *Roberts WC*. Frequency and significance of mitral anular calcium in hypertrophic cardiomyopathy: analysis of 200 necropsy patients. *American Journal of Cardiology* 1987;60:877–844.
770. *Roberts WC*, Siegel RJ, McManus BM. Idiopathic dilated cardiomyopathy: analysis of 152 necropsy patients. *American Journal of Cardiology* 1987;60:1340–1355.
778. Kragel AH, *Roberts WC*. Sudden death and cardiomegaly unassociated with coronary, valvular, congenital or specific myocardial disease. *American Journal of Cardiology* 1988;61:659–660.
792. Mann JM, *Roberts WC*. Acquired ventricular septal defect during acute myocardial infarction: analysis of 38 unoperated necropsy patients and comparison with 50 unoperated necropsy patients without rupture. *American Journal of Cardiology* 1988;652:8–19.
793. Potkin BN, *Roberts WC*. Significance of cardiac weight in patients having coronary artery bypass grafting for angina pectoris. *American Journal of Cardiology* 1988;62:36–40.
794. Potkin BN, *Roberts WC*. Effects of percutaneous transluminal coronary angioplasty on atherosclerotic plaques and relation of plaque composition and arterial size to outcome. *American Journal of Cardiology* 1988;62:41–50.
798. Wilensky RL, Yudelman P, Cohen AI, Fletcher RD, Atkinson J, Virmani R, *Roberts WC*. Serial electrocardiographic changes in idiopathic dilated cardiomyopathy confirmed at necropsy. *American Journal of Cardiology* 1988;62:276–283.

805. Kragel AH, *Roberts WC*. Anomalous origin of either the right or left main coronary artery from the aorta with subsequent coursing between aorta and pulmonary trunk: analysis of 332 necropsy cases. *American Journal of Cardiology* 1988;62:771–777.
808. Mann JM, *Roberts WC*. Rupture of the left ventricular free wall during acute myocardial infarction: analysis of 138 necropsy patients and comparison with 50 necropsy patients with acute myocardial infarction without rupture. *American Journal of Cardiology* 1988;62:847–859.
811. Potkin BN, *Roberts WC*. Location of an acute myocardial infarct in patients with a healed myocardial infarct: analysis of 129 patients studied at necropsy. *American Journal of Cardiology* 1988;62:1017–1023.
816. *Roberts WC*, Kragel AH. Anomalous origin of either the right or left main coronary artery from the aorta without coursing of the anomalistically arising artery between aorta and pulmonary trunk. *American Journal of Cardiology* 1988;62:1263–1267.
829. Kragel AH, McIntosh CM, *Roberts WC*. Morphologic changes in coronary artery seen late after endarterectomy. *American Journal of Cardiology* 1889;63:893–896.
832. Reddy SG, *Roberts WC*. Frequency of rupture of the left ventricular free wall or ventricular septum among necropsy cases of fatal acute myocardial infarction since introduction of coronary care units. *American Journal of Cardiology* 1989;63:906–911.
835. Dressler FA, Roberts WC. Infective endocarditis in opiate addicts: Analysis of 80 cases studied at necropsy. *American Journal of Cardiology* 1989;63:1240–1257.
838. *Roberts WC*. Qualitative and quantitative comparison of amounts of narrowing by atherosclerotic plaques in the major epicardial coronary arteries at necropsy in sudden coronary death, transmural acute myocardial infarction, transmural healed myocardial infarction and unstable angina pectoris. *American Journal of Cardiology* 1989;64:324–328.
849. Dressler FA, *Roberts WC*. Modes of death and types of cardiac diseases in opiate addicts: analysis of 168 necropsy cases. *American Journal of Cardiology* 1989;64:909–920.
851. Dollar AL, *Roberts WC*. Usefulness of total 12-lead QRS voltage compared with other criteria for determining left ventricular hypertrophy in hypertrophic cardiomyopathy: analysis of 57 patients studied at necropsy. *American Journal of Medicine* 1989;87:377–381.
852. Malekzadeh S, *Roberts WC*. Growth rate of left atrial myxoma. *American Journal of Cardiology* 1989;64:1075–1076.
854. Roberts CS, *Roberts WC*. Hypertrophic cardiomyopathy as a cause of massive cardiomegaly (>1000 g). *American Journal of Cardiology* 1989;64:1209–1210.
857. Kragel AH, Reddy SG, Wittes JT, *Roberts WC*. Morphometric analysis of the composition of atherosclerotic plaques in the four major epicardial coronary arteries in acute myocardial infarction and in sudden coronary death. *Circulation* 1989;80:1747–1756.
860. *Roberts WC*, Potkin BN, Solus DE, Reddy SG. Mode of death, frequency of healed and acute myocardial infarction, number of major epicardial coronary arteries severely narrowed by atherosclerotic plaque, and heart weight in fatal atherosclerotic coronary artery disease: analysis of 889 patients studied at necropsy. *Journal of the American College of Cardiology* 1990;15:196–203.
864. Dressler FA, Malekzadeh S, *Roberts WC*. Quantitative analysis of amounts of coronary arterial narrowing in cocaine addicts. *American Journal of Cardiology* 1990;65:536–537.
877. Kalan JM, *Roberts WC*. Morphologic findings in saphenous veins used as coronary arterial bypass conduits for longer than 1 year: necropsy analysis of 53 patients, 123 saphenous veins and 1865 five-millimeter segments of veins. *American Heart Journal* 1990; 119:1164–1184.
883. Kragel AH, Reddy SG, Wittes JT, *Roberts WC*. Morphometric analysis of the composition of coronary arterial plaques in isolated unstable angina pectoris with pain at rest. *American Journal of Cardiology* 1990;66:562–567.
887. Gertz SD, Kragel AH, Kalan JM, Braunwald E, *Roberts WC*, and the TIMI Investigators. Comparison of coronary and myocardial morphologic findings in patients with and without thrombolytic therapy during fatal first acute myocardial infarction. *American Journal of Cardiology* 1990;66:904–909.
889. Antecol DH, Roberts WC. Sudden death behind the wheel from natural disease in drivers of four-wheeled motorized vehicles. *American Journal of Cardiology* 1990;66:1329–1335.
892. Antecol DH, *Roberts WC*. Aortic dissection with the entrance tear in transverse aorta: analysis of 12 autopsy patients. *Annals of Thoracic Surgery* 1990;50:762–766.
894. *Roberts WC*, Kragel AH, Potkin BN. Ages at death and sex distribution in age decade in fatal coronary artery disease. *American Journal of Cardiology* 1991;66:1379–1381.
901. Kragel AH, *Roberts WC*. Composition of atherosclerotic plaques in the coronary arteries in homozygous familial hypercholesterolemia. *American Heart Journal* 1991;121:210–211.
905. Roberts CS, *Roberts WC*. Dissection of the aorta associated with congenital malformation of the aortic valve. *Journal of the American College of Cardiology* 1991;17:712–716.
906. Dollar AL, *Roberts WC*. Morphologic comparison of patients with mitral valve prolapse who died suddenly with patients who died from severe valvular dysfunction or other conditions. *Journal of the American College of Cardiology* 1991;17:92–931.
908. Roberts CS, *Roberts WC*. Aortic dissection with the entrance tear in the descending thoracic aorta. Analysis of 40 necropsy patients. *Annals of Surgery* 1991;213:356–358.
910. Dollar AL, Kragel AH, Fernicola DJ, Waclawiw MA, *Roberts WC*. Composition of atherosclerotic plaques in coronary arteries in women <40 years of age with fatal coronary artery disease and implications for plaque reversibility. *American Journal of Cardiology* 1991;67:1223–1227.
911. Gertz SD, Malekzadeh S, Dollar AL, Kragel AH, *Roberts WC*. Composition of atherosclerotic plaques in the four major epicardial coronary arteries in patients 90 years of age. *American Journal of Cardiology* 1991;67:1228–1233.
927. Kragel AH, Gertz SD, *Roberts WC*. Morphologic comparison of frequency and types of acute lesions in the major epicardial coronary arteries in unstable angina pectoris, sudden coronary death and acute myocardial infarction. *Journal of American College of Cardiology* 1991;18:801–808.
928. Klues HG, *Roberts WC*, Maron BJ. Anomalous insertion of papillary muscle directly into anterior mitral leaflet in hypertrophic cardiomyopathy. Significance in producing left ventricular outflow obstruction. *Circulation* 1991;84:1188–1197.
930. *Roberts WC*, Kragel AH, Gertz SD, Roberts CS, Halan JM. The heart in fatal unstable angina pectoris. *American Journal of Cardiology* 1991;68:22B–227B.
931. Roberts CS, *Roberts WC*. Combined thoracic aortic dissection and abdominal aortic fusiform aneurysm. *Annals of Thoracic Surgery* 1991;52:537–540.
937. Roberts CS, Gertz SD, Klues HG, Cannon RO III, Maron BJ, McIntosh CL, *Roberts WC*. Appearance of or persistence of severe mitral regurgitation without left ventricular outflow obstruction after partial ventricular septal myotomy-myectomy in hypertrophic cardiomyopathy. *American Journal of Cardiology* 1991;68: 1726–1728.
943. *Roberts WC*, Kishel JC, McIntosh CL, Cannon RO III, Maron BJ. Severe mitral or aortic valve regurgitation, or both, requiring valve replacement for infective endocarditis complicating hypertrophic cardiomyopathy. *Journal of the American College of Cardiology* 1992;19:365–371.
946. *Roberts WC*. Morphologic aspects of cardiac valve dysfunction. *American Heart Journal* 1992;123:1610–1632.
948. *Roberts WC*, Shirani J. The four subtypes of anomalous origin of the left main coronary artery from the right aortic sinus (or from the right coronary artery). *American Journal of Cardiology* 1992; 70:119–121.
951. Mautner GC, *Roberts WC*. Reported frequency of coronary arterial narrowing by angiogram in patients with valvular aortic stenosis. *American Journal of Cardiology* 1992;70:539–540.
955. Glick BN, *Roberts WC*. Usefulness of total 12-lead QRS voltage in diagnosing left ventricular hypertrophy in clinically isolated, pure, chronic, severe mitral regurgitation. *American Journal of Cardiology* 1992;70:1088–1092.
957. Mautner GC, Berezowski K, Mautner SL, *Roberts WC*. Degrees of coronary arterial narrowing at necropsy in men with large fusiform abdominal aortic aneurysm. *American Journal of Cardiology* 1992;70:1143–1146.

958. Mautner GC, Mautner SL, *Roberts WC*. Amounts of coronary arterial narrowing by atherosclerotic plaque at necropsy in patients with lower extremity amputation. *American Journal of Cardiology* 1992;70:1147–1151.
959. Mautner GC, Mautner SL, *Roberts WC*. Composition of atherosclerotic plaques in the epicardial coronary arteries in juvenile (type I) diabetes mellitus. *American Journal of Cardiology* 1992; 70:1264–1268.
963. Mautner SL, Mautner GC, Hunsberger SA, *Roberts WC*. Comparison of composition of atherosclerotic plaques in saphenous veins used as aortocoronary bypass conduits with plaques in native coronary arteries in the same men. *American Journal of Cardiology* 1992;70:1380–1387.
969. *Roberts WC*. Ninety-three hearts ≥90 years of age. *American Journal of Cardiology* 1993;71:599–602.
972. *Roberts WC*, Oluwole BO, Fernicola DJ. Comparison of active infective endocarditis involving a previously stenotic versus a previously nonstenotic aortic valve. *American Journal of Cardiology* 1993;71:1082–1088.
975. Vaslef SN, *Roberts WC*. Early descriptions of aortic valve stenosis. *American Heart Journal* 1993;125:1465–1474.
976. Vaslef SN, *Roberts WC*. Early descriptions of aortic regurgitation. *American Heart Journal* 1993;125:1475–1483.
977. Mautner SL, Lin F, Mautner GC, *Roberts WC*. Comparison in women versus men of composition of atherosclerotic plaques in native coronary arteries and in saphenous veins used as aortocoronary conduits. *Journal of the American College of Cardiology* 1993;21:1312–1318.
978. Fernicola DJ, *Roberts WC*. Clinicopathologic features of active infective endocarditis isolated to the mitral valve. *American Journal of Cardiology* 1993;71:1186–1197.
979. Shirani J, Roberts WC. Subepicardial myocardial lesions. *American Heart Journal* 1993; 125:1346–1352.
981. Shirani J, Roberts WC. Clinical electrocardiographic and morphologic features of massive fatty deposits ("lipomatous hypertrophy") in the atrial septum *Journal of the American College of Cardiology* 1993;22:226–238.
983. Mautner GC, Mautner SL, Cannon RO III, Hunsberger SA, *Roberts WC*. Clinical factors useful in predicting aortic valve structure in patients >40 years of age with isolated valvular aortic stenosis. *American Journal of Cardiology* 1993;72:194–198.
991. Shirani J, Maron BJ, Cannon RO III, Sheyda S, *Roberts WC*. Clinicopathologic features of hypertrophic cardiomyopathy managed by cardiac transplantation. *American Journal of Cardiology* 1993;72:434–440.
997. Shirani J, Freant LJ, *Roberts WC*. Gross and semiquantitative histologic findings in mononuclear cell myocarditis causing sudden death, and implications for endomyocardial biopsy. *American Journal of Cardiology* 1993;72:952–957.
1007. Shirani J, *Roberts WC*. Status of the major epicardial coronary arteries at necropsy in paraplegia and quadriplegia. *American Journal of Cardiology* 1994;73:207–208.
1009. Glick BN, *Roberts WC*. Congenitally bicuspid aortic valve in multiple family members. *American Journal of Cardiology* 1994; 73:400–404.
1019. *Roberts WC*, Kragel AH, Gertz SD, Roberts CS. Coronary arteries in unstable angina pectoris, acute myocardial infarction, and sudden death. *American Heart Journal* 1994;127:1588–1593.
1036. Shirani J, Yousefi, J, *Roberts WC*: Major cardiac findings at necropsy in 366 American octogenarians. *American Journal of Cardiology* 1995;75:151–156.
1046. Shirani J, Berezowski K, *Roberts WC*. Quantitative measurement of normal and excessive (cor adiposum) subepicardial adipose tissue, its clinical significance, and its effect on electrocardiographic QRS voltage. *American Journal of Cardiology* 1995;76: 414–418.
1059. Maron BJ, Shirani J, Poliac LC, Mathenge R, *Roberts WC*, Mueller FO. Sudden death in competitive athletes. Clinical demographic, and pathological profiles. *JAMA* 1996;276: 199–204.
1066. Arbustini E, Bello BD, Morbini P, Grosso M, Diegoli M, Fasani R, Pilotto A, Bellini O, Pellegrini C, Martinelli L, Campana C, Gavazzi A, Specchia G, Vigano M, *Roberts WC*. Frequency and characteristics of coronary thrombosis in the epicardial coronary arteries after cardiac transplantation. *American Journal of Cardiology* 1996;78:795–800.
1072. Stephan PJ, Henry AC III, Hebeler RF Jr, Whiddon L, *Roberts WC*. Comparison of age, gender, number of aortic valve cusps, concomitant coronary artery bypass grafting, and magnitude of left ventricular-systemic arterial peak systolic gradient in adults having aortic valve replacement for isolated aortic valve stenosis. *American Journal of Cardiology* 1997;79:166–172.
1109. Waller TA, Hiser WL, Capehart JE, *Roberts WC*. Comparison of clinical and morphologic cardiac findings in patients having cardiac transplantation for ischemic cardiomyopathy, idiopathic dilated cardiomyopathy, and dilated hypertrophic cardiomyopathy. *American Journal of Cardiology* 1998;81:884-894.
1123. *Roberts WC*, Shirani J. Comparison of cardiac findings at necropsy in octogenarians, nonagenarians, and centenarians. *American Journal of Cardiology* 1998;82:627–631.
1138. *Roberts WC*, High ST. The heart in systemic lupus erythematosus. *Current Problems in Cardiology* 1999;24(#1):1–56, January.
1209. *Roberts WC*. Neoplasms involving the heart, their simulators, and adverse consequences of their therapy. *Baylor University Medical Center Proceedings* 2000;14:358–376.
1246. Yoon DHA, *Roberts WC*. Sex distribution in cardiac myxomas. *American College of Cardiology* 2002;90:563–565.
1279. *Roberts WC*, Laborde NJ III, Pearl GJ. Comparison of ages between men and women and their distribution across five age decades among patients undergoing carotid endarterectomy. *American Journal of Cardiology* 2003;92:762–763.
1288. *Roberts WC*, Ko JM. Weights of operatively-excised stenotic unicuspid, bicuspid, and tricuspid aortic valves and their relation to age, sex, body mass index, and presence or absence of concomitant coronary artery bypass grafting. *American Journal of Cardiology* 2003;92:1057V1065.
1319. *Roberts WC*, Ko JM. Weights of individual cusps in operatively-excised stenotic congenitally *bicuspid* aortic valves. *American Journal of Cardiology* 2004;94:678-681.
1320. *Roberts WC*, Ko JM. Weights of individual cusps in operatively-excised stenotic congenitally *three-cuspid* aortic valves. *American Journal of Cardiology* 2004;94:681–684.
1325. *Roberts WC*. Ko JM. Relation of weights of operatively excised stenotic aortic valves to preoperative transvalvular peak systolic pressure gradients and to calculated aortic valve areas. *Journal of the American College of Cardiology* 2004;44:1847–1855.
1332. *Roberts WC*, Ko JM. Frequency by decade of unicuspid, bicuspid, and tricuspid aortic valves in adults having isolated aortic valve replacement for aortic stenosis, with or without associated aortic regurgitation. *Circulation* 2005;111:920–925.
1351. *Roberts WC*, Ko JM, Hamilton C. Comparison of valve structure, valve weight, and severity of the valve obstruction in 1849 patients having isolated aortic valve replacement for aortic valve stenosis (with or without aortic regurgitation) studied at 3 different medical centers in 2 different time periods. *Circulation* 2005;112: 3919–3929.
1377. *Roberts WC*, Ko JM, Moore TR, Jones WH III. Etiology of pure aortic regurgitation in patients having isolated aortic valve replacement at a single US tertiary hospital (1993–2005). *Circulation* 2006;114:422–429.
1385. *Roberts WC*, Ko JM, Matter GJ. Aortic valve replacement for aortic stenosis in nonagenarians. *American Journal of Cardiology* 2006;98:1251–1253.
1386. *Roberts WC*, Ko JM, Pearl GJ. Relation of weights of intraaneurysmal thrombi to maximal right-to-left diameters of abdominal aortic aneurysms. *American Journal of Cardiology* 2006;98: 1519–1524.

From the Editor Columns in the *American Journal of Cardiology*

1. A few words from the Journal's second editor. (50:A3), July 1982 (485).
2. Blind reviews. (50:A45), August 1982 (492).
3. Brief reports. (50:A3), September 1982 (498).
4. The editorial board. (50:A3), October 1982 (501).

5. Reviewing manuscripts: occasionally a test of character. (50:A3), November 1982 (505).
6. Speeding up the manuscript review process. (50:A3), December 1982 (507).
7. Getting the manuscript accepted: think like a lawyer and cover the flanks. (51:A3), January1983 (513).
8. Paper accepted/abstract rejected or vice versa: differences in the grading of abstracts and the reviewing of manuscripts. (51:A3), February 1983 (515).
9. Author-editor-reviewer: how the triumvirate is working at the AJC. (51:A9–A10), March 1, 1983 (521).
10. Author-advertiser: their dependency on one another. (51:A3), March 15, 1983 (524).
11. Abbreviations in the AJC. (51:A9–A10), April 1983 (528).
12. References: a clue to scholarship. (51:A9–A10), May 1, 1983 (532).
13. Oslerian advice. (51:A10-A11), May 15, 1983 (536).
14. Changes in the AJC since June 1982. (1:A9–A10), June 1983 (537).
15. The summary: the manuscript's bottom line. (52:A3), July 1983 (539).
16. Mitral commissurotomy – still a good operation. (52:A9–A10), August 1983 (544).
17. Animal behavior-human behavior-cardiac behavior. (52:A14), September 1983 (547).
18. Who was Holter? (52:A17), October 1983 (554).
19. The "blessing" of angina pectoris. (52:1154), November 1, 1983 (561).
20. Season's greetings and the best for 1984. (52:1356), December 1, 1983 (569).
21. An agent with lipid-lowering, antihypertensive, positive inotropic, negative chronotropic, vasodilating, diuretic, anorexigenic, weight-reducing, cathartic, hypoglycemic, tranquilizing, hypnotic and antidepressive qualities. (53:261–262), January 1, 1984 (573).
22. Studying the "Instructions to Authors" before final typing of a manuscript for submission to a medical journal. (53:398), January 15, 1984 (575).
23. Reducing the blood cholesterol level reduces the risk of heart attack. (53:649), February 1, 1984 (577).
24. The AJC in '83. (53:729), March 1, 1984 (579).
25. Can rest and relaxation be obtained by combining a "vacation" with a medical meeting or a medical meeting with a "vacation"? (53: 987), March 15, 1984 (582).
26. The 2 most common congenital heart diseases. (53:1198), April 1, 1984 (583).
27. When I have an acute myocardial infarction take me to the hospital that has a cardiac catheterization laboratory and open cardiac surgical facilities. (53:1410), May 1, 1984 (584).
28. The AJC editorial board meeting—1984. (53:1483-1485), May 15, 1984 (588).
29. Forces changing America. (52:1737–1738), June 1, 1984 (590).
30. Extreme hypercholesterolemia = malignant atherosclerosis. (54: 242–243), July 1, 1984 (596).
31. Further comments on the "Instructions to Authors". (54:470), August 1, 1984 (601).
32. Editorial board changes. (54:704), September 1, 1984 (606).
33. Writing versus editing. (54:934), October 1984 (608).
34. The worst heart disease. (54:935), November 1984 (611).
35. A good year—1984. (54:1395), December 1, 1984 (618).
36. A suggestion to lighten the load of manuscript reviewers. (55:247), January 1, 1985 (627).
37. Enticing real and potential cardiovascular researchers away from research. (55:503), February 1, 1985 (632).
38. Brief reports in the AJC in 1984. (55:870), March 1, 1985 (637).
39. I still prefer ventricular premature complex. (55:1117), April 1, 1985 (639).
40. The AJC editorial meeting – 1985. (55:1451–1452), May 1, 1985 (644).
41. The "hot eye" and the "cold eye". (55:1663), June 1, 1985 (646).
42. The article's title. (56:210–212), July 1985 (648).
43. Country of origin of articles in the AJC in 1984. (56:380), August 1, 1985 (650).
44. The silver anniversary of cardiac valve replacement. (56:503–506), September 1985 (655).
45. Mitral valve prolapse and systemic hypertension. (56:703), October 1, 1985 (657).
46. How long do physicians live? (56:838), November 1, 1985 (659).
47. Some good cardiologic books. (56:1001–1002), December 1, 1985 (664).
48. The most powerful cause of sudden death. (57:190), January 1, 1986 (671).
49. Effects of antihypertensive therapy on blood lipid levels. (57:379–380), February 1, 1986 (675).
50. The AJC in 1985. (57:711–712), March 1, 1986 (682).
51. Cardiac rupture, abdominal aneurysmal rupture and dissecting aortic rupture: a preventive trio. (57:892–893), April 1, 1986 (684).
52. AJC editorial board meeting – 1986. (57:1209–1211), May 1, 1986 (688).
53. Sudden cardiac death: definitions and causes. (57:1410–1413), May 1, 1986 (691).
54. In one day in the USA. (58:193–194), July 1, 1986 (695).
55. A simple histologic classification of pulmonary arterial hypertension. (58:385–386), August 1, 1986. (697).
56. The senile cardiac calcification syndrome. (58:572–574), September 1, 1986 (702).
57. Justifying a cardiac catheterization laboratory. (58:860–862), October 1, 1986 (714).
58. Characteristics of long-term successful physician researchers. (58: 1052–1053), November 1, 1986 (718).
59. Some good cardiologic books published in 1986. (58:1271–1272), December 1, 1986 (722).
60. Good-bye to thoracotomy for cardiac valvulotomy. (59:198–202), January 1, 1987 (731).
61. The AJC in 1986. (59:391–392), February 1, 1987 (734).
62. Fast foods and quick plaques. (59:721–723), March 1, 1987 (738).
63. Reviews of classic books and ineptness of reviewers: lessons for judges of medical manuscripts. (59:922–923), April 1, 1987 (742).
64. Annual AJC editorial board meeting March 1987. (59:1226–1229), May 1, 1987 (747).
65. Examining operatively excised cardiac valves. (59:1434–1436), June 1, 1987 (749).
66. China and Chinese cardiology. (60:201–202), July 1, 1987 (753).
67. Japan and Japanese medicine. (60:427–429), August 1, 1987 (758).
68. The search for the masterful figure. (60:633–634), September 1, 1987 (759).
69. The malpractice dream. (60:938), October 1, 1987 (766).
70. Publishing manuscripts faster than abstracts. (60:1133), November 1, 1987 (769).
71. Some good cardiologic books published in 1987. (60:1423–1424), December 1, 1987 (773).
72. The Kingdom of Saudi Arabia, oil, money and cardiology. (61:410–412), February 1, 1988 (776).
73. The AJC in 1987. (61:672–674), March 1, 1988 (780).
74. The logic of using either two mechanical valves or two bioprosthetic valves for replacement of both mitral and aortic valves. (61:871), April 1, 1988 (782).
75. AJC editorial board meeting – March 1988. (61:1161–1164), May 1, 1988 (789).
76. Stone agers in the atomic age. Lessons from the Paleolithic life-style for modern man. (61:1365–1366), June 1, 1988 (791).
77. Argentina and Argentine cardiology. (62:167–169), July 1, 1988 (797).
78. The Friedewald-Levy-Frederickson formula for calculating low-density lipoprotein cholesterol, the basis for lipid-lowering therapy. (62:345–346), August 1, 1988 (800).
79. Factors linking cholesterol to atherosclerotic plaques. (62:495–499), September 1, 1988 (803).
80. Drug developers and drug dispensers. Their dependency on one another. (62:840), October 1, 1988 (807).
81. Brazil and Brazilian cardiology. (62:991–993), November 1, 1988 (810).
82. India and Indian cardiology. (62:1326–1329), December 1, 1988 (818).
83. Some good cardiologic books published in 1988. (63:153–154), January 1, 1989 (824).
84. The medical book with the most information for the price. (63:390–391), February 1, 1989 (826).
85. Defining idiopathic dilated cardiomyopathy. A courtroom discussion. (63:893–896), April 1, 1989 (830).

86. Editorial board meeting of *The American Journal of Cardiology* – March 1989. (63:1159–1165), May 1, 1989 (834).
87. Sensitive areas between physicians and pharmaceutical companies. (63:1421), June 1, 1989 (837).
88. Atherosclerotic risk factors—are there ten or is there only one? (64:552–554), September 1, 1989 (841).
89. Lipid-lowering therapy after an atherosclerotic event. (64:693–695), September 15, 1989 (846).
90. Clogged arteries and clogged roads (64:959–960), October 15, 1989 (850).
91. The echocardiographic diseases. (64:1084), November 1, 1989 (853).
92. Living with a congenitally bicuspid aortic valve. (64:1408–), December 1, 1989 (856).
93. Some good cardiologic books published in 1989. (65:116–118), January 1, 1990 (861).
94. Limited research funds and cardiac medicine without cardiac surgery. (65:536–537), February 15, 1990 (865).
95. Bombay and a congress on coronary artery disease. (65:824–825), March 15, 1990 (867).
96. Editorial board meeting of *AJC* – March 1990. (65:1162–1168), May 1, 1990 (876).
97. Making clinical studies involving many patients useful to the single patient. (65:1408), June 1, 1990 (880).
98. Coronary "lesion," coronary "disease," "single-vessel disease" — "two-vessel disease": word and phrase misnomers providing false impressions of the extent of coronary atherosclerosis in symptomatic myocardial ischemia. (66:121–123), July 1, 1990 (881).
99. We think we are one, we act as if we are one, but we are not one. (66:896), October 1, 1990 (885).
100. The best antiarrhythmic agent will be a lipid-lowering agent. (66: 1402), December 1, 1990 (895).
101. Some good cardiologic books published in 1990. (67:106-108), January 1, 1991 (898).
102. "Anything to be done right has got to be done by people that make their living at it" (67:445–446), February 15, 1991 (903).
103. Comparison of the four major USA cardiology journals in 1990: a look at 51 kilograms (112 pounds) of journals and over 15,000 editorial pages. (67:551–554), March 1, 1991 (904).
104. Editorial board meeting of the *AJC* – 5 March 1991. (67:1033–1037), May 1, 1991 (909).
105. Singapore and Singaporean cardiology. (67:1298–1302), June 1, 1991 (912).
106. The government is in your office and listening to their script. (68:143–144), July 1, 1991 (922).
107. Human records and a tribute to the Guinness Book of World Records. (68:288–289), July 15, 1991 (924).
108. Benjamin Franklin's Poor Richard's Almanack and its maxims on physicians, Medicine and Nutrition. (68:703–706), September 1, 1991 (926).
109. Oft-repeated requests to authors from an editor of a cardiology journal. (68:1121–1122), October 15, 1991 (934).
110. What medical students are asking. (68:1260-1261), November 1, 1991 (935).
111. Alkaline paper and preserving the record. (68:1729–1732), December 15, 1991 (938).
112. Some good cardiologic books published in 1991. (69:141–144), January 1, 1992 (941).
113. Doctors, save your money because there will be less in the future. (69:432), February 1, 1992 (942).
114. Editorial board meeting of the *AJC* on 14 April 1992. (69:1645–1649), June 15, 1992 (947).
115. More on fast foods and quick plaques. (70:268–270), July 15, 1992 (950).
116. Cardiologic books published in 1992. (71:126–130), January 1, 1993 (966).
117. The best anti-heart failure agent will be a lipid-lowering agent. (71:628), March 1, 1993 (971).
118. Editorial board meeting of the *AJC* in March 1993. (71:1500–1504), June 15, 1993 (980).
119. The best hospitals in the USA for patients with heart disease. (72:626–627), September 1, 1993 (992).
120. Getting cardiologists interested in lipids. (72:744–745), September 15, 1993 (993).
121. Good cardiologic books appearing in 1993. (73:98–101), January 1, 1994 (1006).
122. The ineffectiveness of a commonly recommended lipid-lowering diet in significantly lowering the serum total and low-density lipoprotein cholesterol levels. (73:623–624), March 15, 1994 (1012).
123. Calculating the percentage of fat and the grams of fat consumed daily to maintain an ideal body weight. (73:719–720), April 1, 1994 (1013).
124. Proceedings of the editorial board meeting of the *AJC* on March 14, 1994, (73:926-931), May 1, 1994 (1016).
125. A son's book on his father's father. (74:518–529), September 1, 1994 (1022).
126. Mexican food: olé. (74:974–975), November 1, 1994 (1028).
127. Ruby Viola Holbrook Roberts. (74:1078), November 15, 1994 (1030).
128. Retail costs of the statin lipid-lowering drugs. (74:1181), December 1, 1994 (1031).
129. Good cardiologic books appearing in 1994. (75:106–109), January 1, 1995 (1035).
130. Proceedings of the editorial board meeting of the *AJC* on March 21, 1995. (75:1075–1080), May 15, 1995 (1042).
131. Personal finances. (76:427), August 15, 1995 (1047).
132. Day-to-day cardiology in Bombay, India. (76:3019-3020), December 15, 1995 (1051).
133. Good cardiologic books appearing in 1995.(77:111-114), January 1, 1996 (1053).
134. Proceedings of the editorial board meeting of the *AJC* on March 26, 1996. (77:1138-1144), May 15, 1996 (1055).
135. The underused miracle drugs: The statin drugs are to atherosclerosis what penicillin was to infectious disease. (78:377–378), August 1, 1996 (1061).
136. Tobacco. (78:1084–1085), November 1, 1996 (1069).
137. The best hospitals in the USA for patients with heart disease. (78:652), November 15, 1996 (1070).
138. Good books on cardiovascular disease appearing in 1996. (79:248–252), January 15, 1997 (1073).
139. Proceedings of the editorial board meeting of the *AJC*. (79:1716–1720), June 15, 1997. (1084).
140. The rule of 5 and the rule of 7 in lipid-lowering by statin drugs. (80:106-107), July 1, 1997 (1086).
141. A unique heart disease associated with a unique cancer: carcinoid heart disease. (80:251–256), July 15, 1997 (1087).
142. Longitude, the longitude act, scurvy, and the beginning of government-supported research. (80:540–541), August 15, 1997 (1089).
143. Primary and secondary neoplasms of the heart. (80:671–682), September 1, 1997 (1090).
144. Papillary fibroelastomas of the heart. (80:973–975), October 1, 1997 (1092).
145. Floating in fat: fat kids and fat adults. (80:1117–1119), October 15, 1997 (1093).
146. The best hospitals in the USA for heart disease—1997. (80:1258–1259), November 1, 1997 (1097).
147. Good books on cardiovascular disease appearing in 1997. (81:524–529), February 15, 1998. (1102).
148. Fewer hearts than earlier predicted. (81:660–662), March 1, 1998 (1104).
149. Proceedings of the editorial board of the *AJC* on 30 March 1998. (81:1512–1517), June 15, 1998 (1116).
150. Good books on cardiovascular disease appearing in 1998. (83:470–474), February 1, 1999 (1137).
151. Obtaining and maintaining an ideal body weight. (83:639), February 15, 1999 (1139).
152. Shifting from decreasing risk to actually preventing and arresting atherosclerosis. (83:816–817), March 1, 1999 (1140).
153. Proceedings of the editorial board meeting of the *AJC* on 9 March 1999 (83:1588–1591), June 1, 1999 (1149).
154. An address to the Dallas, Texas, Rotary Club on 19 May 1999. (84:493–495), August 15, 1999 (1157).
155. Good books in cardiovascular disease appearing in 1999. (85:275–279), January 15, 2000 (1170).
156. Proceedings of the editorial board meeting of the *AJC* on 14 March 2000. (85:1507–1509), June 15, 2000 (1179).
157. Good books in cardiovascular disease appearing in 2000. (87:251–255), January 15, 2001 (1200).

158. Proceedings of the editorial board meeting of the *AJC* on 19 March 2001. (87:1332–1334), June 1, 2001 (1204).
159. High salt intake, its origins, its economic impact, and its effect on blood pressure. (88:1338–1346), December 1, 2001 (1215).
160. Good books in cardiovascular disease appearing in 2001. (89:785–790), March 15, 2002 (1227).
161. Proceedings of the editorial board meeting of the *AJC* on 18 March 2002. (89:1145–1148), May 1, 2002 (1235).
162. The heart at necropsy in massive obesity (>300 pounds or >136 kilograms) (89:145), June 15, 2002 (1237).
163. Getting more people on statins. (90:683–685), September 15, 2002 (1248).
164. Good books in cardiovascular disease appearing in 2002. (91:649–653) March 1, 2003 (1262).
165. Measuring the meter and using the metric system. (91:922–923), April 1, 2003 (1269).
166. Proceedings of the Editorial Board Meeting of the *AJC* on 31 March 2003. (91:1526–1531), June 15, 2003 (1273).
167. Infections. (92:1010–1012), October 15, 2003 (1287).
168. Krakatoa—the ultimate heart attack. (92:1140), November 1, 2003 (1290).
169. Singapore. (92:1254–1256), November 15, 2003 (1291).
170. Life's master molecule and James Watson. (92:1377), December 1, 2003 (1292).
171. Sudden death in Chicago. (92:1495–1496), December 15, 2003. (1293).
172. Miscellany. (93:124–128), January 1, 2004 (1295).
173. The metabolic syndrome. (93:274), January 15, 2004 (1297).
174. Good books in cardiology appearing in 2003. (93:520–523), February 15, 2004 (1298).
175. Two more drugs for dyslipidemia. (93:809–911), March 15, 2004 (1299).
176. Proceedings of the editorial board meeting of the *AJC* on 8 March 2004. (93:1328–1331), May 15, 2004 (1308).
177. The Amish, body weight, and exercise. (94:1221), November 1, 2004 (1324).
178. Over-the-counter statin drug. (94:1362), November 15, 2004 (1326).
179. Good books in cardiovascular disease appearing in 2004. (95:814–816), March 15, 2005 (1334).
180. Proceedings of the editorial board meeting of the *AJC* on 7 March 2005. (95:1273–1276), May 15, 2005 (1340).
181. Design changes in the AJC. (96: 1) July 1, 2005 (with David Dionne, publisher) (1341).
182. Managing patients with high blood pressure before the introduction of antihypertensive drugs. (96:1465–1466), November 15, 2005. (1347).
183. Systemic hypertension: some observations. (96:1610–1611), December 1, 2005 (1349).
184. Saving money and investing money. Advice from a cardiologist. (96:1750–1752), December 15, 2005 (1350).
185. Good books in cardiology appearing in 2005. (97:430–433), February 1, 2006 (1356).
186. Proceedings of the editorial board meeting of the *AJC* on 13 March 2006. (97:1670–1675), June 1, 2006 (1373).
187. Revising manuscripts after studying reviewers' comments (98(7): 989). October 1, 2006 (1380).
188. Atherosclerosis: Its cause and its prevention. (98:1550–1555). December 1, 2006 (1387).

Books

1. DuShane JW, Kirklin JW, Lester RG, van Mierop LHS, Mitchell SC, *Roberts WC*, Bossina KK, van der Haiwaert I, Kamaras J, Keck E, Michaelson M, Pernot C, Real F, Watson H: Classification of Heart Disease in Childhood, VRB Offsetdrukkerji, 1970, 70 pp.
2. DuShane JW, Kirklin JW, Lester RG, Mitchell SC, Rashkind WJ, *Roberts WC*, van Mierop LHS: A Manual Of Nomenclature And Coding Of Cardiovascular Disease In Children: A Supplement To The Systematized Nomenclature Of Pathology, 1970, 69 pp.
3. *Roberts WC*, editor, Congenital Heart Disease:In Adults, FA Davis Co, Philadelphia, 1979, 574 pp.
4. *Roberts WC*, Mason DT, Engle MA, Cohn LH: Cardiology 1981. Yorke medical Books, New York, NY, 1982 (May), 364 pp.
5. *Roberts WC*, Mason DT, Engle MA, Cohn LH: Cardiology 1982. Yorke Medical Books, New York, NY, 1982 (April) 464 pp.
6. *Roberts WC*, Rackley CE, Willerson JT, Mason DT, Karp RB, Pacifico AD, Graham TP, Jr: Cardiology 1983. Yorke Medical Books, New York, NY, 1983 (June), 516 pp.
7. *Roberts WC*, Rackley CE, Mason DT, Willerson JT, Graham TP, Jr, Pacifico AD, Karp RB: Cardiology 1984. Yorke Medical Books, New York, NY, 1984 (June), 479 pp.
8. *Roberts WC*, Mason DT, Rackley CE, Willerson JT, Graham TP, jr, Pacifico AD, Karp RB: Cardiology 1985. Yorke Medical Books, New York, NY, 1985 (September 20), 495 pp.
9. *Roberts WC*, Mason DT, Rackley CE, Willerson JT, Grham TP, Jr, Pacifico AD, Karp RB: Cardiology 1986. Yorke Medical Books, new York, NY, 1986 (June 3), 444 pp.
10. *Roberts WC*, Rackley CE, Mason DT, Willerson JT, Pacifico AD, Graham TP, Jr, Karp RB: Cardiology 1987. Yorke Medical Books, The Cahners Publishing Company, New York, NY, 1987 (July 9), 518 pp.
11. *Roberts WC*, editor. Adult Congenital Heart Disease. Philadelphia: F.A. Davis 1987:752.
12. *Roberts WC*, Rackley CE, Mason DT, Willerson JT, Pacifico AD, Graham TP, Jr, Karp RB: Cardiology 1988: Butterworth, Boston, 1988 (June 22), 505 pp.
13. *Roberts WC*, Mason DT, Rackley CE, Willerson JT, Graham TP, Jr, Karp RB: Cardiology 1989. Butterworth, Boston, 1989 (June), 523 pp.
14. *Roberts WC*, Mason DT, Rackley CE, Willerson JT, Graham TP, Jr, Karp RB: Cardiology 1990. Butterworth-Heinemann, Boston, 1990 (July 3), 494 pp.
15. *Roberts WC*, Willerson JT, Mason DT, Rackley CE, Graham TP, Jr: Cardiology 1991. Butterworth-Heinemann, Boston, 1991 (June), 494 pp.
16. *Roberts WC*, Willerson JT, Rackley CE, Graham TP, Jr: Cardiology 1992. Butterworth-Heinemann, Boston, 1992 (June 30), 480 pp.
17. *Roberts WC*, Willerson JT, Rackley CE, Graham TP, Jr: Cardiology 1993. Butterworth-Heinemann, Boston, 1993 (June 30), 490 pp.
18. *Roberts WC*, Rackley CE, Willerson JT, Mason DT, Parmley WW, Graham TP, Jr: Cardiology 1994. Butterworth-Heinemann, Boston, 1994 (July), 504 pp.
19. *Roberts WC*, Rackley CE, Willerson JT, Mason DT, Parmley WW, Graham TP, Jr: Cardiology 1995. Futura, Armonk, New York, 1995 (June), 499 pp.
20. *Roberts WC*, Willerson JT, Graham TP, Jr, Parmley WW, Rackley CE, Mason DT: Cardiology 1996. Futura, Armonk, New York, 1996 (October 1), 513 pp.
21. Willerson JT, *Roberts WC*, Rackley CE, Graham TP, Jr, Mason DT, Parmley WW. Cardiology 1997. Futura, Armonk, New York, 1997 (October), 624 pp.
22. Willerson JT, *Roberts WC*, Rackley CE, Graham TP, Jr, Mason DT, Parmley WW. Cardiology 1998. Futura, Armonk, New York, 1998 (September), 611 pp.
23. Willerson JT, *Roberts WC*, Rackley CE, Graham TP, Jr, Mason DT, Parmley WW. Cardiology 1999. Futura, Armonk, New York, 1999 (October), 774 pp.
24. *Roberts WC*. Facts and Ideas from Anywhere. Armonk, New York: Futura 2000: 172. A collection of 25 from-the-editor columns discussing 560 different topics and appearing in the *Baylor University Medical Center Proceedings* from April 1994 to April 2000.
25. *Roberts WC*. Facts and Ideas from Anywhere 2000-2005, Dallas: Baylor Health Care System 2006: 180. A collection of 22 from-the-editor columns discussing 433 separate topics and appearing in the *Baylor University Medical Center Proceedings* from July 2000 to October 2005.

William Clifford Roberts, MD: an interview by Charles Stewart Roberts, MD. *Am J Cardiol.* 2007;100(2):338-390. doi:10.1016/j.amjcard.2007.04.009

Brief Biography of Author

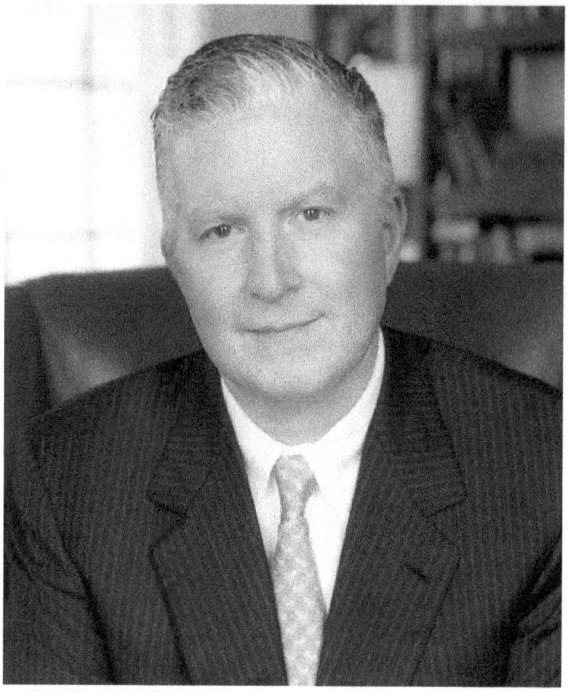

The author is a cardiovascular surgeon and author of several books. Born in Washington, DC, and educated at Vanderbilt (BA, 1981) and Emory (MD, 1986) universities, he was trained in cardiothoracic surgery at the University of North Carolina at Chapel Hill and the Royal Brompton Hospital in London. He began his practice in 1997 and currently serves as Chief of Cardiovascular Quality at Baylor University Medical Center in Dallas, Texas.